T0249006

Recent Progress in Cystic Fibrosis Research

Recent Progress in Cystic Fibrosis Research

Edited by **Jeffrey Swann**

FOSTER
ACADEMICS

New Jersey

Published by Foster Academics,
61 Van Reypen Street,
Jersey City, NJ 07306, USA
www.fosteracademics.com

Recent Progress in Cystic Fibrosis Research
Edited by Jeffrey Swann

© 2015 Foster Academics

International Standard Book Number: 978-1-63242-349-8 (Hardback)

This book contains information obtained from authentic and highly regarded sources. Copyright for all individual chapters remain with the respective authors as indicated. A wide variety of references are listed. Permission and sources are indicated; for detailed attributions, please refer to the permissions page. Reasonable efforts have been made to publish reliable data and information, but the authors, editors and publisher cannot assume any responsibility for the validity of all materials or the consequences of their use.

The publisher's policy is to use permanent paper from mills that operate a sustainable forestry policy. Furthermore, the publisher ensures that the text paper and cover boards used have met acceptable environmental accreditation standards.

Trademark Notice: Registered trademark of products or corporate names are used only for explanation and identification without intent to infringe.

Printed in the United States of America.

Contents

Preface

Every book is initially just a concept; it takes months of research and hard work to give it the final shape in which the readers receive it. In its early stages, this book also went through rigorous reviewing. The notable contributions made by experts from across the globe were first molded into patterned chapters and then arranged in a sensibly sequential manner to bring out the best results.

This book presents recent progress in cystic fibrosis research. Living a healthy life is one's ultimate goal, but the genetics behind the creation of each human is not same. As a curse of human suffering, certain people are born with congenital defects in their menu of the genome. The complexity of cystic fibrosis condition has impacts on several organ systems of the human body perplexing further with secondary infections. It is a complicated disease and scientists across the globe are still trying to comprehend it and formulate a cure because though they narrowed it down to a single target gene, the effects of this disease reach several unfamiliar corners of the human body. Decades of scientific research in the field of chronic diseases has certainly escalated the level of life expectancy. Scientists and researchers from across the globe have contributed significant information in this all-inclusive book which covers two broad sections: therapeutic options and disease management.

It has been my immense pleasure to be a part of this project and to contribute my years of learning in such a meaningful form. I would like to take this opportunity to thank all the people who have been associated with the completion of this book at any step.

Editor

Part 1

Therapeutic Options

Channel Replacement Therapy for Cystic Fibrosis

John M. Tomich, Urška Bukovnik, Jammie Layman and Bruce D. Schultz
Departments of Biochemistry and Anatomy and Physiology
Kansas State University, Manhattan, Kansas
USA

1. Introduction

Epithelial monolayers act as barriers to the movement of small solute molecules – including both inorganic ions and drugs – between body compartments. Ions traverse epithelial apical and basolateral membranes *via* a combination of tightly regulated ion-specific transporters and channels. Compromised function of any component leads to electrolyte and fluid imbalances resulting in morbidity and potentially, mortality. In the case of cystic fibrosis (CF) the defect lies in various genotypes that result in suboptimal synthesis, folding, transport, or gating of the CF transmembrane conductance regulator (CFTR; an anion channel that has other reported cellular functions). Many of the current therapies involve palliative interventions that address infections, inflammation, nutrition and mucus viscosity issues in patients. While these approaches have increased the life span of CF patients by reducing the rate of decline in lung functions or other health issues, none of them addresses the underlying cause of the disease at the cellular or tissue level, namely reduced anion conductance that sets the chemiosmotic driving force for both paracellular and transcellular fluid movement.

Many recent studies focus on small molecule approaches to rescue some forms of CFTR that are defective with respect to folding, intracellular trafficking, or activity. Of particular note has been the identification of VX-770, a small molecule that restores CFTR activity in patients harboring the G551D mutation. Results of a phase 3 clinical trial showed that VX-770 improved lung function by 10.5 percent over the placebo and achieved all secondary goals of the study (Accuroso et al., 2010). This is the first drug to show improvement in lung function in patients with the G551D mutation. Unfortunately, such profound effects of this drug have not been realized when tests were conducted with patients harboring other CFTR mutations. Other small molecules that may affect other forms of CFTR (e.g., ataluren for premature stop codons) are in the pipeline, although none appears to be as advanced as VX-770.

The idea of using small pore-forming peptides to treat various channelopathies has been an ongoing objective since identifying the pore-defining M2 transmembrane (TM) segment in the α-subunit of the spinal cord glycine receptor (GlyR) Cl⁻ channel in the early 1990's (Reddy et al., 1993). The parent sequence, M2GlyR, is the pore-forming segment of the Cl⁻

selective human spinal cord glycine receptor. In Wallace et al., (1992), we first suggested that inserting exogenous Cl- channel-forming peptides into the apical membranes of airway epithelial cells of CF patients may aid in restoring the ability of these cells to secrete fluid. This was the rationale for developing synthetic Cl--conducting channel-forming peptides as potential therapeutic agents. We have since developed synthetic peptides that form pores with varying degrees of anion conduction and selectivity. A guiding goal has been the *de novo* generation of a pore that could be used as a general therapeutic for CF since it would not require genotyping of individual patients. This novel therapeutic intervention, which would provide a new conductance pathway for selected anions, lies midway between conventional drug therapy and gene therapy. The primary target tissue, airway epithelium is accessible to aerosolized formulations such that the therapeutic peptides could be delivered easily.

The ideal therapeutic channel-forming peptide should: 1) have high aqueous solubility as a monomer; 2) have no detectable antigenicity; 3) bind to and then partition into biological membranes rapidly at low solution concentrations; 4) undergo supramolecular assembly in the membrane to form pores with measurable ion throughput; and 5) show physiologically relevant anion selectivity. All of these targeted outcomes have been achieved with the exception of the final goal, anion selectivity. In this regard, we are exploring distinct approaches to raise the permselectivity for Cl- (P_{Cl}) relative to both Na+ and K+.

Cells exposed to our *de novo* peptides that form membrane pores appear to tolerate them well, with net anion flux controlled by the natural regulation of counter-ion transport and/or anion loading. Using a combination of peptide synthesis, electrophysiology, structural biology and computer simulations we are endeavoring to prepare highly anion-selective channels. Numerous studies have been performed that switch anion to cation selectivity and vice-versa (see review-Keramidasa et al., 2004). Our studies targeting enhanced anion selectivity are novel and will yield a lead compound for treating CF as well as aid in our understanding of anion selectivity in channel proteins. The work is being accomplished by preparing sequences with rational alterations to the residues that dictate the chemical composition and structure of the pore.

This chapter will review our extensive exploration of the permissible amino acid replacements in the M2GlyR sequence based on knowledge of Cl- binding motifs and channel architecture. Modifications to the channel forming peptides were based on a wealth of data obtained from the fields of inorganic chemistry, channel physiology, structural determinations and computer modeling. The channel-forming peptides discovered during this project are remarkable in several ways: 1) they are small and easily synthesized; 2) they are water soluble and can be delivered to membrane surfaces without added organic solvents; 3) most are predominantly monomeric in solution; 4) when inserted into membranes, all peptides are expected to be oriented in the same direction due to the highly positively charged N-terminus; 5) all assembled pores are composed with a parallel orientation of the helices; 6) functional ion conducting pores are formed that can provide information on various channel properties; and 7) the small size of the peptides and the assembled pores facilitate concerted efforts for structural analyses and computer modeling that can produce informative structures.

To our knowledge no other membrane/peptide system offers such flexibility for design and analysis. Many TM sequences have been and are being studied by others (Marsh, 1996). However, for the most part, incorporation into bilayers leads to a mixed orientation with helical dipoles present in both directions. Such mixing of dipole orientations is prevented in our oligo-lysine adducted M2GlyR peptide system. This review will describe our understanding of how these peptides form channels with a range of anion selectivity and conductance properties, through a combination of electrophysiology, biophysical structural studies and computer simulations.

2. Current CF therapies

While a number of therapies for CF are currently in development, many of the treatment options presently available to patients are palliative in nature, addressing one or more symptoms of the condition and acting to reduce the severity of these effects and their associated risks.

Diet/nutritional supplements Proper diet and nutrition may reduce the impact and risk of CF-related conditions such as diabetes and osteoporosis. The lungs of CF patients appear to have fewer natural antioxidants than those without the condition, which may contribute to repeated infection and persistent inflammation. Patients may benefit from an increase in their intake of antioxidants through diet or supplements to fight this inflammation. Further promise may lie in drugs that work to build antioxidants in the lungs. AquADEKs® by Yasoo Health, Inc. is a vitamin supplement specifically formulated to meet the antioxidant needs of those with CF, and is commercially available. It has been shown to improve lung function, normalize vitamin levels in plasma and reduce neutrophilic inflammation (Sagel et al., 2011).

Enzyme replacement therapies Pancreatic enzyme products work to increase the digestion and absorption of fats, proteins, and starches while promoting the absorption of certain vitamins in those with CF, who often suffer from malnutrition due to enzyme deficiencies. The U.S. Food and Drug Agency (FDA) has approved a number of these products, including Zennen® (Eurand Pharmaceuticals), Creon® (Abbott Laboratories) and Pancreaze™ (Ortho-McNeil Pharmaceutical), while others, such as Pancrecarb® (DCI) and Ultrase® (Axcan Scandipharm) are still awaiting clinical trials. Liprotamase® (Alnara Pharmaceuticals) is a non-porcine pancreolipase enzyme therapy, which has completed a phase 3 clinical trial. However, the new drug application submitted by Alnara was rejected by the FDA on the grounds of insufficient data demonstrating the efficacy of the drug (Lowry, 2011).

Antibiotics/anti-infectives Due to the increased risk of disease caused by the excess and/or viscous mucus that is characteristic of CF, patients are often treated with antibiotics to circumvent chronic infections, such as that of *Pseudomonas aeruginosa*. Antibiotics can be administered orally, intravenously, via inhalation through devices such as metered dose inhalers (MDIs), or through implanted devices such as a port or Peripherally Inserted Central Catheter (PICC) (Gibson et al. 2003). TOBI® (tobramycin solution for inhalation) and recently developed Cayston® (aztreonam solution for inhalation) are two approved and commonly prescribed antibiotics for patients with CF, and both are effective against *P. aeruginosa*. TOBI® is approved to treat P. aeruginosa infections by concentrating the delivery of the antibiotic to the airways. Developed by Novartis Pharmaceuticals and widely used worldwide since its FDA approval in 1997, TOBI® has been successful in improving overall lung function while reducing hospital stays for CF patients (Cheer et al., 2003). TIP (TOBI® Inhalation Powder) is a new form of tobramycin that takes less time to administer via a Podhaler® and exhibits the same efficacy as the original formulation. It has been approved for use in Canada (http://www.pharmiweb.com/pressreleases/pressrel.asp? ROW_ID=23942 and http://www.novartis.com/newsroom /media-releases/en/2010/ 1446760.shtml). Cayston® (formerly GS9310/11) by Gilead Sciences is a newly developed version of the antibiotic aztreonam lysine in aerosol form. It was approved by the FDA and has been available to CF patients since February of 2010 (http://www.accessdata.fda.gov/ scripts/cder/drugsatfda/ index.cfm?fuseaction=Search.DrugDetails).

The macrolide antibiotic azithromycin (Pfizer, Inc.) has been shown, when administered orally, to fight *P. aeruginosa* infection and improve pulmonary function in CF patients aged 6 years and older. Further studies are required to determine efficacy of prolonged treatment and in treating those under 6 years of age (Saiman et al., 2003). Further, azithromycin (Delete "the common antibiotic") was shown in phase 3 trials to preserve healthy lung function in CF patients (Saiman et al., 2010). Several other anti-infective agents, which are presently being evaluated, are discussed in brief below. Mpex Pharmaceuticals has recently developed MP-376, an aerosol form of levofloxacin, used to treat *P. aeruginosa* infections in the lungs. Phase 3 trials are currently underway (http://www.mpexpharma.com/mp-376.html). Insmed Incorporated recently completed phase 2 trials of Arikace™, a version of the FDA-approved antibiotic amikacin in a liposomal formulation that is inhaled using a nebulizer. It was shown in animal studies to decrease the pathogenicity of *P. aeruginosa* and has demonstrated success in permeating human sputum in the lungs. Phase 3 trials are set to begin in late 2011 (http://www.insmed.com/arikace.php). Bayer Schering Pharmaceuticals' BAY Q3939, was developed as a new inhaled version of the drug ciprofloxacin to more effectively treat infections in air passages. Phase 2 trials for the drug are currently underway (http://clinicaltrials.gov/ct2/show/NCT00645788).

Mucolytics/Airway-Rehydrating Agents Since viscous mucus build-up in the lungs can promote bacterial infections, many therapies are directed toward reducing the symptom by restoring the liquid necessary to hydrate the mucus or the underlying layer to facilitate expectoration (Pettit and Johnson, 2011) or, in the case of Pulmozyme® and other agents, to reduce mucus viscosity. Pulmozyme® by Genentech is a Dornase alfa (recombinant human deoxyribonuclease) treatment used to break down the DNA responsible for thickening pulmonary mucus and thus to reduce viscosity, promote mucus clearing, and ultimately restrict (delete "to", replace "reduce" with "restrict") the environment that supports bacterial growth. Approved in 1993 and introduced in 1994, Pulmozyme® is currently in use as a mucolytic for patients with CF and has been shown to increase lung function by about 6% and reduce the risk of infection by 27% (Fuchs et al., 1994; http://www.pulmozyme.com/hcp/prescribing-info.jsp#table1). Moli1901 by Lantibio stimulates alternative Cl⁻ channels in order to compensate for the deficiencies of CFTR in the pulmonary epithelium of patients. In phase 2 European trials, Moli1901 was well tolerated in most patients (one participant experienced a transient decrease in pulmonary function). Those receiving treatment of 2.5 mg daily of inhaled Moli1901 showed significant improvement in lung function measured as forced expiratory volume in one second (FEV_1; Grasemann et al., 2007).Initially promising, Denufosol, a P2Y2 agonist developed by Inspire, was believed to rehydrate the airway surface liquid, bypassing the basic CFTR protein defect, producing improvement in pulmonary function (Kellerman et al., 2008). However, the most recent clinical trial found it to be without effect. GS9411 by Gilead is an epithelial Na^+ channel (ENaC) inhibitor, which blocks Na^+ absorption in airways to reduce mucus dehydration. A phase 1 trial of GS9411 has been completed and the drug was shown to be safe and well tolerated (Sears et al., 2011; http://clinicaltrials.gov/ct2/show/ NCT00999531).

An Australian clinical trial showed that a mist of hypertonic saline delivered via nebulizer twice daily for one year helped to improve lung function and reduce lung infections. The study included participants 6 years of age and older with mild or moderate lung disease (however, those with *Burkholderia cepacia* were not included in the study). The study tested two groups, one receiving "normal saline" solution at 0.9%, and the other receiving the "hypertonic saline" solution at 7% salt. While both groups showed improvement in pulmonary function during the study, those receiving hypertonic saline exhibited significantly greater improvement than those on normal saline. Elkins et al. (2006) reported that hypertonic saline also caused a reduction in exacerbations from the lungs, and Donaldson et al. (2008) hypothesized that this was due to the "protection" by hypertonic saline of non-obstructed airways from further mucus build-up and bacterial infection.

Similarly, an inhaled version of mannitol was shown to help clear CF airways and improve pulmonary function by an average of 7.3% (FEV_1) and forced airway flow by 15.5%. Mannitol works by drawing water into the lungs osmotically and thus helping to clear mucus. No serious adverse side effects were observed and it appeared to be well tolerated by patients (Jaques et al., 2008; Bilton et al., 2011). Phase 3 trials have been completed and the therapy is currently being marketed in Europe, and Pharmaxis hopes to submit a new drug application for Bronchitol to the FDA (http://www.pharmaxis.com.au/assets/pdf/2010/15122010).

Anti-Inflammatories Due to the recruitment of macrophages and neutrophils during rounds of bacterial infection, collateral damage to host airway cells by nuclear factor (NF)-*kappa* B activation and elevated pro-inflammatory cytokines leads to scarring and fibrosis. A number of anti-inflammatory agents are currently being used or studied to determine their efficacy in reducing inflammation in the pulmonary passages of CF patients. The over-the-counter drug, ibuprofen, taken orally twice daily at dosages adjusted to give peak plasma concentrations of 50 to 100 micrograms per milliliter, reportedly reduced the decline of lung function (Konstan et al., 1995). Oral N-acetylcysteine (PharrmaNAC, BioAdvantex Pharma, Inc.) was shown in clinical trials to reduce inflammation and increase pulmonary function by restoring glutathione in neutrophils. A phase 2 trial has completed enrolling subjects recently (Tirouvanziam et al., 2006; Atkuri et al., 2007). In a similar approach, inhaled doses of glutathione have completed phase 2 trials in Germany and data will be available in late 2011 (Retsch-Bogart, 2007). A University of Massachusetts study was conducted to test the efficacy of adding the fatty acid docosahexaenoic acid (DHA) to fortify infant formula in reducing CF pathogenicity. This work is based on the observation that an imbalance in fatty acids can lead to inflammation. It is hypothesized that an increase in DHA can help reduce inflammation that occurs with CF-related imbalances. Results of the study will be available in 2011. Genzyme Corp., which has licensed the patent as a treatment for CF, is considering new and more effective means of delivering DHA (Freedman et al., 1999; 2004). KB001 produced by Kalobios Pharmaceuticals reduces local inflammation from the virulence factor of *P. aeruginosa*. *P. aeruginosa* uses the structure of its Type Three Secretion System (TTSS) to break through cellular membranes and release toxins. KB001 binds to the PcrV protein essential to TTSS and inhibits its activity, reducing pathogenicity and preserving the immune defense of the host against *P. aeruginosa*. Though KB001 may reduce pathogenicity of *P. aeruginosa*, thereby preventing inflammation, it does not appear to affect in vivo growth of the bacteria, and thus is not classified as an anti-infective (Baer et al., 2008; http://www.kalobios.com/kb_pipeline_001.php). A recent report showed that an inhaled phosphodiesterase type 5 inhibitor, sildenafil, increased Cl- transport in mice (Lubamba et al., 2011). Further research at the University of Wales suggested that sildenafil may assist in intracellular trafficking of the ΔF508-CFTR gene protein (Dormer et al., 2005). The corticosteroid, GSK SB 656933 manufactured by GlaxoSmithKline is an inhaled dose of fluticasone propionate used to treat lung inflammation was shown to be safe and tolerated in CF patients in phase 1 clinical trials (Lazar et al., 2011; http://www.clinicaltrials.gov/ct2/show/NCT00903201?term=656933&rank=5NLM Identifier: NCT00903201). The drug is currently used to reduce pulmonary inflammation in chronic obstructive pulmonary disease (COPD).

Experimental CF Therapies Aside from gene therapy, some new experimental approaches are aimed at modifying the folding or translocation of the endogenous mutant CFTR proteins in order to generate a functional channel protein at the cell surface. Correcting these defects would re-establish transcellular flow of Cl-, Na+, and water to clinically relevant levels to provide appropriate airway surface liquid volume and composition (http://www.cff.org/treatments/Pipeline/).

CF Gene Therapy is directed toward correcting the channelopathy by incorporating DNA that encodes for the full-length wild-type CFTR protein. Research suggests that CFTR gene expression is required at a mere 5% of the normal level in order to improve pulmonary function (Ramalho et al., 2002). There are a number of gene therapy protocols currently under investigation with the frontrunners discussed below.

Compacted DNA (PLASmin®): (unbold. Inconsistent) One problem in developing a treatment for CF through gene therapy is that non-viral DNA must be condensed, which is commonly achieved through the use of polycations. However, this often results in a complex that is too large to cross the cellular membrane effectively and deliver DNA to the affected cells. Cleveland-based Copernicus Therapeutics, Inc. developed a compacted DNA/DNA nanoparticle therapy (PLASmin®) that decreases the volume of the complex by up to 1000-fold, to a single molecule small enough to permeate the membrane and nuclei of target cells. The complex contains only one copy of the DNA to be delivered, increasing the stability and efficacy of the treatment (Chen et al., 2007). In phase 1a trials, plasmid DNA nanoparticles with the gene responsible for encoding CFTR were applied intra-nasally with lysine peptides substituted with polyethylene glycol. About two-thirds of the participants in the study showed a significant improvement and results persisted for up to 6 days. No adverse side effects of considerable severity were observed as a result of the compacted DNA. However, this trial presented no demonstration of gene expression (Konstan et al., 2004). More recently, Copernicus has experienced greater success with the level and duration of CFTR expression in animal models

(http://www.thefreelibrary.com/Copernicus+
Receives+Milestone+Payment+from+Cystic+ Fibrosis+Foundation...-a0172302400).

VX-770 (Ivacaftor; Vertex Pharmaceuticals) is a novel therapy that seeks to augment CFTR activity in patients harboring the G551D mutation. This small molecule is a CFTR "potentiator" that increases function of faulty CFTR proteins by holding the defective channels in the open conformation. This treatment has completed phase 1 and phase 2 trials, which have shown efficacy in reducing sweat Cl- concentrations and increasing nasal potential difference measures as well as improvements in general lung health. VX-770 replicated these results in two phase 3 trials – one for ages 12 and above (adult) and one for ages 6-11 (child). Both trials showed relevant increases in FEV_1 of 10.6% and 12.5% for each age group respectively over the placebo groups. VX-770 also helped patients in the trials gain weight – nearly 7 pounds on average for the adult trial and about 8 pounds for the children's trial. Finally, the phase 3 trials also showed increases in general lung health, indicated the treatment was well tolerated, and demonstrated lower sweat Cl- levels. This closer to normal Cl- range is very important to note as it provides empirical evidence that VX-770 is effectively treating the cause of CF and not just its symptoms. Vertex plans to submit a new drug application (NDA) to the FDA in late 2011 for VX-770 (Sheridan, 2011).

VX-809 in conjunction with VX-770: VX-809 is a novel small molecule CFTR "corrector" being developed by Vertex Pharmaceuticals that seeks to augment channel activity in CF patients with the ΔF508 CFTR mutation when used in conjunction with VX-770. The ΔF508 mutation affects 87% of CF patients in the United States (48% of patients have both mutant alleles while 39% have one). Misfolding of the mutated protein interferes with cytosolic trafficking such that the protein never reaches the apical membrane, precluding any anion secretion. VX-809 partially corrects the defect by promoting the trafficking of CFTR proteins to its proper location in the apical membrane. ΔF508 CFTR has a reduced open probability. Thus, VX-809 is paired with VX-770, the CFTR "potentiator", in the hopes of increasing total protein function for maximum effect on the disease. A phase 2 trial testing various dose combinations of the two compounds met its primary endpoints of safety and efficacy in the first part of the trial. Patients harboring the ΔF508 mutation were given VX-809 or a placebo for 14 days and then a combination VX-809 and VX-770 or a placebo for 7 more days. The drugs were well tolerated, though about half of patients did report some adverse respiratory events, none of which were deemed serious. Furthermore, the most effective combination regiment showed significant total reductions in the sweat Cl- levels of 13 mmol/L from a baseline of ~100 mmol/L. The 14 days of solely VX-809 reduced sweat Cl- by 4 mmol/L. This is strong evidence that, first, VX-809 is able to direct CFTR to its operational location and, second, that VX-770 is able to increase the function of this most common mutated form of CFTR once it has been moved to that location. The final part of this study will begin at the end of 2011 (Pollack, 2011; and http://investors.vrtx.com/releasedetail.cfm?releaseid= 583683).

Ataluren (formerly known as PTC124®) is a protein restoration therapy that helps produce working copies from mutated forms of CFTR that harbor nonsense mutations (nmCF). Pioneered by PTC Therapeutics, Ataluren® is a small molecule compound that has shown clinical promise through phase 2 trials in the alleviation of several genetic disorders caused by nonsense mutations, including nmCF. Exclusively targeting nonsense mutations, ataluren® overrides the premature stop codons symptomatic of these mutations to allow for the completion of the desired protein. In the case of nmCF, a small (19 participant) phase 2 trial showed an ability to produce viable, working copies of CFTR via this "ribosomal read through" mechanism. The study showed significant improvements in total Cl- channel activity, measured by nasal transepithelial potential difference, which increased over time and led to improved pulmonary function and coughing. Ataluren was able to do this without interfering with other properly functioning stop codons, allowing the CFTR protein to be translated as initially designed and making the compound safe to administer. All trials of the compound have shown it to be well tolerated in humans with side effects mild and sparse to date. Ataluren®is currently in a 48 week CF phase 3 trial seeking statistically significant increased lung function, measured by FEV_1 as its primary endpoint with safety and drug activity as secondary endpoints. Ataluren has orphan status from the FDA and European Commission as well as Subpart E for expedited development from the FDA. The phase 3 trial data will become available in the first half of 2012 (Wilschanski et al., 2011; and http://www.ptcbio.com/3.1.1_genetic_disorders.aspx).

3. Channel replacement therapy

As indicated above, there are numerous approaches to treating this channelopathy. Combinations of these treatment modalities have increased the lifespan of those afflicted from 4, to now greater than 35 years of age. Perhaps the most significant of these therapies has been the use of pancreatic enzyme replacements, anti-inflammatories and powerful antibiotics. While restoration of CFTR activity has been an ultimate goal through CFTR rescue and in particular gene therapy, these therapeutic approaches have helped only limited numbers of patients. We have advocated another approach: *peptide-based channel replacement therapy*. Under this scenario a channel-forming peptide is applied to the apical surface of CF airway tissues to promote anion secretion and surface hydration. Gene therapy, to date, has involved the delivery of a CFTR-encoding DNA segment encased in a viral capsid to the affected epithelial tissues. There are serious problems with the gene therapy delivery vectors, transformation efficiency and CFTR production and delivery. Also airway epithelial cells have limited half-lives and the airway would need to undergo gene therapy on a regular basis to maintain expression. The new approach described here is much simpler (administered at home) and places the therapeutic directly on the target membrane (**Fig. 1**). Our efforts have been focused on developing a membrane-active peptide that can be delivered efficiently, assemble into a Cl-selective pore, trigger fluid secretion and elicit no detectable immune or inflammatory responses. The remainder of this chapter traces the development of this treatment modality. While many of the desired properties have been incorporated into this therapy some hurdles remain. These will be discussed later in the chapter.

Chloride Channels Ion channels are usually multi-subunit protein molecules that have gated water-lined pores and an ion selectivity filter. Channels are individually gated by a variety of signals including ligands, non-covalent and covalent modifications, voltage, and/or mechanical stimuli. In most biological fluids, the most relevant physiological cations and anions are Na^+, K^+, and Ca^{2+}; and Cl^-, and HCO_3^-, respectively. An extensive literature is available to clearly document the high selectivity of naturally occurring cation channels in both excitable and non-excitable tissues (e.g., K_v, Na_v, ENaC, Ca_v, etc.). Three major classes of Cl- channels have been cloned and studied. These include 1) the ligand gated channels typified by inhibitory post-synaptic glycine, glutamate and GABA receptors; 2) CFTR, which is an ABC transporter family member exhibiting complex nucleotide-dependent gating; and 3) ClC channels, which appear to be ubiquitous and are both voltage and metabolically gated. Ion channel classes display significant structural differences in the conductive pathway.

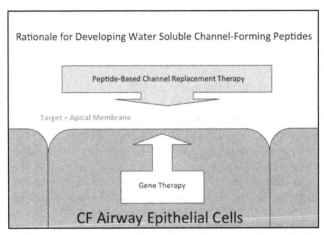

Fig. 1. The channel-forming peptide is delivered as an aerosol to the apical surface of CF airway cells. Upon binding to the surface it assembles to form an anion selective pathway to raise fluid secretion into the airway lumen thus rehydrating the airway surface fluid layer to allow proper cilia mediated airway clearance.

Class 1, the cys-loop ligand-gated ion channel superfamily of neurotransmitter receptors, includes the anion-selective inhibitory post-synaptic glycine (GlyR) and γ–aminobutyric acid type A (GABAAR) receptors, as well as cation selective nicotinic acetylcholine (nAChR), and 5-hydroxytryptamine type 3 (5-HT3R) receptors (Jensen et al., 2005; Sine and Engel, 2006) and the invertebrate post-synaptic glutamate receptor (Sunesen et al., 2006). These related structures all have a simple central pore defined by the parallel association of the second TM or 'M2' segments contributed by each of the five assembled subunits. Structural features common across members of this superfamily include the presence of heteropentameric bundles of subunits that are each composed of four hydrophobic TM segments, M1-M4, along with various sizes of intracellular and extracellular domains. Each M2 contributes a pore lining helix to form the channel. Unwin and co-workers (Unwin, 2003; Miyazawa et al., 2003; Unwin, 2005) published a 4 Å density map of the nAChR from *Torpedo marmorata*. The pentameric pore forms an hourglass-shaped pathway with the narrowest part at the middle of the lipid bilayer. The cation-conducting pathway, which is 40 Å long and extends beyond the lipid bilayer, is formed by parallel helices that are aligned, in registry, such that the same residues in different helices form rings that define discrete microenvironments. S266, E262, T244, E241, S248, and S252 form polar rings and hydrophobic residues V255 and L251 form the narrowest portion of the pore. It is important to note that in this barrel and stave type pore, amino acids possessing R-groups with a full charge are present. These negatively charged R groups are located as sites where the hourglass geometry is more open. McCammon and co-workers (Ivanov et al., 2007) modeled the α1-GlyR pore by threading the GlyR M2 helical segments onto the Unwin structure. Then, using molecular dynamics, they simulated the water density profile and Cl- translocation. A number of relevant conclusions were presented: the GlyR M2 pore is fully hydrated indicating that permeating Cl- is fully hydrated as well, no hydrophobic barrier was observed that would help in dehydrating the anion, and that the pore at its narrowest had a radius of 2.5 Å. These observations are in agreement with data that we have observed with our anion selective pores, which will be presented later. The McCammon group did not take into account any contribution of the M1-M2 loop toward anion selectivity. This extracellular loop, through mutational analyses, has been implicated in selectivity by several groups (Gunthorpe and Lummis, 2001; Jensen et al., 2005).

Hilf and Dutzler (2008) published the first x-ray structure of a bacterial cys-loop channel at 3.3 Å resolution in a presumed "closed-state". This channel protein shares 16% sequence identity with the *Torpedo* nAChRα protein. It is strictly a cation channel although there is little selectivity between Na+, K+, and Ca^{2+}. It differs significantly from the mammalian cys-loop channels in that no helical cytoplasmic domain is present. The authors were unable to identify any ion binding sites within the pore itself. This structure is of great significance since it provides key parameters such as the handedness of the helical bundle (left) and the tilt angle of the helices. The TM pore-forming helix is 25 residues in length with the pore lined by residues S226, E229, T233, T236, T240, A243, Y247 and I251. This structure provides key spatial coordinates for our modeling studies.

GlyR α_1-subunits alone have been shown to form homopentameric channels, when expressed in *Xenopus* oocytes, with properties similar to the parent channels (Schmeiden et al., 1989). The ability of this channel to function as a homo-pentameric array made it an attractive candidate for probing ion selectivity and permeation.

Class 2 is represented by CFTR, the only channel member of the ABC transporter superfamily, which has 12 TM segments divided between two different halves each containing a nucleotide binding domain and linked by a regulatory domain (Riordan, 2008; Zhang et al., 2011). In a collaborative study with M. Montal, we identified four segments (M2, M6, M10, and M12) that assembled in synthetic bilayers to form a Cl- conducting pore (Montal, et al., 1994). Since that time other TM segments (M1, M3, M5 and M11) have been implicated in participating in pore assembly (Zhang et al., 2000; Linsdell, 2006). Others have suggested that the active channel is composed of a homo-dimer (Zerhusen et al., 1999). The selectivity filter is believed to reside in the M6 segment (Zhou et al., 2002). Mutational studies in M6 support this assignment (Beck et al., 2008; Alexander et al., 2009). Clearly, this channel structure is more complex than that observed for the GlyR in that the CFTR pore requires the assembly of multiple non-identical TM segments.

Dawson and co-workers (Mansoura et al., 1998; Dawson et al., 1999; Smith et al., 2001; Liu et al., 2001) examined the selectivity properties of the CFTR channel, and proposed that reducing the dielectric of the pore is enough to cause anion selectivity. They prefaced their remarks by saying that the CFTR channel is probably a more primitive channel than the Class 1 channel types. CFTR exhibits lyotropic anion selectivity such that anions that are more readily dehydrated than Cl- are preferentially selected and show higher permeability rates. Their model predicts that larger anions, like SCN-, although they experience weaker interactions (relative to Cl-) with water and the channel, are more permeant than Cl- (but with a smaller conductance). They appear to have a smaller net energy cost entering the channel relative to that of Cl-. That is, the reduced energy of hydration allows the net transfer energy (the well depth) to be more negative. The net positive charge of the pore lining residues also contributes to selectivity.

Class 3 is the ClC channel family, which includes ClC-0, through ClC-7 in vertebrate species. This is the only family for which detailed structural assignments have been generated. Several bacterial ClC channels have been crystallized and analyzed with regard to the pore structure and the Cl- selectivity filter (Dutzler, et al., 2002; Dutzler et al., 2003). The active protein is a homo-dimer assembled from subunits that contain two identical anti-parallel domains. Each subunit contributes one channel to make a double-barreled channel structure. Each pore is made up of numerous anti-parallel helices of various lengths and contains two gating regions and a Cl- binding site. More recent crystallographic and mutational data suggest that there are three anion-binding sites within the open state of each pore in the highly conserved ClC family of channels and transporters (Lobet and Dutzler, 2006). The proposed central selectivity filter is composed, in part, using amide nitrogens from three different helices (N, F and D) pointing toward the anion-binding site. These amides are more positively charged because of the helix dipoles. The site also contains S107 and T445 (Corry and Chung, 2006). The amides and hydroxyls of these atoms are oriented such that they could form hydrogen bonds with Cl-. The serine side chain appears to be activated since the serine hydroxyl oxygen is also hydrogen bound to the amide nitrogen of I109. The anion never appears to interact with full positive charge from residues such as lysine or arginine. More recently three other residues have been implicated in selectivity through mutational studies K149, G352, and H401 in ClC-0 (Zhang et al., 2006). This class of channels is structurally distinct from the class 1 ligand-gated channels that contain a single pentameric array of parallel M2 helices of identical length. Despite these significant differences, the central ClC Cl- selectivity filter offers insight into the types of binding interactions that are utilized by Cl- selective channels.

4. M2GlyR studies

Early studies regarding first generation M2GlyR sequences When it became apparent that CFTR was a Cl- selective channel, finding and inserting an alternative Cl- conductive pathway into airway epithelia as a potential treatment modality became a realizable goal. Having already observed Cl- selectivity in synthetic phospholipid bilayers (Reddy et al., 1993) with the M2 segment from the glycine receptor as both the free peptide (M2GlyR) and as a four-helix bundle (T$_4$-M2GlyR) built with a template strategy (Mutter et al., 1989; Iwamoto et al., 1994), this sequence was an obvious choice to begin studying its effects on epithelial monolayers. Due to the complexity of synthesizing and purifying the template sequence, the studies focused on the more tractable monomeric form.

The initial ion permeation studies in epithelial monolayers were conducted with the sequence PARVGLGITTVLTMTTQSSGSRA, corresponding to amino acids 250-272 in the glycine receptor protein, using confluent Madin-Darby canine kidney (MDCK) monolayers. When suspended at 100 μM in water containing 1% DMSO, the peptide caused a 1 μAcm^{-1} increase in short circuit current (I_{sc}), an extremely sensitive indicator of net ion flux. The increase in I_{SC}

occurred slowly with the net change being observed 30 minutes after peptide addition and this increase was observed only in 24 of 37 monolayers tested, suggesting inconsistencies in delivering the sequence to the membrane and then having it insert properly. In addition to the poor efficiency value, other drawbacks included limited solubility of the sequence and the inability to control the orientation of the inserted peptide in the bilayer.

To decrease these deficiencies, the M2GlyR sequence was modified systematically by adding up to six lysyl or diaminopropionic acid (DAP) residues to either the C- or N-terminus (Tomich et al., 1998). This study examined a number of physical, pharmacological and physiological characteristics of the adducted sequences. Increasing the positive charge at either terminus increased solubility dramatically and also directed the orientation of the peptide within the bilayer. The effect was more dramatic for the C-terminus additions (**Fig. 2**) with 5 lysines giving a peptide that showed solubility at saturation, in Ringer solution, of 56.1 mM. Placing four lysines at either the C- or N-terminus appeared to be optimal in that these modified sequences yielded larger I_{SC} values, greater aqueous solubility and exhibited nearly 100 percent efficiency in generating measurable changes in I_{SC}. The resulting I_{SC} was sensitive to bumetanide, a diuretic that blocks the activity of the $Na^+/K^+/2Cl^-$ cotransporter that is responsible for anion loading at the basolateral membrane, and to a non-selective Cl^- channel blocker, DPC. The aqueous solubility increased from 1.4 mM for the unmodified sequence to 27.5 and 13.4 mM for the CK_4- and NK_4-M2GlyR sequences, respectively. I_{SC} for CK_4- and NK_4-M2GlyR were larger by 2.7- and 1.2-fold, respectively.

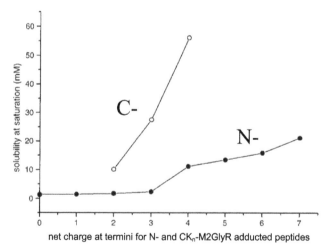

Fig. 2. Solubility as a function of net charge by the addition of lysines to either the C- or N-terminus of M2GlyR

Given the fact that adding lysines to either end improved solubility and showed increased magnitudes of net ion transport, studies were initiated to more fully describe the effects of CK_4-M2GlyR on MDCK cell monolayers primarily because placing lysines at the C-terminus yielded a pore that had an orientation, relative to the cell membrane, that was identical to the native GlyR channel. Additionally, the presence of the C-terminal lysines would be expected to stabilize the helix dipole. The helix dipole is important in the packing of adjacent helices such as those found in the helical bundle formed by the supramolecular assembly of the M2 peptides.

CK_4-M2GlyR significantly increased I_{SC}, hyperpolarized transepithelial potential difference, and induced fluid secretion. In 28 monolayers, CK_4-M2GlyR (100 µM) significantly increased I_{SC} from 0.8 ± 0.1 to 3.3 ± 0.4 µAcm^{-2} and hyperpolarized transepithelial voltage (V_{te}) from 1.5 ± 0.4 to 3.5 ± 0.6 mV (apical bath negative). Transepithelial electrical resistance (R_{te}; a composite indicator of the transcellular and paracellular permeation pathways) decreased from $1{,}399 \pm 341$ to $1{,}013 \pm 171$ Ω cm^2. In other experiments the increase in I_{SC} was inhibited by bumetanide (100 µM) and by some Cl⁻ channel inhibitors. The effectiveness of the channel blockers followed the sequence niflumic acid ≥ 5-nitro-2- (3-phenylpropylamino) benzoate (NPPB) > diphenylamine-2-carboxylate (DPC) > glibenclamide. The effect of the peptide was not inhibited by 4,4'- diisothiocyanostilbene-2, 2'-disulfonic acid (DIDS). Removing Cl⁻ from the bathing solutions also abrogated the effect of the peptide. The Cl⁻ efflux pathway induced by CK_4-M2GlyR differs from the native adenosine 3', 5'-cyclic monophosphate (cAMP)-mediated pathway that can be activated by adrenergic agonists and by forskolin. First, intracellular cAMP levels were unaffected and second, the concentration of DPC required to inhibit the effect of the peptide was much lower than that needed to block the forskolin response (100 µM vs. 3 mM). These results support the hypothesis that the synthetic peptide, CK_4-M2GlyR, can form Cl⁻-selective channels in the apical membrane of secretory epithelial cells and can induce sustained transepithelial Cl⁻ secretion that can drive fluid secretion. I_{SC} remained relatively constant for the first 2 h after the addition of the peptide. After 3 h, the CK_4-M2GlyR-stimulated current was 90% of the current recorded at 60 min and decreased to 55% after 4 h. In washout experiments (n = 3), I_{SC} was measured after removing CK_4-M2GlyR from the bath. One hour after removal of the peptide, 39% of the CK_4-M2GlyR-induced current remained, and, after 2 h, there was no persisting effect of the peptide.

In a separate series of experiments (Wallace et al., 2000), transport of Cl⁻ through the CK_4-M2GlyR conductive pathway was modulated by basolateral K⁺ efflux through Ca^{2+}-dependent K⁺ channels. Application of CK_4-M2GlyR to the apical surface of T84 cell monolayers (derived from human colon) generated a sustained increase in I_{SC} and caused net fluid secretion. The current was reduced by clotrimazole, an inhibitor of SK and IK channels, and by charybdotoxin, a more selective and potent inhibitor of the KCNN4 gene product, KCa3.1, a Ca^{2+}-dependent K⁺ channel. Direct activation of these channels with 1-ethyl-2-benzimidazolinone (1-EBIO) greatly amplified the Cl⁻ secretory current induced by CK_4-M2GlyR. The effect of the combination of CK_4-M2GlyR and 1-EBIO on I_{SC} was significantly greater than the sum of the individual effects of the two compounds and was independent of cAMP. Treatment with 1-EBIO also increased the magnitude of fluid secretion induced by the peptide. The cooperative action of CK_4-M2GlyR and 1-EBIO on I_{SC} was attenuated by Cl⁻ transport inhibitors, by removing Cl⁻ from the bathing solution, and by basolateral treatment with K⁺ channel blockers. These results indicate that apical membrane insertion of Cl⁻ channel-forming peptides such as CK_4-M2GlyR and direct activation of basolateral K⁺ channels with benzimidazolones may coordinate the apical Cl⁻ conductance and the basolateral K⁺ conductance, thereby providing a pharmacological approach to modulate Cl⁻ and fluid secretion by human epithelia deficient in CFTR.

Changes in the electrical properties of epithelial monolayers exposed to both 1-EBIO and CK$_4$-M2GlyR were observed. Basolateral addition of 1-EBIO (600 µM) induced a small increase in I_{SC} and doubled V_{te} with only a nominal decrease in R_{te}. Apical exposure of the 1-EBIO-treated monolayers to CK$_4$-M2GlyR (100 µM) caused an eight-fold increase in I_{SC} from 2.1 ± 0.2 to 16.5 ± 0.9 µAcm^{-2}, hyperpolarized V_{te} hyperpolarized by 7.3 ± 0.5 mV and reduced R_{te} by 1.53 ± 0.33 KΩcm^2. In two experiments, the response to 1-EBIO and CK$_4$-M2GlyR was monitored for 5 h. I_{SC} remained relatively constant during the first 60 min; however, I_{SC} had decreased to 73% of this current at 2 h, 53% at 3 h, 41% at 4 h and 29% of the current at 5 h. In washout experiments (n=2), the current generated by the additions of 1-EBIO and CK$_4$-M2GlyR was monitored for a set period of time, then CK$_4$-M2GlyR was washed out of the chamber. The removal of CK$_4$-M2GlyR from the medium decreased I_{SC} by 39%, whereas the subsequent removal of 1-EBIO decreased I_{SC} to the control level.

The addition of 1-EBIO increases the secretion of fluid induced by the apical application of CK$_4$-M2GlyR to T84 cell monolayers. T84 cell monolayers were grown in four groups of 10 monolayers, to test for the effects on the rate of transcellular fluid transport. Group I was incubated for 12 h in control medium, group II was exposed apically to CK$_4$-M2GlyR (500 µM), group III was exposed to 1-EBIO (300 µM) and group IV was exposed to both CK$_4$-M2GlyR and 1-EBIO. Monolayers incubated in control medium secreted fluid at a rate of 130 ± 40 nLh^{-1}cm^{-2}, a value that was not significantly different from monolayers exposed to 1-EBIO (180 ± 30 nLh^{-1}cm^{-2}). Monolayers exposed to just CK$_4$-M2GlyR exhibited a significantly greater rate of fluid secretion, 250 ± 20 nLh^{-1}cm^{-2} and a combination of CK$_4$-M2GlyR and 1-EBIO increased the rate of fluid secretion further to 330 ± 20 nLh^{-1}cm^{-2}. These results demonstrated that anion secretion induced by the apical membrane insertion of CK$_4$-M2GlyR drives the secretion of fluid and that the direct activation of basolateral K$^+$ channels by 1-EBIO potentiates this effect on the rate of secretion.

In other experiments, it was determined that the increase in Cl$^-$ and fluid secretion induced by combining CK$_4$-M2GlyR and 1-EBIO was independent of intracellular cAMP levels since the addition of the two compounds did not significantly affect cAMP content. This implies that CK$_4$-M2GlyR and 1-EBIO had minimal effect on CFTR Cl$^-$ conductance or other cAMP-dependent processes. Therefore, we propose that the major action of 1-EBIO is to activate the Ca^{2+}-dependent K$^+$ channels and that the increase in the Cl$^-$ secretory current is due to increasing the electrochemical driving force for Cl$^-$ efflux through synthetic Cl$^-$ channels generated by the membrane insertion of CK$_4$-M2GlyR. In summary, we have demonstrated that the synthetic Cl$^-$ channel-forming peptide, CK$_4$-M2GlyR, induces Cl$^-$ and fluid secretion by T84 cells, which are derived from human intestine. Activators and inhibitors of a basolateral Ca^{2+}-dependent K$^+$ conductance modulated the magnitude of this response. We propose that the combination of the novel synthetic Cl$^-$ channel-forming peptide, CK$_4$-M2GlyR, and agents like 1-EBIO may have pharmacological benefits for inducing and modulating transepithelial Cl$^-$ and fluid secretion independent of the cAMP-dependent Cl$^-$ secretion that is impaired in CF.

In a subsequent study we examined whether CK$_4$-M2GlyR could exert effects on whole cell Cl$^-$ conductance in isolated epithelial cells, and if the observed effects were the result of formation of a novel Cl$^-$ conductance pathway, modulation of endogenous Cl$^-$ channel activity, or a combination of these effects. The outcomes indicated that extracellular application of CK_4-M2GlyR to isolated MDCK, T84, and IB3-1 cells resulted in increased permeability of the cells to Cl^-. The experimental evidence suggested a direct mechanism of action. Studies looking at the effects of the oligo-lysine portion of the sequence suggested that a poly-lysine modified K_4-helical peptide was not sufficient to activate endogenous CFTR through an electrostatic mechanism.

The ability of CK_4-M2GlyR to induce a time- and voltage-independent current in the IB3-1 cell line, which lacks functional CFTR, suggested that CK_4-M2GlyR does not increase Cl^- current by activating CFTR. Furthermore, the pharmacological profile of the induced current supports this conclusion. Specifically, the CK_4-M2GlyR-induced currents do not share biophysical characteristics of the hyperpolarization activated current associated with ClC-2 as determined with and without antisense ClC-2 cDNA, the swelling-activated current associated with Volume-Sensitive Organic Osmolyte/Anion Channels (VSOAC), with and without tamoxifen, and the Ca^{2+}-dependent Cl^- current activated by CaM Kinase II, with and without KN-62. Together, these results support the premise that the M2GlyR peptides increase I_{SC} across epithelial monolayers by forming a novel permeation pathway for Cl^- rather than by activation of endogenous Cl^- conductances.

In some of the most compelling work done to test the validity of the peptide-based channel replacement therapy, nasal potential difference (PD) studies were performed at the Gregory Fleming James Cystic Fibrosis Center at the University of Alabama, Birmingham, under the direction of Dr. Eric Sorscher. More than 40 mice were tested for effects of either CK_4-M2GlyR or NK_4-M2GlyR. A standardized protocol that employs transitions to amiloride, Cl^--free medium, and exposure to adrenergic stimuli was employed. The ΔF508 homozygous transgenic mouse nasal epithelia exhibit ion transport defects identical to those in CF human airways and, thus, are an excellent model to test for potential therapeutic effects. Ion transport was assessed by repeated nasal PD measurements in both transgenic and wild-type mice (Brady et al., 2001). Key data from a double-blind study employing both CK_4-M2GlyR and NK_4-M2GlyR are summarized in **Fig. 3**. As expected, isoproterenol, in a Cl^--free medium containing amiloride, caused a positive shift in nasal PD of CF mice (CF control) while causing a negative shift in the nasal PD of wild-type (WT) littermates. Importantly, following exposure of CF nasal epithelia to either CK_4-M2GlyR or NK_4-M2GlyR (500 µM) the effect of isoproterenol more closely resembled the effect in the WT animals than in the CF animals that received no peptide or were exposed to either of two control peptides that were expected to have no effect. Control #1 was too short to span the bilayer of a cell membrane and Control #2 (NK_4-Sc) has its transmembrane segment randomized, although computer modeling was employed to maximize helical propensities while minimizing the amphipathic character of the helix. Sustained Cl^- conductance was observed for up to 6 h after a single application of peptide in solution. While this outcome is very encouraging, this type of treatment would have to be administered one or more times per day for optimal clinical results.

Concurrent exposure to 1-EBIO changed the direction for the development of M2GlyR channel-forming peptides. Initially, most studies were performed using CK_4-M2GlyR. However, CK_4-M2GlyR and NK_4-M2GlyR behaved differently in the presence of the K^+-channel opener. N-terminal modification of a channel-forming peptide increases capacity for epithelial anion secretion. In Ussing chamber experiments, apical exposure of MDCK and T84 cell monolayers to NK_4-M2GlyR (250 µM) increased I_{SC} by 7.7 ± 1.7 and 10.6 ± 0.9 µAcm-

[2], respectively (Broughman et al., 2001). These values are significantly greater than those previously reported for the same peptide modified by adding the lysines at the C- terminus (Wallace et al., 1997). NK_4-M2GlyR caused a concentration-dependent increase in I_{SC} ($k_{1/2}$ = 190 μM) that was potentiated two- to threefold by 1-EBIO (300 μM). NK_4-M2GlyR-mediated increases in I_{SC} were insensitive to changes in apical cation species. Pharmacological inhibitors of endogenous Cl^- conductances (glibenclamide, DPC, NPPB, DIDS, and niflumic acid) had little effect on NK_4-M2GlyR-mediated I_{SC}. Whole cell membrane patch-voltage clamp studies revealed an NK_4-M2GlyR-induced anion conductance that exhibited modest outward rectification and modest time- and voltage-dependent activation. Planar lipid bilayer studies indicated that NK_4-M2GlyR forms a 50-pS anion conductance with a $k_{1/2}$ for Cl^- of 290 mEq. NK_4-M2GlyR was similar to the previously characterized analog, CK_4-M2GlyR, in that both sequences elicited increases in the anion-selective current in lipid bilayers, whole cell membrane patches, and epithelial monolayers. When employed at similar concentrations, NK_4-M2GlyR provided for greater anion secretion across epithelial cell monolayers than any related channel-forming peptide tested to this point. Effects for NK_4-M2GlyR were observed with as little as 25–30 μM, and maximal effects were observed with about 500 μM (**Table 1** and **Fig. 4**; Broughman et al., 2002a).

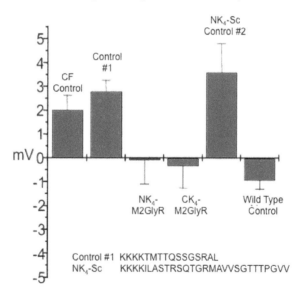

Fig. 3. Isoproterenol-induced change in nasal PD of ΔF508 homozygous mice and wild-type littermates in the absence or presence of indicated peptides.

Sequence	name	Mr (Da)	Sol.(mM)	n	I_{MAX} (μA/cm2)	$k_{1/2}$ (μM)
1. PARVGLGITTVLTMTTQSSGSRA	M2GlyR	2304.7	1.4	N/A	N/A	N/A
2. PARVGLGITTVLTMTTQSSGSRAKKKK	CK_4-M2GlyR	2817.4	27.5	2.7 ± 0.9	102.5	>500
3. KKKKPARVGLGITTVLTMTTQSSGSRA	NK_4-M2GlyR	2817.4	13.4	1.52 ± 0.55	24.3 ± 0.5	319 ± 192

Table 1. Characterization of M2GlyR peptides with C- and N-terminal oligo-lysine adducts.

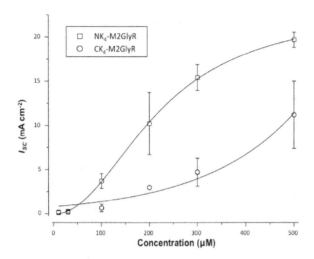

Fig. 4. The dependence of I_{SC} of MDCK monolayers on NK$_4$-M2GlyR and CK$_4$-M2GlyR concentration in the presence of 1-EBIO. Solid lines represent the best fit of a modified Hill equation to the data sets.

The resulting parameters for NK$_4$-M2GlyR (I_{max} = 25.2 ± 10.4 µAcm^{-2}, $k_{1/2}$ = 319 ± 192 µM, n (Hill coefficient) = 1.52 ± 0.55) are similar to those reported above , I_{max} = 24.3 ± 0.5 µAcm^{-2}, $k_{1/2}$ = 208 ± 6 µM, and n = 2.6 ± 0.1). This degree of cooperativity suggests that a multi-step process is required to form functional channel assemblies. Whether the cooperative step involves membrane partitioning, assembly of the helical bundles into structures, or a combination of these necessary steps for channel formation is not known. The concentration dependence of CK$_4$-M2GlyR is right-shifted compared to that of NK$_4$-M2GlyR, with the response at the greatest concentration tested (500 µM) showing no indication of saturation. The experimental data for CK$_4$-M2GlyR, when fitted by the modified Hill equation, resulted in a substantially greater value for I_{max} than that observed for a variety of agonists and pore-forming peptides (25–30 µA cm^{-2}). When employed at similar concentrations, NK$_4$-M2GlyR provides for greater anion secretion across epithelial cell monolayers than any related channel-forming peptide tested thus far. These results indicate that NK$_4$-M2GlyR forms an anion-selective channel in epithelial monolayers and again showed its therapeutic potential for the treatment of hyposecretory disorders such as CF.

One of the early applications of NK$_4$-M2GlyR included a study looking at the effect of exogenously applied peptide to the surface of immortalized human tracheal epithelial cells from a homozygous ΔF508 CFTR CF patient (Yankaskas et al., 1993). CF is characterized by defective epithelial Cl$^-$ transport with damage to the lungs occurring, in part, via chronic inflammation and oxidative stress. Glutathione, a major antioxidant in the airway lining fluid, is decreased in CF airway due to reduced glutathione efflux (Gao et al., 1999). This observation prompted a study to examine the question of whether exposure to channel-forming peptides would also restore glutathione secretion (Gao et al., 2001). Addition of the Cl$^-$ channel-forming NK$_4$-M2GlyR (500 µM) and a K$^+$ channel activator (chlorzoxazone, 500 µM) increased Cl$^-$ secretion, measured as bumetanide-sensitive I_{SC}, and/or glutathione efflux, measured by high-performance liquid chromatography, in a human CF airway epithelial cell line (CFT1). Addition of the peptide alone increased glutathione secretion (181 ± 8% of the control value), whereas chlorzoxazone alone did not significantly affect glutathione efflux; however, chlorzoxazone potentiated the effect of the NK_4-M2GlyR on glutathione release (359 ± 16% of the control value). CK_4-M2GlyR has decreased efficacy compared with NK_4-M2GlyR in both I_{SC} and GSH efflux assays. The addition of 1-EBIO also amplified the effect of NK_4-M2GlyR (500 μM) on GSH efflux (286 ± 1 % of control values). These studies demonstrated that glutathione efflux can be modulated by channel-forming peptides and is likely associated with Cl- secretion, not necessarily with CFTR per se, and the defect of glutathione efflux in CF can be overcome pharmacologically.

Both orientations of the M2GlyR helix within the membrane form anion-selective pores. However, differences in solubility, solution associations and channel-forming activity for the oligo-lysyl adducted forms were observed. While deciding on which of the oligo-lysine adducted M2GlyR peptides to develop further, we began a study utilizing chemical cross-linking, NMR and molecular modeling to determine how the positioning of the lysyl residues affected the channel properties and structural characteristics. These sequences are amphipaths with distinct clusters of hydrophobic and hydrophilic residues. In aqueous solution, hydrophobic patches associate and hydrophilic ones are solvent exposed. This property generally leads to aggregation through a concentration dependent process. This model predicts that multiple higher molecular weight assemblies, which do not readily interact with membranes, would be formed (**Fig. 5**). Evidence indicating aggregate formation is discussed below. A preferred outcome, however, would be to have a peptide that remained predominantly monomeric in solution while retaining its membrane binding and insertion activities. The actual sequence of insertion and assembly events leading to a functional channel are still unresolved. We do know that much of the process is slowly reversible based on perfusion washout experiments (indicated by the double ended arrows). Two possible routes are shown. One (right) has the peptide inserting and folding as a single step followed by assembly. The second (left) has peptide folding occurring at the surface followed by assembly as a prerequisite for insertion. A mixture of the two pathways could also be possible. Optimization of the channel-forming structure included modifications to reduce solution oligomerization and thereby increase the concentration of peptide that could insert and form active assemblies. CK_4-M2GlyR and NK_4-M2GlyR formed aggregates in aqueous solutions to differing degrees, as shown in **Fig. 6**. A cross-linking reagent was used to trap solution aggregates that were visualized using sodium dodecyl sulfate – polyacrylamine gel electrophoresis (SDS-PAGE) (Broughman et al., 2002b). Bis [Sulfosuccinimidyl] suberate (BS^3), a water-soluble homo-bifunctional cross-linking reagent that reacts with free amino groups in the lysine adducts was employed. The cross-linking reactions were carried out in 10 mM 4-(2-hydroxyethyl) piperazine-1-ethanesulfonic acid (HEPES) buffer, pH 6.5, at selected peptide concentrations in the presence of a 40-fold molar excess of cross-linking reagent. The results from a typical experiment are shown in **Fig. 6**. Lanes 5 and 9, show the electrophoretic mobility of non-cross-linked CK_4-M2GlyR and NK_4-M2GlyR boiled in 10% SDS, respectively. Under these conditions both sequences are monomeric, indicating that the solution associations that are trapped with the cross-linking reagent (in the adjoining lanes) are dissociated in the presence of the anionic detergent. The cross-linked molecular weight profiles for the two sequences are strikingly different. CK_4-M2GlyR forms lower molecular weight associations with monomer through trimer being the most prevalent. NK$_4$-M2GlyR forms many more associated forms, starting with monomer and going beyond 20-mers. Comparing the relative concentration of monomer to the higher species for each of the sequences, monomer is the most abundant species for CK$_4$-M2GlyR while in NK$_4$-M2GlyR the monomer accounts for less than 50% of the captured species. This result was somewhat surprising since NK$_4$-M2GlyR has considerably more activity per peptide concentration even though there is apparently a smaller percentage of monomer able to bind and insert into the membrane.

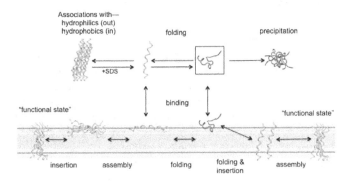

Fig. 5. Solution and membrane inserted states for channel-forming peptides.

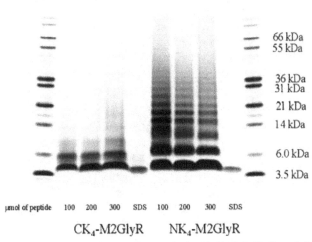

Fig. 6. Silver-stained polyacrylamide gel of cross-linked NK$_4$-M2GlyR and CK$_4$-M2GlyR.

Assuming that the energy barrier for the translocation of the four-lysyl residues across the hydrophobic membrane is prohibitive (Vogt et al., 2000), either orientation (NH$_2$ or COOH terminal towards extracellular surface) can insert into the membrane and assemble into an anion-conducting pore. However, based on the observation that the concentration required to produce 50% of the maximum increase in I_{SC} (k$_{1/2}$) for NK$_4$-M2GlyR is one-third less than that required for CK$_4$-M2GlyR (319 µM vs. 553 µM, respectively), the efficiency of the insertion or the assembly of these two peptides into channel-forming structures is not equivalent. Furthermore, the concentration-dependent effects of the peptides on I_{SC} show a smaller Hill coefficient for NK4-M2GlyR than CK4-M2GlyR (n = 1.5 vs. 2.3, respectively). This suggests that one or more of the steps required for channel assembly (e.g., insertion, oligomerization) is/are more cooperative in the case of CK4-M2GlyR. Alternatively, as NK4-M2GlyR is less soluble than CK4-M2GlyR in aqueous solution, the hydrophobic driving force for the insertion of NK4-M2GlyR into the membrane is greater. In either case, structural differences between the lysine-modified peptides result in altered channel-forming activity.

A series of one- and two-dimensional NMR experiments were performed on NK4- and CK4-M2GlyR. TOCSY NMR spectra were recorded for each (Broughman et al., 2002b). Data presented in **Fig. 7** show the fingerprint region (NH to Cα and side chain proton connectivity) for 500 MHz 1H 2D-experiments for both peptides recorded in water containing 30% deuterated trifluoroethanol (TFE) at 30°C (assignments are shown for the lysine residues). The extent of chemical-shift dispersion of the backbone proton resonances, particularly of the lysine residue amide protons (in spite of the oligomeric nature of the lysines in these sequences), suggest that such a spread of chemical shift can be induced only by secondary structure. However, in comparing the chemical shifts for the lysine residues in the two TOCSY spectra, it is clear that the environments for these basic amino acids in the two peptides are distinct. For the NH2-terminal lysine adducted peptide the dispersion range of the TOCSY chemical shifts for 3 of the 4 lysines was 8.55 to 8.1 ppm. The fourth lysine could not be assigned. In contrast, the COOH-terminal-adducted peptide had a dispersion range of chemical shifts that spanned 8.15–7.72 ppm. All four of the CK4-M2GlyR lysine resonances were assigned. Greater dispersion in the chemical shift pattern observed with NK4-M2GlyR indicates that these residues are more mobile and solvent exposed while the lysine residues adducted to the COOH-terminus are hydrogen bonded intramolcularly.

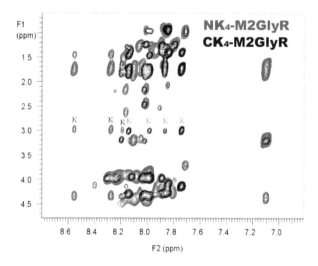

Fig. 7. TOCSY NMR spectra (500 MHz) of NK4-M2GlyR and CK4-M2GlyR.

The NMR coordinates for CK$_4$-M2GlyR and NK$_4$-M2GlyR were modeled using a combination of energy based minimizations and molecular-dynamics simulations. The lysine residues of CK$_4$-M2GlyR form a C-cap by extensive H-bonding interactions with the helix backbone, which remain fairly static throughout the molecular dynamics simulation period. The side chain ε-amino group of K24 of CK$_4$-M2GlyR forms a capping structure that stabilizes the helix by forming H-bonds with the backbone carbonyl groups of S21, R22 and A23, fulfilling H-bonding interactions that are absent in the COOH terminal residues of an α-helix. The ε-amino group of K25 of CK$_4$-M2GlyR forms H-bonds with the backbone carbonyl groups of T16 and K-27 and the hydroxyl side chain of T16. The ε-amino groups of K26 and K27 of CK$_4$-M2GlyR form hydrogen bonds to the backbone carbonyl of K25 and the side chain carbonyl of Q17, respectively. The side chain ε-amino groups of K1 and K4 of NK$_4$-M2GlyR do not form H-bonds, as the lysyl residues' side chains extend away from the helix backbone. There was very little motion of the helix backbone of CK$_4$-M2GlyR during the simulation period. In contrast, the lysine residues of NK$_4$-M2GlyR remained mostly extended away from the helix during the simulation, interacting minimally with the M2GlyR backbone. These differences in dynamics could affect the rates of assembly and pore geometries. Large differences are predicted for the dipoles of NK$_4$-M2GlyR and CK$_4$-M2GlyR (**Fig. 8** left and right structures, respectively). Note the similarities, both in magnitude and in orientation, between the dipoles of the unmodified M2GlyR sequence and NK$_4$-M2GlyR. The dipole of CK$_4$-M2GlyR is shifted by nearly 90 degrees and is less than 2% of the magnitude of the dipole for the parent compound. This perturbation of the dipole could play a role in the differences observed in peptide-peptide association and channel activity of the CK$_4$-M2GlyR peptide.

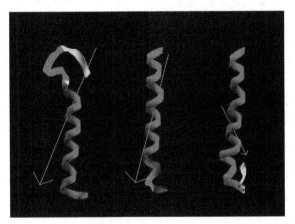

Fig. 8. The dipole moments of NK$_4$-M2GlyR (left), M2GlyR (center) and CK$_4$-M2GlyR (right) are shown as ribbon structures (magenta is helix and cyan is random coil) with the dipoles represented by green arrows. For this representation, the dipoles of NK$_4$-M2GlyR and M2GlyR were scaled down by a factor of 20, while the dipole for CK$_4$-M2GlyR was scaled up by a factor of 3.

To identify the portion of the M2GlyR molecule that was promoting the solution assemblies of NK$_4$-M2GlyR, channel activity and cross-linking experiments were performed on various truncated forms of CK$_4$-M2GlyR and NK$_4$-M2GlyR. The results (**Figs. 9 and 10**) suggested that a nucleation site for self-association of the peptide is located near the COOH-terminus of the M2GlyR sequence since removal of five residues (SGSRA) from the C-terminus of NK$_4$-M2GlyR resulted in a reduction of higher molecular weight species. Importantly, there was little loss of ion transport activity. Removal of additional C-terminal residues led to a progressive decrease in I_{SC}, although there was a slight reduction in apparent solubility to 11.1 mM. Measurable activity was observed with even 11 residues removed from the C-terminus. In contrast, the nucleation site is likely masked by the oligo-lysine tail at the COOH-terminus, which prevents formation of higher order assemblies by CK$_4$-M2GlyR and removal of residues from the N-terminus of CK$_4$-M2GlyR had little effect on the various low molecular weight associations. However, these truncated forms exhibited substantially less ion transport activity. The truncated NK$_4$ sequence, referred to as NK$_4$-M2GlyR-p22, became the lead compound for further development. Removing the five residues greatly reduced the cost of synthesizing a purer peptide with fewer failed sequences.

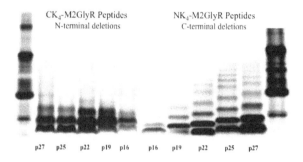

Fig. 9. Silver-stained Tricine polyacrylamide gel of cross-linking patterns for truncated CK$_4$-M2GlyR and NK$_4$-M2GlyR treated with a 40-fold excess of crosslinking reagent.

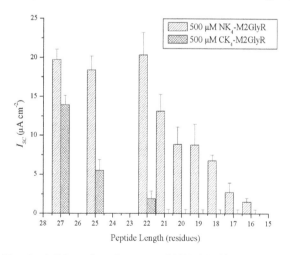

Fig. 10. I_{SC} induced by the full length and truncated NK$_4$-M2GlyR and CK$_4$-M2GlyR peptides (500 µM) on MDCK epithelial monolayers. Symbols represent the mean and standard error of three to seven observations.

Results described thus far indicate that the native M2 sequence that forms the GlyR pore can be employed to form de novo anion selective channels in epithelial cell membranes. Further, the structure can be optimized to enhance aqueous solubility and to decrease solution aggregation, which increases effective bioavailable concentration. Lysyl-adduction at the amino terminus appeared to be preferred based upon outcomes with truncated peptides. An additional and exciting outcome of these truncation studies was that shorter peptides might be used to achieve the therapeutic goal, which provides for many potential benefits in design and delivery of this therapeutic modality.

Studies on the second generation of NK$_4$-M2GlyR-p22 sequences In the process of truncating the NK$_4$-adducted M2GlyR sequence, a number of hydrophilic residues were eliminated as defined by the Wimley and White hydrophobicity scales developed for TM sequences (Wimley and White, 1996; Wimley and White, 1999; Wimley and White, 2000; Jayasinghe et al., 2001). The increase in hydrophobicity was reflected in reduced solubility for the deletion peptides. Among the residues removed was R22 in the C-terminus of the parent M2 sequence. It has been postulated, based on solution NMR studies in dodecyl phosphatidylcholine micelles, that the registry of the wild-type TM segment is defined by residues R3 and R22, thereby defining an 18-residue TM segment (Tang et al., 2002; Yushmanov et al., 2003). Arginine is often located at the water/lipid interface in TM segments (Vogt et al., 2000; Harzel and Bechinger, 2000; Mitaku et al., 2002). Without the C-terminal R in the NK$_4$-M2GlyR-p22 sequence, both ion selectivity and positioning, and registry of the TM segment within the acyl lipid core are potentially compromised. Therefore, a study was initiated to evaluate the effects on channel transport properties of reintroducing an R at positions near the new carboxyl-terminus. Arginine residues were introduced individually at positions 18 through 22 and in subsequent experiments double amino acid replacements were generated with aromatic amino acids placed at or near the C-terminus along with R at positions 19-22. MDCK monolayers were used to assess peptide-dependent ion transport.

A series of five individual C-terminal R substitutions were made placing R at the following positions: M18R, T19R, T20R, Q21R and S22R (Shank et al., 2006). With the exception of M18R, the substituted peptides generally exhibited similar concentration dependent I_{SC} profiles in MDCK monolayers (**Table 2**). Substitution of an R enhanced solubility by 50% or more, did not affect the Hill coefficient (**n**), showed similar half maximal activity ($k_{1/2}$) values and had similar helical content as judged by circular dichroism recorded using 50 μM peptide in 10 mM sodium dodecyl sulfate (SDS). Cross-linking experiments using BS^3 revealed that all of these substituted sequences showed solution aggregation patterns similar to that seen for NK$_4$-M2GlyR-p22 (e.g., see **Fig. 9**).

Rather than rely simply on an R to define the lipid-water boundary at the truncated end of M2GlyR, a W was used to replace the C-terminal serine. A propensity for tryptophans residing at the aqueous/lipid interface also had been observed and tested by others (Braun and von Heijne, 1999; Mall et al., 2000; Demmers et al., 2001; de Planque et al., 2003; Granseth et al., 2005; van der Wel et al., 2007; Hong et al., 2007). Placing a W at the C-terminus sets the registry of the TM segment that spans the bilayer. In the absence of an R or aromatic residue at or near the C-terminus, the peptide could rise up and down within the fluid bilayer thereby affecting the depth of peptide insertion into the membrane and tilt angle of the peptide. By limiting mobility, the degrees of freedom for the TM registry of the peptide are reduced. During the assembly process this allows the annealing peptides to find their preferred interfacial contacts faster and at a lower concentration. **Fig. 11** shows the concentration dependence on I_{SC} for the full length and the truncated M2GlyR peptides when applied to the apical membrane of MDCK cells in the presence of 1-EBIO (Cook et al., 2004). The solid lines represent the best fit of a modified Hill equation to each data set. In paired monolayers both NK$_4$-M2GlyR-p27 and NK$_4$-M2GlyR-p22 peptides (previously characterized in Broughman et al., 2002a) displayed similar concentration dependency curves and induced similar I_{SC} at each concentration tested. Introduction of the W in NK$_4$-M2GlyR-p22 S22W yielded a curve with a reduced I_{MAX} (13.0 ± 1.0 µAcm^{-2}) but more importantly a significantly reduced $k_{1/2}$ (44 ± 6 µM) with a considerably greater Hill coefficient of 5.4 ± 2.9. The sum effect of changes in the three kinetic parameters (I_{MAX}, $k_{1/2}$, and Hill coefficient) is a substantial reduction in the peptide concentration required to yield maximal anion secretion.

Sequence	Substitution	Mr (Da)	Sol.(mM)	n	I_{MAX} (µA/cm²)	$k_{1/2}$ (µM)
1. KKKKPARVGLGITTVLTMTTQS	none	2358.9	11.1	1.9 ± 0.6	23.7 ± 5.6	210 ± 70
2. KKKKPARVGLGITTVLTMTTQR	S22R	2427.9	15.6	2.7 ± 0.9	24.1 ± 5.3	290 ± 60
3. KKKKPARVGLGITTVLTMTTRS	Q21R	2387.0	19.7	2.2 ± 1.1	31.0 ± 18.0	390 ± 220
4. KKKKPARVGLGITTVLTMTRQS	T20R	2414.0	18.7	1.3 ± 0.5	28.5 ± 14.8	310 ± 227
5. KKKKPARVGLGITTVLTMRTQS	T19R	2414.0	18.3	0.7 ± 0.6	16.3 ± 3.5	120 ± 40
6. KKKKPARVGLGITTVLTRTTQS	M18R	2383.9	23.3	0.6 ± 2.6	3.0 ± 4.0	840 ± 200

Table 2. Characterization of M2GlyR-p22 derived peptides with C-terminal Arginines.

We then assessed the solution associations of the selected NK$_4$-M2GlyR peptides using a silver-stained gel following cross-linking reactions. In **Fig. 12**, lane 1 (consistent with 34:9-11) contained a mobility standard to indicate relative molecular weights. Lanes 2 through 9 contain the indicated peptides that were suspended in aqueous buffer in the absence and presence of a twenty-fold excess of BS3, as indicated The cross-linker revealed the presence of higher molecular weight homo-oligomers. Without the addition of cross-linker and after boiling the sample in SDS containing loading buffer, only monomer was observed. The W substituted sequence, however, appeared to be predominantly monomeric in solution under either experimental condition. These results indicated that NK$_4$-M2GlyR-p22 S22W (150 µM) forms essentially no aggregates in aqueous solution and the entire suspended mass is capable of membrane interaction.

It is unclear whether the left shift in $k_{1/2}$ observed for the W containing peptide in **Fig. 11** is due solely to an increase in concentration of the membrane active monomeric species or includes a contribution from the C-terminal W limiting the possible orientations of the peptide within the bilayer. The change in the Hill coefficient is likely due to the addition of the membrane anchor that facilitates the supramolecular assembly of the peptides into an active oligomeric pore. We speculated that the anchor reduces the degrees of freedom for the TM segment making alignment more favorable during assembly. An alternative explanation could be that in the absence of the tryptophan there is both positive and negative cooperativity. Addition of the tryptophan eliminates the negative cooperativity and we see the level of positive cooperativity that might be expected for the assembly of a pentameric structure. The presence of the fluorescent tryptophan also provides both a convenient method for determining the concentration of the peptide solution and a sensitive tool for probing the environment surrounding the indole.

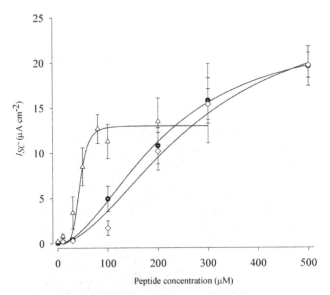

Fig. 11. Concentration-dependence of I_{SC} induced by NK_4-M2GlyR derived peptides on MDCK epithelial monolayers. The NK_4-M2GlyR derived peptides concentration dependent I_{SC} curves are as follows: NK_4-M2GlyR p27(◊), NK_4-M2GlyR p22 WT (●) and NK_4-M2GlyR p22 S22W (△).

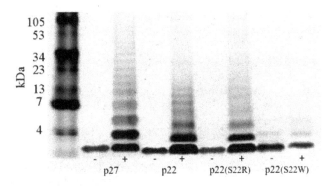

Fig. 12. NK_4-M2GlyR and derivative peptide solutions (150 µM) mixed without (-) and with (+) a 20-fold excess of BS^3 cross-linker.

NMR structural and computer modeling studies were carried out on 40% deuterated TFE solutions of NK_4-M2GlyR-p22 and NK_4-M2GlyR-p22 S22W to determine how the substituted C-terminal W potentially influences solution associations of the peptide (Cook et al., 2004). A measurement of the NK_4-M2GlyR-p22 (WT) peptide structure shows that the length of the entire TM segment is greater than 32 Å, more than enough to span the hydrophobic core of the membrane (**Fig. 13,** left structure). This structure is similar to the results shown in micelle studies done on the wild-type glycine receptor α_1 subunit (Tang et al., 2002; Yushmanov et al., 2003). An identical segment of the peptide was determined to be helical when incorporated in SDS micelles. The rest of the peptide was unstructured and flexible, including the C-terminus. The outcomes indicated that the structured portion of the peptide is restricted to residues 8 to 22 regardless of the length of the peptide. The WT structure resembles other TM segments observed in the x-ray crystal structure of a ClC chloride channel. In that structure, the Cl⁻ binding TM segments are made up of shorter helices that do not completely span the width of the membrane (Dutzler et al., 2002; Esrévez and Jentsch, 2002).

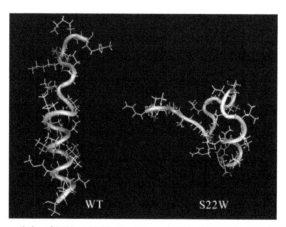

Fig. 13. Calculated models of NK_4-M2GlyR-p22 and NK_4-M2GlyR-p22 S22W in TFE.

The structured C-terminus of NK_4-M2GlyR-p22 S22W is made up of a single-turn helix (residues 11 - 14), a stretched beta-like turn (residues 14 - 17), and then another two-turn helix (residues 15 - 21). The observed structure indicated a helical content of about 40%, which was in good agreement with CD data for the S22W containing 22-residue peptide. This backbone structure allows the peptide to loop or fold over into a closed structure (**Fig. 13**). This fold sequesters the hydrophobic residues such that the acyl side chains have reduced solvent exposure. The structure likely has little relevance to a TM segment where the aliphatic side chains would be fully exposed and interacting with the lipid acyl chains in the membrane bilayer. Nonetheless, the C-terminal fold of NK_4-M2GlyR-p22 S22W explains why the peptide remains in the monomeric form in solution, since the hydrophobic groups are less exposed and unable to associate with hydrophobic groups from other peptides. While TFE is not added to peptide stock solutions used for assessing channel activity, it is clear that this monomer-inducing fold is sampled with enough frequency that the higher molecular weight forms do not occur. Based on the CD spectra obtained using 10 mM SDS micelles, the peptide is able to adopt a more helical structure, much like the WT peptide.

NMR studies in SDS (**Fig. 14**) confirmed the CD results (Herrera et al., 2010). These atomic structures clearly show that both NK$_4$-M2GlyR-p22 (WT) and NK$_4$-M2GlyR-p22 S22W are linear and mostly helical from residues 6–20 in SDS micelles. The N-terminal lysines are largely unstructured and apparently exhibit substantial flexibility. These lysine residues are expected to be out of the micelle floating in the aqueous environment and/or interacting with the sulfate groups. The hydrophobic and hydrophilic side chains are segregated to different sides of the helix, as expected for channel forming TM segments.

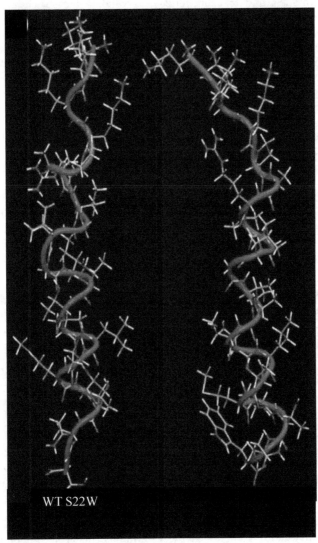

WT S22W

Fig. 14. Average structures of NK$_4$-M2GlyR-p22 and NK$_4$-M2GlyR-p22 S22W after MD refinement in an implicit membrane. Backbones are shown as a blue tube with licorice side chains.

NMR structures, along with a range of additional experimental data and theoretical considerations, were utilized to assemble the monomer structure into channels, including oligomerization state, pore-lining interface, helix packing distance, and tilt angle. In particular, experimental identification of the pore-lining residues greatly reduces uncertainty of the channel assembly and allows the construction of reliable initial structural models. All-atom molecular dynamics (MD) simulations in fully solvated 1-palmitoyl-2-oleoyl-*sn*-glycero-3-phosphocholine (POPC) bilayers were subsequently carried out to refine these structural models and to characterize and validate the structural and dynamical properties of the channels (**Fig. 15**). The results demonstrate that the channel structures as constructed are adequately stable within the simulation time frame (up to 20 ns) and remain sufficiently open for ion conductance. All initial structures relax to transiently stable structures within a few nanoseconds. Analysis of the relaxed structures of NK_4-M2GlyR-p22 WT and NK_4-M2GlyR-p22 S22W reveal important differences in their structural and dynamical properties, providing a basis for understanding the differences in channel activities. Specifically, the structural characterization supports the initial postulation that the S22W substitution in NK_4-M2GlyR-p22 helps to anchor the peptide in the membrane and reduces the flexibility of the whole assembly. The implied increased stability of the NK_4-M2GlyR-p22 S22W channel potentially explains the steeper short circuit current-concentration slope measured experimentally. Furthermore, introduction of the C-terminal W appears to lead to global changes of the channel structure. The NK_4-M2GlyR-p22 S22W channel maintains a smaller opening at the narrowest region and throughout the rest of the pore compared with the NK_4-M2GlyR-p22 channel. The smaller size of NK_4-M2GlyR-p22 S22W could effectively reduce its ion throughput or conductance by a magnitude that is consistent with a nearly 50% reduction in measured I_{MAX}. The ability to recapitulate these differences in key physiological properties observed experimentally is an important validation of the proposed structural models.

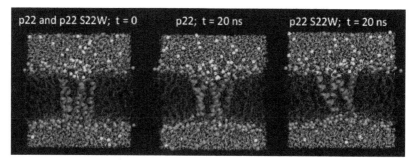

Fig. 15. Snapshots of NK_4-M2GlyR-p22 and NK_4-M2GlyR-p22 S22W left-handed channels in a fully solvated POPC bilayer before and after the 20 ns production simulation. Both peptides have identical structures at t = 0.The protein is shown in purple cartoon and lipid molecules shown in the grey licorice with phosphorus atoms shown as orange spheres.

Development of third generation NK_4-M2GlyR-p22 derived sequences From a drug delivery perspective, adding the W at the C-terminus yields a compound that can be delivered from solution at a stable accurate concentration and at considerably lower dosages. Both having the peptide predominantly as the monomer and treating with lower dosages dramatically reduce the cost of the treatment. For the third generation sequences substitutions were made based on increasing conductance and anion selectivity. In an attempt to enhance anion selectivity by reintroducing a charged residue at or near the C-terminus of the W-substituted sequence, a series of doubly substituted peptides were prepared. Restoration of a positive charge near the C-terminus of the 22-residue peptide was first tested with regard to increasing throughput rates. A helical wheel projection of the M2GlyR-p22 helix revealed an even distribution of the polar residues. Not knowing where to optimally substitute an R, a series of M2GlyR peptides was prepared with R replacing one amino acid in each of the four C-terminal sequence positions.

NK$_4$-M2GlyR-p22 displayed concentration-response relationships similar to those observed with the 27 residue full-length CK$_4$-M2GlyR and NK$_4$-M2GlyR peptides. **Table 3** presents the summarized ion transport kinetic constants associated with the fitted lines presented in **Fig. 16**. NK$_4$-M2GlyR-p22 displayed a concentration-dependent response similar to that observed with the 27 residue full-length CK$_4$-M2GlyR and NK$_4$-M2GlyR peptides. NK$_4$-M2GlyR-p22 provided benchmark values for I_{MAX} of 23.7 ± 5.6 µAcm^{-2}, $k_{1/2}$ of 210 ± 70 µM, and Hill coefficient of 1.9 ± 0.6.

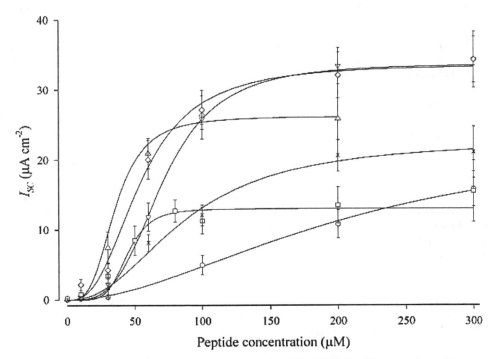

Fig. 16. Concentration-dependence of I_{SC} induced by NK$_4$-M2GlyR-p22 derived peptides with W and R amino acid substitutions on MDCK epithelial monolayers. Symbols represent the mean and standard error of 6 or greater observations for each concentration tested. Solid lines represent the best fit of a modified Hill equation to each data set. The NK$_4$-M2GlyR derived peptides concentration dependent I_{SC} curves are as follows: NK$_4$-M2GlyR-p22 (O), NK$_4$-M2GlyR-p22 S22W (□), NK$_4$-M2GlyR-p22 Q21R,S22W(Δ), NK$_4$-M2GlyR-p22 T20R,S22W(×), NK$_4$-M2GlyR-p22 T19R, S22W (∇) and NK$_4$-M2GlyR-p22 Q21W, S22R(◊).

Sequence	Replace-ment	Mr (Da)	Sol.(mM)	n	I_{MAX} (μA/cm^2)	$k_{1/2}$ (μM)
KKKKPARVGLGITTVLTMTTQS	none	2358.9	11.1	1.9 ± 0.6	23.7 ± 5.6	210 ± 70
KKKKPARVGLGITTVLTMTTQW	S22W	2458.0	1.9	5.4 ± 2.9	13.0 ± 1.0	45
KKKKPARVGLGITTVLTMTTRW	Q21R, S22W	2486.1	4.9	3.3 ± 1.6	26.5 ± 3.2	36 ± 5
KKKKPARVGLGITTVLTMTRQW	T20R, S22W	2513.1	5.2	2.3 ± 0.8	22.7 ± 2.7	87 ± 15

Table 3. Characterization of M2GlyR derived peptides with W and R substitutions.

Introduction of a W in the presence and absence of the added R had a dramatic effect on the concentration required for half-maximal ion transport activity. The left-shifted $k_{1/2}$ values ranged from 36 to 87 μM as compared with the 210 μM observed for NK$_4$-M2GlyR-p22. Three of the doubly substituted sequences exhibited similar left shifts in the $k_{1/2}$ for anion transport when compared to NK$_4$-M2GlyR-p22 S22W. NK$_4$-M2GlyR-p22 T20R, S22W did not show this dramatic left-shift. The simplest interpretation is that the sequences with left-shifted $k_{1/2}$ values form homo-oligomeric supramolecular assemblies at lower concentrations than the benchmark peptide.

With regard to I_{MAX}, the doubly substituted sequences exhibited greater maximal transport rates relative to either NK$_4$-M2GlyR-p22 or C-terminal W substituted NK$_4$-M2GlyR-p22 S22W peptides. In the doubly substituted sequences the position of the R relative to the W also had an effect on I_{MAX}. The sequences which introduced R at positions 20 or 21, exhibited a greater I_{MAX} (22.7 ± 2.7 and 26.2 ± 3.2 μAcm^{-2}, respectively) than was observed with the W alone substituted sequence. These I_{MAX} values are similar to that seen for M2GlyR-p22. Introduction of the R at position 19 and inverting the R - W pair of sequence NK$_4$-M2GlyR-p22 Q21R, S22W to W - R resulted in even larger I_{MAX} values of 33.7 ± 1.3 and 33.6 ± 2.2 μAcm^{-2}, respectively. Most importantly, R substituted sequences showed greatly enhanced efficacy with I_{SC} values equaling I_{MAX} for M2GlyR-p22 with concentrations at or below 50 μM. The sum effect of changes in the kinetic parameters (I_{MAX} and $k_{1/2}$) is a substantial reduction in the peptide concentration required to attain ion transport rates that will likely be relevant in future basic and applied applications. With the exception of NK$_4$-M2GlyR-p22 T20R, S22W all of the other W and R containing sequences have greater Hill coefficients (3.3 ± 1.6 to 5.4 ± 2.9) than that calculated for NK$_4$-M2GlyR-p22 (2.1 ± 0.8). M2GlyR-p22 T20R, S22W had a Hill coefficient (2.8 ± 0.8) similar to that seen with NK$_4$-M2GlyR-p22. The increase in the Hill coefficients to values approaching five suggests that association/dissociation mechanisms in the bilayer are sensitive to structural changes in the peptide and consistent with the prediction that the channel pore is a homo-oligomeric supramolecular assembly that assembles by a complex or multistep mechanism.

As assessed in the Ussing chamber experiments, reintroduction of an R near the C-terminus in conjunction with the added W contributes another factor that influences the minimum concentrations required for assembly of a functional channel. Introduction of an R at, at any of the tested positions slightly decreases the Hill coefficient, suggesting that there is an energetic cost in forcing the R (transiently) across the acyl core of the phospholipids. Placing R either at position 19 or just outside the membrane appears to be optimal with regard to I_{MAX}, while an R placed at position 21 appears to be optimal with regard to $k_{1/2}$. Placing R at position 20 seems to be the least optimal position since the Hill coefficient, $k_{1/2}$ and I_{MAX}

show the lowest values within this peptide series. Computer modeling studies indicated that the R in any of the internal C-terminal positions could snorkel back toward the membrane to form a second membrane anchor. There is no evidence that the R in any of these substituted peptides is positioned with the side chain pointed into the water-filled lumen of the assembled pore.

In a parallel set of experiments designed to assess the role of the indole group in altering n, I_{MAX} and $k_{1/2}$ values (Derived from **Fig. 17** and summarized in **Table 4**), sequences were prepared that replaced the W with either F or Y. The F or Y substituted sequences, which also contain a second R substitution, exhibited greater solubility compared to their W-containing counterparts, with the exception of NK$_4$-M2GlyR-p22 Q21F, S22R. All of the aromatic amino acid containing sequences had lesser amounts of higher molecular weight associations in aqueous environments compared to the aromatic-free sequence. Predominantly monomer, with some dimer, is present in the cross-linked aromatic sequences.

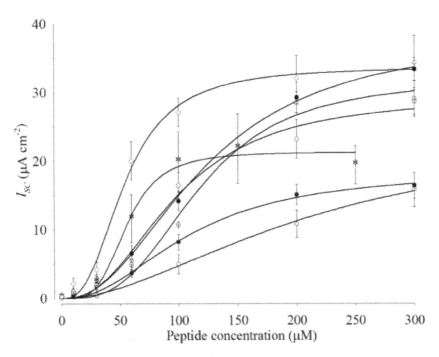

Fig. 17. Concentration-dependence of I_{SC} induced by NK$_4$-M2GlyR-p22 derived peptides with either F or Y and W amino acid substitutions on MDCK epithelial monolayers. Symbols represent the mean and standard error of 4 or greater observations for each concentration tested. Solid lines represent the best fit of a modified Hill equation to each data set. The NK$_4$-M2GlyR derived peptides dose dependent I_{SC} curves are as follows: NK$_4$-M2GlyR-p22 (O), NK$_4$-M2GlyR-p22 Q21W, S22R (◊), NK$_4$-M2GlyR-p22 Q21R, S22F (*), NK$_4$-M2GlyR-p22 T19R, S22F (closed hexagon), NK$_4$-M2GlyR-p22 Q21F, S22R (⊕), NK$_4$-M2GlyR-p22 Q21R, S22Y (open hexagon) and NK$_4$-M2GlyR-p22 T19R, S22Y (●).

Sequence	Replacement	Mr (Da)	Sol.(mM)	n	I_{MAX} (μA/cm^2)	$k_{1/2}$ (μM)
KKKKPARVGLGITTVLTMTTRF	Q21R, S22F	2447.1	6.1	3.8 ± 2.5	21.3 ± 2.5	56 ± 8
KKKKPARVGLGITTVLTMRTQF	T19R, S22F	2474.1	12.2	2.3 ± 0.3	38.0 ± 2.3	120 ± 14
KKKKPARVGLGITTVLTMTTFR	Q21F, S22R	2447.1	21.0	3.1 ± 0.6	31.8 ± 3.6	120 ± 10

Table 4. Characterization of M2GlyR derived peptides with F/Y and R Substitutions.

The secondary structures of these peptides were measured in SDS micelles. CD spectra contained minima at 208 and 222 nm, similar to those seen for all other sequences, which indicate predominantly helical structures. Considering the lack of solution aggregation and similar CD profiles, we concluded that these sequences formed a similar hydrophobic fold (in solution) that prevents association or aggregation in aqueous solution, similar to that described above for other structures. In addition to stabilizing the concentration of monomer in aqueous solutions, inclusion of any C-terminal aromatic residue provided a lipid/water interfacial anchor. As was seen with W, F residues are commonly present (and Y to a lesser extent) at the hydrophobic/hydrophilic interface for TM segments of membrane proteins (Braun and von Heijne, 1999; Mall et al., 2000; Demmers et al., 2001; de Planque et al., 2003; Granseth et al., 2005; van der Wel et al., 2007; Hong et al., 2007). The data for sequences NK4-M2GlyR-p22 and NK4-M2GlyR-p22 Q21W, S22R are included as reference values. Comparing the F substituted sequences to those containing the paired W, the F-containing peptides displayed similar I_{MAX} but have right-shifted $k_{1/2}$ values. The Y variants gave mixed results relative to their W counterparts. NK4-M2GlyR-p22 Q21R, S22Y showed a higher I_{MAX}, but had a right-shifted $k_{1/2}$ value while sequence NK4-M2GlyR-p22 T19R, S22Y was inferior in both respects. With the exception of NK4-M2GlyR-p22 Q21R, S22F, the $k_{1/2}$ values for the Y and F containing peptides are right-shifted relative to the W-containing peptides but left-shifted relative to the unmodified M2GlyR-p22.

Comparing all of the summarized data in **Tables 3 and 4** and the profiles shown in **Figs. 16 and 17**, the sequences displaying the highest ion transport activity and the second and third most left-shifted $k_{1/2}$ values are both W containing peptide sequences, NK4-M2GlyR-p22 T19R, S22W and NK4-M2GlyR-p22 Q21W, S22R. Based on the concentrations required for $k_{1/2}$, a rank ordering of the assembly-promoting effects of the C-terminal aromatic substitutions are as follows W > F >>Y. Given that when the R is placed at the C-terminus in NK4-M2GlyR-p22 Q21W, S22R will most likely cause further thinning of the membrane upon insertion (see **Fig. 17**), the sequence NK4-M2GlyR-p22 T19R, S22W was chosen as a lead sequence for further analysis and modification.

Before committing to *in vivo* animal studies and preclinical trials, a few questions had to be addressed – did the lysine adduction and amino acid substitutions at T19R and S22W of the peptide alter its selectivity as an anion channel and did these modifications generate a potentially immunogenic structure?

NK$_4$-M2GlyR-p22 T19R, S22W was administered at clinically relevant dosages to the nasal passages of specific-pathogen-free female C57/BL6 mice to test for the induction of an immune response with or without cholera toxin (CT) a strong mucosal adjuvant. Lipopolycaccharide (LPS)-free peptide, when administered alone, induced very little peptide-specific immunity based on analyses of peptide-specific antibodies by enzyme-linked immunosorbent and enzyme-linked immunospot assays, induction of cytokine production, and delayed-type hypersensitivity (DTH) responses. The administration of NK$_4$-M2GlyR-p22 T19R, S22W with CT induced peptide-specific immunoglobulin G (IgG) antibodies, DTH responses and a Th2-dominant cytokine response. Co-administration of CT induced a systemic NK$_4$-M2GlyR-p22 T19R, S22W-specific IgG response but not a mucosal peptide-specific antibody response. The lack of peptide-specific immunity and specifically mucosal immunity should allow repeated NK$_4$-M2GlyR-p22 T19R, S22W peptide applications to epithelial surfaces to correct ion channelopathies (van Ginkel et al., 2008).

Results indicate that additional modifications are necessary to achieve the desired anion selectivity. NK$_4$-M2GlyR-p22 T19R, S22W was tested in artificial bilayers composed of **1-palmitoyl-2-oleoyl-sn-glycero-3-phosphocholine:1-palmitoyl-2-oleoyl-sn-glycero-3-phospho-L-serine** (POPC:POPS, 70:30) and in *Xenopus* oocytes. In both cases the selectivity for monovalent anions relative to monovalent cations had dropped to a value slightly above unity, indicating that the pore formed was only slightly anion selective. Computer simulations were employed as an initial strategy to determine the most promising structures for synthesis and testing. Before those simulations could be conducted, the identity of the pore-forming residues had to be established. The structure of NK$_4$-M2GlyR-p22 T19R, S22W was analyzed by solution NMR as a monomer in detergent micelles and simulated as five-helix bundles in a membrane environment. Details of helix packing and residue distribution of the pore were analyzed. Results summarized in **Fig. 18a** demonstrate that the pore is mainly lined with A6, R7, L10, T13, T14, T17, T20 and Q21. Note the N- and C-terminal residues, K1-4 and W22, should not be considered as pore lining, even though they are indicated to have high pore-lining probabilities based on their contacts with (bulk) water molecules. The predicted pore-lining interface is largely consistent with the one derived from consideration of amphipathicity. However, the predicted pore-lining interface is broader due to substantial fluctuations of the pore. Participation of residues in helix-helix packing is characterized by calculating the average burial areas of side-chains, shown in **Fig. 18b**. Clearly, most residues with the structured region contribute to helix-helix interactions, except G9, G11, I12, V15 and R19. These residues either lack side chains (G9 and G11) or are fully membrane exposed. (I12, V15, L16 and R19). L10 and Q21 appear to be particularly important for stabilization of the pore assembly with the largest buried surface areas. Ongoing studies are guided by the hypothesis that alterations in one or more of the following parameters-- hydrogen bonding potentials of pore lining residues, electrostatics of pore lining residues, pore length or pore rigidity--will affect anion selectivity. By defining which of these elements increase selectivity we will elucidate how selectivity filters and permeation rates might be modulated so that an optimal sequence to allow for highly-selective Cl$^-$ permeation can be developed. Current experiments are designed to examine the effect of adding the positively charged amino acid L-diaminopropionic acid (DAP; R= CH$_2$-$^+$NH$_3$). Computer Modeling studies were performed on both singly and doubly DAP-substituted sequences (**Fig. 19**). Modeling the Potential of Mean Force (PMF) for moving different ions from one side of the channel to the other predicted similar permeabilities through NK$_4$-M2GlyR-p22 T19R, S22W for both Cl$^-$ and Na$^+$, while introduction of the cationic DAP residues favored the passage of Cl⁻. The double-substituted T13Dap, T20Dap sequence shows the smallest energy wells where Cl⁻ could become trapped, suggesting that it could be a preferred sequence.

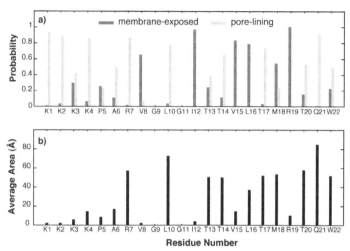

Fig. 18. **a.** Probabilities of a residue being either a pore-lining one or a membrane-exposed one. **b.** Average surface area of burial due to peptide-peptide interactions. The results are calculated from the last 80 ns of 100 ns production simulation of the left-handed channel.

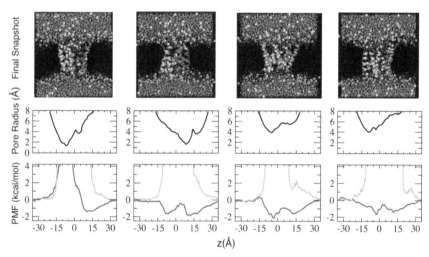

Fig. 19. Summary of the preliminary simulations of NK_4-M2GlyR-p22 T19R, S22W (lane 1) and its several singly (lane 2, T17Dap) and doubly Dap substituted sequences (lane 3, T13Dap,T17Dap; lane 4, T13Dap,T20Dap). The lengths of the simulations are at least 20 ns. The pore profiles were computed using the HOLE program based on the last snapshots shown. The PMFs were computed from equilibrium ion densities. The red line signifies chloride and the green line sodium.

Surprisingly, in generating more cationic channel-forming sequences, assembly, as assessed *in silico*, was not hampered by the presence of inter-peptide charge repulsion between the amino groups on adjacent helical segments. This repulsion appears to be accommodated by a widening of the pore. It might also cause the helices to adopt a staggered registry; however, these modeling studies have not indicated that outcome. Computer modeling of the M2GlyR-p22 T19R, S22W pore predicts the diameter to be about 4-5 Å at the narrowest portion of the channel (position T17). As stated above, modeling indicates that widening of the pore by the introduction of cationic residues results in a shift of the narrowest part of the pore to L10 with about the same pore diameter. The sequences containing multiple DAP residues appear to increase the diameter of the pore to ~8 Å, potentially leading to the passage of larger anions that were previously impermeable (glutamate, isethionate, etc.) and/or increased conductance. Preliminary results indicate that all of the DAP substituted sequences generate ion fluxes both across MDCK monolayers and in *Xenopus* oocytes. Permselectivity, however, remains to be determined.

NK$_4$-M2GlyR p-22 peptides with both W and R substitutions near the C terminus appear to be optimal structures for ongoing development of a therapeutic agent. These structures exhibited the greatest net ion flux and were among the most potent of the peptides assessed. Importantly, a mucosal immune response was not observed following exposure to these structures. The greatest challenge for ongoing development is the establishment of high anion to cation selectivity. Pore and lipid interfacial side chains have been identified to provide key information that is being used to build new structures in silico. These new structures are now being tested for ion throughput and selectivity. In addition to developing a potentially therapeutic structure, the outcomes of these experiments will provide a wealth of information regarding the contributions of hydrogen bonding, electrostatics, and pore rigidity to ion selectivity.

5. Summary

Nearly seventy-five years have passed since cystic fibrosis of the pancreas was first described as a unique clinical syndrome that was associated with failure to thrive and death in early childhood. The underlying cause of the disease, the absence of an epithelial anion conductance, was determined in the early 1980s and the gene coding for this anion channel was identified by the end of that decade. Even though the underlying cause has been known for more than twenty years, a curative treatment has not been developed, even at the tissue or organ level. Through the years, numerous therapies have been implemented – some with more positive outcomes than others. The commonality of all therapies is their palliative nature – there is no cure for CF although there are promising therapies in the pipeline for some subsets of the patient population (e.g., VX-770 for patients harboring G551D mutations). Supplemental pancreatic enzymes, more potent antibiotics and targeted delivery systems, daily respiratory therapy and the use of anti-inflammatory agents have added years to the typical lifespan and have greatly enhanced the quality of life of those suffering from CF. Nonetheless, additional therapeutic options are needed to address both tissue-specific and generalized disease progression. A synthetic anion-selective channel that can be delivered directly to epithelial cell membranes will provide one such option for improved health.

This line of investigation has as its primary goal to create a therapeutic channel-forming peptide that can be delivered from aqueous solution, insert itself into cell membranes and provide a pathway that is selective for the permeation of anions. The synthetic peptide should be effective at low aqueous concentrations, persistent in the membrane, and should not be antigenic. A particular benefit of this approach is that the therapy could be effective independent of the genetic mutation(s) expressed by each patient.

The development of synthetic channel-forming peptides has progressed through a series of stages including discovery, initial implementation or proof of concept, and optimization for various physical, biochemical and physiological endpoints. The glycine receptor, a naturally occurring anion selective channel, was selected as the simplest chassis from which to start the process. The M2 segment, which constitutes the pore of the pentameric receptor, was used to demonstrate that exogenously applied peptides could support anion movement across an epithelium. This peptide was modified with the addition of lysine residues to increase aqueous solubility and a truncated version was found to be equally effective, which reduced a portion of the burden of peptide synthesis. The truncated version was further modified to establish an anchor at the membrane:water interface. Together, these modifications yielded a peptide that is effective at aqueous concentrations below 50 micromolar and that persists in the epithelium for hours. At various stages in this project, results have shown that the peptides have the desired effects on electrophysiology when tested in murine nasal epithelia and the peptides appear not to induce a mucosal immune response, even when administered with cholera toxin as an adjuvant. Although the underlying mechanism remains to be determined, channel forming peptides were also associated with an increase in glutathione release from CF cells, which also constitutes a therapeutic outcome. Overall, the line of investigation has yielded much new knowledge regarding the design and construction of ion channels. Ongoing studies are focused to modify the ion selectivity of the channel, i.e., to build an anion selective channel for therapeutics and to determine the contribution of structural elements to channel ion selectivity. Clearly, there continues to be a need for new and novel therapies to treat the many aspects of CF. Synthetic anion selective channels constitute a therapeutic modality that has great potential to improve the lives of these patients.

6. Acknowledgements

We thank Gary Radke, Takeo Iwamoto Ph.D., Robert Brandt and Ryan Carlin for their technical assistance. We thank Professor Jianhan Chen for his assistance in redrawing computer simulation figures. This article is contribution no. 12-054-B from the Kansas Agricultural Experiment Station. Manhattan, KS-66506. This study has been supported in part by United States of America PHS grants form the National Institutes of Health to JMT: DK61866, GM43617 and GM074096.

7. References

Accurso, F.J., Rowe, S.M., Clancy, J.P., Boyle, M.P., Dunitz, J.M., Durie, P.R., Sagel, S.D., Hornick, D.B., Konstan, M.W., Donaldson, S.H., Moss, R.B., Pilewski, J.M., Rubenstein, R.C., Uluer, A.Z., Aitken, M.L., Freedman, S.D., Rose, L.M., Mayer-Hamblett, N., Dong, Q., Zha, J., Stone, A.J., Olson, E.R., Ordoñez, C.L., Campbell, P.W., Ashlock, M.A., Ramsey, B.W. (2010) Effect of VX-770 in persons with cystic fibrosis and the G551D-CFTR mutation. *N Engl J Med.* 363(21):1991-2003.

Alexander, C., Ivetac, A., Liu, X., Norimatsu, Y., Serrano, J.R., Landstrom, A., Sansom, M., Dawson, D.C. (2009) Cystic fibrosis transmembrane conductance regulator: using differential reactivity toward channel-permeant and channel-impermeant thiol-reactive probes to test a molecular model for the pore. Biochemistry. 2048(42):10078-10088.

Atkuri, K.R., Mantovani, J.J., Herzenberg, L.A., Herzenberg, L.A. (2007) N-Acetylcysteine-a safe antidote for cysteine/glutathione deficiency. Current Opinion in Pharmacology 7:355-359.

Baer, M., Sawa, T., Flynn, P., Luehrsen, K., Martinez, D., Wiener-Kronish, J.P., Yarranton, G., Bebbington, C. (2009) An engineered human antibody Fab fragment specific for Pseudomonas aeruginosa PcrV antigen has potent anti-bacterial activity. Infect Immun. 77(3):1083-1090.

Beck, E.J., Yang, Y., Yaemsiri, S., Raghuram, V. (2008) Conformational changes in a pore-lining helix coupled to cystic fibrosis transmembrane conductance regulator channel gating. J Biol Chem. 283:4957-4966.

Bilton, D., Robinson, P., Cooper, P., Gallagher, C., Kolbe, J., Fox, H., Jaques, A., Charlton, B. (2011) Inhaled dry powder mannitol in cystic fibrosis: An efficacy and safety study. Eur Respiratory J. 38(5):1071-1080.

Brady, K.G., Kelley, T.J., Drumm, M.L. (2001) Examining basal chloride transport using the nasal potential. Am J Physiol Lung Cell Mol Physiol. 281(5):L1173-1179.

Braun, P., von Heijne, G. (1999) The aromatic residues Trp and Phe have different effects on the positioning of a transmembrane helix in the microsomal membrane. Biochemistry 38:9778-9782.

Broughman, J.R., Shank, L.P., Iwamoto, T., Prakash, O., Schultz, B.D., Tomich, J.M., Mitchell, K.E. (2002) Structural implications of placing cationic residues at either the NH2- or COOH- terminus in a pore-forming synthetic peptide. J Membrane Biol. 190:93-103.

Broughman, J.R., Shank, L.P., Takeguchi, W., Iwamoto, T., Mitchell, K.E., Schultz, B.D., Tomich, J.M. (2002) Distinct structural elements that direct solution aggregation and membrane assembly in the channel-forming peptide M2GlyR. Biochemistry 41:7350-7358.

Broughman, J.R., K. Mitchell, T. Iwamoto, B.D. Schultz, J.M. Tomich. (2001) Amino-terminal modification of a channel forming peptide increases capacity for epithelial anion secretion. Am. J. Physiol: (Cell Physiol.) 280:C451-458.

Cheer, S.M., Waugh, J., Noble, S. (2003) Inhaled tobramycin (TOBI): a review of its use in the management of Pseudomonas aeruginosa infections in patients with cystic fibrosis. Drugs 63:2501-2520.

Chen, X., Kube, D.M., Cooper, M.J., Davis, P.M. (2007) Cell Surface Nucleolin Serves as Receptor for DNA Nanoparticles Composed of Pegylated Polylysine and DNA. Molecular Therapy 16:333-342.

Cook, G.A., Prakash, O., Zhang, K., Shank, L.P., Takeguchi, W.A., Robbins, A., Gong, Y.X., Iwamoto, T., Schultz, B.D., Tomich, J.M.. (2004) Activity and structural comparisons of solution associating and monomeric channel-forming peptides derived from the glycine receptor M2 segment. Biophys J. 86(3):1424-1435.

Corry, B., Chung, S.H. (2006) Mechanisms of valence selectivity in biological ion channels. Cell Mol Life Sci. 63:301-315.

Dawson, D.C., Smith, S.S., Mansoura, M.K. (1999) CFTR: Mechanism of anion conduction. Physiol Rev. 79(1 Suppl):S47-75.

de Planque, M.R., Bonev, B.B., Demmers, J.A., Greathouse, D.V., Koeppe, R.E. 2nd, Separovic, F., Watts, A. and Killian, J.A. (2003) Interfacial anchor properties of tryptophan residues in transmembrane peptides can dominate over hydrophobic matching effects in peptide-lipid interactions. *Biochemistry* 42:5341-5348.

Demmers, J.A., van Duijn, E., Haverkamp, J., Greathouse, D.V., Koeppe, R.E. 2nd, Heck, A.J., Killian, J.A. (2001) Interfacial positioning and stability of transmembrane peptides in lipid bilayers studied by combining hydrogen/deuterium exchange and mass spectrometry. *J Biol. Chem.* 276:34501-34508.

Donaldson, S.H., Bennett, W.D., Zeman, K.L., Knowles, M.R., Tarran, R., Boucher, R.C. (2006) Mucus Clearance and Lung Function in Cystic Fibrosis with Hypertonic Saline. *New England Journal of Medicine* 354(3):1848-1851.

Dormer, R.L., Harris, C.M., Clark, Z., Pereira, M.M.C., Doull, I.J.M., Norez, C., Becq F., McPherson, M.A. (2005) Sildenafil (Viagra) corrects ΔF508-CFTR location in nasal epithelial cells from patients with cystic fibrosis. *Thorax* 60:55–59.

Dutzler, R., Campbell, E.B., Cadene, M., Chait, B.T., MacKinnon, R. (2002) X-ray structure of a ClC Cl- channel at 3.0 A reveals the molecular basis of anion selectivity. *Nature* 415(6869):287-294.

Dutzler, R., Campbell, E.B., MacKinnon, R. (2003) Gating the selectivity filter in ClC Cl-channels. *Science* 300:108-112.

Dutzler, R., E.B. Cambell, M. Cadene, B.T. Chait, and R. MacKinnon. (2002) X-ray structure of a ClC chloride channel at 3.0 Å reveals the molecular basis of anion selectivity. *Nature* 415:287-294.

Elkins, M.R., Robinson, M., Rose, B.R., Harbour, C., Moriarty, C.P., Marks, G.B., Belousova, E.G., Xuan, W., Bye, P.T. (2006) A controlled trial of long-term inhaled hypertonic saline in patients with cystic fibrosis. *N Engl J Med.* 354:229-240.

Estévez, R., Jentsch, T. (2002) CLC chloride channels: correlating structure with function. *Current Opinion in Structural Biology* 12:531-539.

Fuchs, H.J., Borowitz, D.S., Christiansen, D.H., Morris, E.M., Nash, M.L., Ramsey, B.W., Rosenstein, B.J., Smith, A.L., Wohl, M.E. (1994) Effect of aerosolized recombinant human DNase on exacerbations of respiratory symptoms and on pulmonary function in patients with cystic fibrosis. *N Engl J Med* 331:637-642.

Freedman, S.D., Katz, M.H., Parker, E.M., Laposata, M., Urman, M.Y., Alvarez, J.G. (1999) A membrane lipid imbalance plays a role in the phenotypic expression of cystic fibrosis in cftr (-/-) mice. *Proc. Natl. Acad. Sci. USA* 96:13995-14000.

Freedman, S.D., Blanco, P.G., Zaman, M.M., Shea, J.C., Ollero, M., Hopper, I.K., Weed, D.A., Gelrud, A., Regan, M.M., Laposata, M., Alvarez, J.G., O'Sullivan, B.P. (2004) Association of cystic fibrosis with abnormalities in fatty acid metabolism. *N Engl J Med.* 350:560-569.

Gao, L., Kim, K.J., Yankaskas, J.R., and Forman, H.J. (1999) Abnormal glutathione transport in cystic fibrosis airway epithelia. *Am J Physiol Lung Cell Mol Physiol* 277:L113–L118.

Gao, L., Broughman, J.R., Iwamoto, T., Tomich, J.M., Venglarik, C.J., Forman, H.J. (2001) Synthetic Cl- channel restores glutathione secretion in airway epithelia. *Am. J. Physiol. (Lung)* 281: L24-L30.

Gibson, R.L., Burns, J.L., Ramsey, B.W. (2003) Pathophysiology and management of pulmonary infections in cystic fibrosis. *Am J Respir Crit Care Med.* 168:918–951.

Granseth, E., von Heijne, G., Elofsson, A. (2005) A study of the membrane-water interface region of membrane proteins. *J Mol. Biol.* 346(1):377-385.

Grasemann, H., Stehling, F., Brunar, H., Widmann, R., Laliberte, T.W., Molina, L., Doring, G., Ratjen, F. (2007) Inhalation of Moli1901 in patients with cystic fibrosis. Chest 131:1461–1466.

Gunthorpe, M.J., Lummis, S.C. (2001) Conversion of the ion selectivity of the 5-HT(3a) receptor from cationic to anionic reveals a conserved feature of the ligand-gated ion channel superfamily. J Biol Chem. 276:10977-10983.

Harzer, U., Bechinger, B. (2000) Alignment of lysine-anchored membrane peptides under conditions of hydrophobic mismatch: a CD, ^{15}N and ^{31}P solid-state NMR spectroscopy investigation. Biochemistry 39:13106-13114.

Herrera, A.I., Al-Rawi, A., Cook G.A., Prakash, O., Tomich, J.M., Chen, J. (2010) Introduction of a C-Terminal Tryptophan in a Pore-Forming Peptide: A Structure/Activity Study. PROTEINS: Structure, Function, and Genetics 78(10): 2238-2250.

Hilf, R.J., Dutzler, R. (2008) X-ray structure of a prokaryotic pentameric ligand-gated ion channel. Nature 452:375-380.

Hong, H., Park, S., Jiménez, R.H., Rinehart, D., Tamm, L.K. (2007) Role of aromatic side chains in the folding and thermodynamic stability of integral membrane proteins. J. Am. Chem. Soc. 129(26):8320-8327.

Ivanov, I., Cheng, X., Sine, S.M., McCammon, J.A. (2007) Barriers to ion translocation in cationic and anionic receptors from the Cys-loop family. J Am Chem Soc. 129:8217-8224.

Iwamoto, T., Grove, A., Montal, M. O., Montal, M., Tomich, J. M. (1994) Chemical synthesis and characterization of peptides and oligomeric proteins designed to form transmembrane ion channels. Int. J. Peptide Protein Res. 43:597-607.

Jaques, A., Daviskas, E., Turton, J.A., McKay, K., Cooper, P., Stirling, R.G., Robertson, C.F., Bye, P.T., Lesouëf, P.N., Shadbolt, B., Anderson, S.D., Charlton, B. (2008) Inhaled mannitol improves lung function in cystic fibrosis.Chest 133(6):1388–1396.

Jayasinghe, S., Hristova, K., White S.H.(2001) Energetics, stability, and prediction of transmembrane helices. J Mol Biol. 312:927-934.

Jensen, M.L., Pedersen, L.N., Timmermann, D.B., Schousboe, A., Ahring, P.K. (2005) Mutational studies using a cation-conducting GABA-A receptor reveal the selectivity determinants of the Cys-loop family of ligand-gated ion channels. J Neurochem. 92:962-972.

Jensen, M.L., Schousboe, A., Ahring, P.K. (2005) Charge selectivity of the Cys-loop family of ligand-gated ion channels. J Neurochem. 92:217-225.

Kellerman, D., Mospan, R., Engels, J., Schaberg, A., Gorden, J., Smiley, L. (2008) Denufosol: A review of studies with inhaled P2Y(2) agonists that led to phase 3. Pulm Pharmacol Ther. 21:600-607.

Keramidasa, A., Moorhousea, A.A., Schofieldb, P.R. and Barry, P.H. (1994) Ligand-gated ion channels: mechanisms underlying ion selectivity. Progress in Biophysics & Molecular Biology 86:161-204.

Konstan, M.W., Byard, P.J., Hoppel, C.L., Davis, P.B. (1995) Effect of high-dose ibuprofen in patients with cystic fibrosis. N Engl J Med. 332:848-854.

Konstan, M.W., Davis, P.B., Wagener, J.S., Hilliard, K.A., Stern, R.C., Milgram, L.J.H., Kowalczyk, T.H., Hyatt, S.L., Fink, T.L., Gedeon, C.R., Oette, S.M., Payne, J.M., Muhammad, O., Ziady, A.G., Moen, R.C., Cooper, M.J. (2004)Compacted DNA nanoparticles administered to the nasal mucosa of cystic fibrosis subjects are safe and demonstrate partial to complete cystic fibrosis transmembrane regulator reconstitution. Hum Gene Ther. 15:1255–1269.

Lazaar, A.L., Sweeney, L.E., MacDonald, A.J., Alexis, N.E., Chen, C., Tal-Singer, R. (2011) SB-656933, a novel CXCR2 selective antagonist, inhibits ex-vivo neutrophil activation and ozone-induced airway inflammation in humans. *British Journal of Clinical Pharmacology.* 72(2):282-293.

Linsdell, P. (2006) Mechanism of chloride permeation in the cystic fibrosis transmembrane conductance regulator chloride channel. *Exp Physiol.* 91:123-129.

Liu, X., Smith, S.S., Sun, F., Dawson, D.C. (2001) CFTR: Covalent modification of cysteine-substituted channels expressed in Xenopus oocytes shows that activation is due to the opening of channels resident in the plasma membrane. *J Gen Physiol.* 118:433-46.

Lobet, S., Dutzler, R. (2006) Ion-binding properties of the ClC chloride selectivity filter. *EMBO J.* 25:24-33.

Lowry, F. (2011) FDA Panel Sends Liprotamase Back to the Drawing Board. Medscape Medical News. http://www.medscape.com/viewarticle/735722

Mall, S., Broadbridge, R., Sharma, R.P., Lee, A.G., East J.M. (2000) Effects of aromatic residues at the ends of transmembrane alpha-helices on helix interactions with lipid bilayers. *Biochemistry* 39:2071-2078.

Mansoura, M.K., Smith, S.S., Choi, A.D., Richards, N.W., Strong, T.V., Drumm, M.L., Collins, F.S., Dawson, D.C. (1998) Cystic fibrosis transmembrane conductance regulator (CFTR) anion binding as a probe of the pore. *Biophys J.* 74:1320-1332.

Marsh, D. (1996) Peptide models for membrane channels. *Biochem J.* 315(Pt 2):345-361.

Mitaku, S., Hirokawa, T., Tsuji T. (2002) Amphiphilicity index of polar amino acids as an aid in the characterization of amino acid preference at membrane-water interfaces. *Bioinformatics* 18:608-616.

Miyazawa, A., Fujiyoshi, Y., Unwin, N. (2003) Structure and gating mechanism of the acetylcholine receptor pore. *Nature* 424:949-955.

Montal, M.O., Reddy, G.L., Iwamoto, T., Tomich, J.M., Montal, M. (1994) Identification of an ion channel-forming motif in the primary structure of CFTR, the Cystic Fibrosis Cl-channel. *Proc. Natl. Acad. Sci. USA* 91:1495-1499.

Mutter, M., Hersperger, R., Gubernator, K., Müller, K. (1989) The construction of new proteins: V. A template-assembled synthetic protein (TASP) containing both a 4-helix bundle and beta-barrel-like structure. *Proteins* 5(1):13-21.

Pettit, R.S. and Johnson, C.E. (2011) Airway-rehydrating agents for the treatment of cystic fibrosis: past, present, and future. *Ann. Pharmacother* 45:49-59.

Pollack, A. (2011) Vertex says trial of Vertex's VX-770, a cystic fibrosis drug, eased breathing - NYTimes.com. The Business of Health Care - Prescriptions Blog - NYTimes.com. http://prescriptions.blogs.nytimes.com/2011/02/23/vertex-says-cystic-fibrosis-drug-helped-patients-breathe-easier/

Ramalho, A.S., Beck, S., Meyer, M., Penque, D., Cutting, G.R., Amaral, M.D. (2002) Five percent of normal cystic fibrosis transmembrane conductance regulator mRNA ameliorates the severity of pulmonary disease in cystic fibrosis. *Am J Respir Cell Mol Biol.* 27:619-627.

Reddy, L.G., Iwamoto, T., Tomich, J.M. and Montal, M. (1993) Synthetic peptides and four-helix bundle proteins as model systems for the pore-forming structure of channel proteins. III. Transmembrane segment M2 of the brain glycine receptor channel is a plausible candidate for the pore-lining structure. *J. Biol. Chem.* 268:14608-14615.

Retsch-Bogart, G. (2011) Role of new therapies in CF lung disease. CF Learning Center http://www.cflearningcenter. com /pdfs/CFLC2011/healthcare/Role_of_New_Therapies_ in_CF_Lung_Disease.pdf

Riordan, J.R. (2008) CFTR Function and Prospects for Therapy. *Annu Rev Biochem.* 77:701-726

Saiman, L., Marshall, B.C., Mayer-Hamblett, N., Burns, J.L., Quittner, A.L., Cibene, D.A., Coquillette, S., Fieberg, A.Y., Accurso, F.J., Campbell, P.W. 3rd. (2003) Azithromycin in patients with cystic fibrosis chronically infected with Pseudomonas aeruginosa: a randomized controlled trial. *J A M A* 290:1749-1756.

Sagel, S.D., Sontag, M.K., Anthony, M.M., Emmett, P., Papas, K.A. (2011). Effect of an antioxidant-rich multivitamin supplement in cystic fibrosis. *J Cystic Fibrosis* 10(1):31-36.

Schmieden, V., Grenningloh, G., Schofield, P.R., Betz, H. (1989) Functional expression in Xenopus oocytes of the strychnine binding 48 kd subunit of the glycine receptor. *EMBO J.* 8:695-700.

Sears, H., Gartman, J., Casserly, P. (2011) Treatment options for cystic fibrosis: State of the art and future perspectives. *Reviews on Recent Clinical Trials* 6(2):94-107.

Shank, L.P., Broughman, J.R., Brandt, R.M., Robbins, A.S., Takeguchi, W., Cook, G.A., Hahn, L., Radke, G., Iwamoto, T., Schultz, B.D., Tomich, J.M. (2006) Redesigning channel-forming peptides: amino acid substitutions in channel- forming peptides that enhance rates of supramolecular assembly and raise ion transport activity. *Biophys J.* 90:2138-2150.

Sheridan, C. (2011) First cystic fibrosis drug advances towards approval. *Nature Biotechnology,* 29(6):465-466.

Sine, S.M., Engel, A.G. (2006) Recent advances in cys-loop receptor structure and function. *Nature* 440:448-455.

Smith, S.S., Liu, X., Zhang, Z.R., Sun, F., Kriewall, T.E., McCarty, N.A., Dawson, D.C. (2001) CFTR: Covalent and noncovalent modification suggests a role for fixed charges in anion conduction. *J Gen Physiol.* 118:407-431.

Sunesen, M., de Carvalho, L.P., Dufresne, V., Grailhe, R., Savatier-Duclert, N., Gibor, G., Peretz, A., Attali, B., Changeux, J.P., Paas, Y. (2006) Mechanism of Cl- selection by a glutamate-gated chloride (GluCl) receptor revealed through mutations in the selectivity filter. *J Biol Chem.* 281:14875-14881.

Tang, P., Mandal, P.K., Xu, Y. (2002) NMR structures of the second transmembrane domain of the human glycine receptor alpha(1) subunit: model of pore architecture and channel gating. *Biophys J.* 83:252-262.

Tirouvanziam, R., Conrad, C.K., Bottiglieri, T., Herzenberg, L.A., Moss, R.B. (2006) High-dose oral N-acetylcysteine, a glutathione prodrug, modulates inflammation in cystic fibrosis. *Proc Natl Acad Sci USA* 103:4628-4633.

Tomich, J.M., Wallace, D.P., Henderson, K., Brandt, R., Ambler, C.A., Scott, A.J., Mitchell, K.E., Radke, G., Grantham, J. J. Sullivan, L.P., Iwamoto, T. (1998) Aqueous solubilization of transmembrane peptide sequences with retention of membrane insertion and function. *Biophys J.* 74:256-267.

Unwin, N. (2003) Structure and action of the nicotinic acetylcholine receptor explored by electron microscopy. *FEBS Lett.* 555:91-95.

Unwin, N. (2005) Refined structure of the nicotinic acetylcholine receptor at 4Å resolution. *J Mol Biol.* 346:967-989.

van der Wel, P.C.A., Reed, N.D., Greathouse, D.V., Koeppe, R.E.II (2007) Orientation and motion of tryptophan interfacial anchors in membrane-spanning peptides *Biochemistry* 46(25):7514-7524.

Vogt, B., Ducarme, P., Schinzel, S., Brasseur, R., Bechinger, B. (2000) The topology of lysine-containing amphipathic peptides in bilayers by circular dichroism, solid-state NMR, and molecular modeling. *Biophys J.* 79:2644-2656.

Vogt, B., Ducarme, P., Schinzel, S., Brasseur, R., Bechinger, B. (2000) The topology of lysine-containing amphipathic peptides in bilayers by circular dichroism, solid-state NMR, and molecular modeling. *Biophys J.* 79:2644-2656.

Wallace, D.P., Tomich, J.M., Eppler, J., Iwamoto, T., Grantham, J.J., Sullivan, L.P. (2000) A Channel forming peptide induces Cl- secretion by T84 cells: Modulation by Ca^{2+}-dependent K$^+$ channels. *Biochem Biophys Acta* 1464:69-82.

Wallace, D.P., Tomich, J.M., Iwamoto, T., Henderson, K., Grantham, J.J., Sullivan, L.P. (1997) A synthetic peptide derived from the glycine-gated Cl- channel generates Cl- and fluid secretion by epithelial monolayers. *Am J Physiol: (Cell Physiol)* 272:C1672-C1679.

Wilschanski, M., Miller, L., Shoseyov, D., Blau, H., Rivlin, J., Aviram, M., Cohen, M., Armoni, S., Yaakov, Y., Pugatch, T., Cohen-Cymberknoh, M., Miller, N.L., Reha, A., Northcutt, V.J., Hirawat, S., Donnelly, K., Elfring, G.L., Ajayi, T., Kerem, E. (2011) Chronic ataluren (PTC124) treatment of nonsense mutation cystic fibrosis. *Eur Respiratory J.* 38(1):59-69.

Wimley W.C., White, S.H. (1996) Experimentally determined hydrophobicity scale for proteins at membrane interfaces. *Nat Struct Biol.* 3:842-848.

Wimley, W.C., White, S.H. (1999) Membrane protein folding and stability: physical principles. *Ann Rev Biomol Struct.* 28:319-365.

Wimley, W.C., White, S.H. (2000) Designing Transmembrane α-Helices That Insert Spontaneously. *Biochemistry* 39:4432-4442.

Yankaskas, J.R., (1993) Papilloma virus immortalized tracheal epithelial cells retain a well-differentiated phenotype. *Am J Physiol Cell Physiol.* 264:C1219–C1230.

Yushmanov, V.E., Mandal, P.K., Liu, Z., Tang, P., Xu, Y. (2003) NMR structure and backbone dynamics of the extended second transmembrane domain of the human neuronal glycine receptor α$_1$ subunit. *Biochemistry* 42:3989-3995.

Zerhusen, B., Zhao, J., Xie, J., Davis, P.B., Ma, J. (1999) A single conductance pore for Cl- ions formed by two cystic fibrosis transmembrane conductance regulator molecules. *J Biol Chem.* 274:7627-7630.

Zhang, L., Aleksandrov, L.A., Riordan, J.R., Ford, R.C. (2011) Domain location within the cystic fibrosis transmembrane conductance regulator protein investigated by electron microscopy and gold labelling. *Biochim Biophys Acta.* 1808(1):399-404.

Zhang, Z.R., McDonough, S.I., McCarty, N.A. (2000) Interaction between permeation and gating in a putative pore domain mutant in the cystic fibrosis transmembrane conductance regulator. *Biophys J.* 79:298-313.

Zhang, X.D., Li, Y., Yu, W.P., Chen, T.Y. (2006) Roles of K149, G352, and H401 in the channel functions of ClC-0: testing the predictions from theoretical calculations. *J Gen Physiol.* 127:435-447.

Zhou, Z., Hu, S., Hwang, T.C. (2002) Probing an open CFTR pore with organic anion blockers. *J Gen Physiol.* 120:647-662.

Fine Tuning of CFTR Traffic and Function by PDZ Scaffolding Proteins

Florian Bossard[1], Emilie Silantieff[2] and Chantal Gauthier[2]
[1]Department of Physiology; McGill University, Montreal, Quebec,
[2]L'Institut du Thorax, INSERM UMR 1087, CNRL UMR 6291,
Université de Nantes; Nantes
[1]Canada
[2]France

1. Introduction

Cystic fibrosis (CF) is the most common lethal genetic disorder in Caucasian population (Welsh et al., 1995). This pathology is due to mutations in the CF transmembrane conductance regulator (CFTR) encoding gene leading to alterations or loss of function of this channel (Kerem et al., 1989; Riordan et al., 1989; Rommens et al., 1989). CF affects several organs such as sweat glands, reproductive system and gastrointestinal tract, but the first cause of morbidity and mortality is respiratory system affections. While gene therapy for replacement of CFTR was a promising curative approach since the discovery of the CFTR gene, it turned to be more difficult than initially thought and no cure has arisen so far. Protein-protein interactions are powerful regulators of both protein trafficking and function, and can be enhanced or prevented by small molecules and short peptides (Zhang et al., 2011). Modulating these protein interactions are becoming a hopeful approach to develop new treatments for various diseases, including CF.

2. CFTR protein localization, structure and functions

CFTR protein is a chloride channel expressed at the apical membrane of polarized cells (Dalemans et al., 1992) and randomly expressed at the plasma membrane of non-polarized cells (Cheng et al., 1990). Moreover, CFTR protein has been also localized at the membrane of organelles such as endoplasmic reticulum (ER) where it is inserted upon biosynthesis (Pasyk & Foskett, 1995), Trans-Golgi network where it matures, endosomes where it interchanges with plasma membrane (Lukacs et al., 1992) and lysosomes where it is degraded (Barasch et al., 1991). CFTR is the only chloride channel of the adenosine triphosphate (ATP) Binding Cassette (ABC) transporters family. As several ABC transporters, CFTR protein is composed of two transmembrane domains (TMD) and two nucleotide binding domains (NBD). Unlike the other ABC transporters, CFTR also possesses a regulatory (R) domain. CFTR gating is controlled by two simultaneous phenomena: (i) the fixation and the hydrolysis of ATP on NBD domains (Anderson et al., 1991) and (ii) the phosphorylation of specific residues on the R domain by different kinases such as the 3'-5' cyclic adenosine monophosphate (cAMP) dependant protein kinase (PKA) (Berger et al., 1991; Tabcharani et al., 1991). In addition to be a chloride channel, CFTR also regulates other transmembrane proteins. Thereby, in several epithelial cells, CFTR expression decreases the epithelial Na^+ channel (ENaC) (Stutts et al., 1995) and Ca^{2+}-dependent Cl^- channel (CaCC) (Kunzelmann et al., 1997; Wei et al., 1999) activities; and increases the function of the outwardly rectifying Cl^- channel (ORCC) (Egan et al., 1992; Gabriel et al., 1993), the $Cl^-/HCO3^+$ exchangers of SLC26 family (Ko et al., 2002), the Renal Outer Medullary K^+ channel (ROMK) (Loussouarn et al., 1996) and some aquaporins (AQP) (Schreiber et al., 1997; Schreiber et al., 1999). Consequently, CFTR loss of function is responsible of a general dysregulation of ion transports in cells. Moreover, the regulation of most of these ion channels by CFTR occurs through interactions with Postsynaptic density-95/ Disc large/ Zonula occludens-1 (PDZ) scaffolding proteins (Lohi et al., 2003; Mohler et al., 1999; Pietrement et al., 2008; Yoo et al., 2004).

3. CFTR interacts with PDZ proteins through its C-terminus tail

PDZ domains are highly conserved sequences of about 80-90 amino acids known to be the most abundant protein-protein interaction modules in the human genome. Their three-dimensional structure is composed of 6 β sheets and 2 α helixes forming a cavity able to receive a protein motif of 3 to 7 amino acids, generally expressed at the C-terminus cytosolic tail of the target proteins (Bezprozvanny & Maximov, 2001; Fanning & Anderson, 1999; Harris & Lim, 2001; Hung & Sheng, 2002). However, intra-protein motifs able to bind PDZ domains have also been described (Hillier et al., 1999; Paasche et al., 2005; Slattery et al., 2011). A single PDZ domain can bind several target proteins with variable affinities. Moreover, a single PDZ motif can be recognized by different PDZ domains. To date, four types of PDZ motifs have been reported (Table 1).

PDZ domain	Protein motif
Type I	S/T-x-Φ
Type II	Φ-x-Φ
Type III	Ψ-x-Φ
Type IV	D-x-V

x: any amino-acid; Φ: hydrophobic amino-acid; Ψ: hydrophilic amino-acid

Table 1. Consensus sequences linking the different PDZ domains.

A PDZ protein can have several PDZ domains and so can interact simultaneously with several partner proteins. In addition, PDZ proteins can also form homo- or hetero multimeric structure (Fouassier et al., 2000; Lalonde & Bretscher, 2009; Lau & Hall, 2001; Shenolikar et al., 2001) thus forming wide submembrane docking networks for multiple transmembrane proteins where they can interact with each other and with anchored cytosolic regulatory proteins. Therefore, PDZ proteins play an important role in protein stability at the plasma membrane (i.e. endocytosis and recycling) and function. Some PDZ proteins are ubiquitous and others have a cell type-specific expression. Considering the organ or the tissue, PDZ proteins can be implicated in cellular morphology, cellular polarity, intercellular contacts, cell migration and cell growth (Altschuler et al., 2003; Hall et al., 1998; Kocher et al., 1999; C. Li et al., 2005; 2007; Naren et al., 2003; Pietrement et al., 2008; Seidler et al., 2009; Short et al., 1998; Singh et al., 2009; Wang et al., 1998; 2000; Yoo et al., 2004). CFTR possesses at its C-terminus a consensus motif, (D/E)-T-(R/K)-L, which belongs to the type I class of PDZ domain-binding motifs and is conserved across species (Table 2).

Species	CFTR C-terminal sequence
Human	SSKCKSKPQIAALKEETEEEVQDTRL
Frog	SSKRKSRPQISALQEETEEEVQDTRL
Rat	SSKQKPRTQITAVKEETEEEVQETRL
Mouse	SSKHKPRTQITALKEETEEEVQETRL
Dogfish	SSKRKTRPKISALQEEAEEDLQETRL
Sheep	SSRQRSRANIAALKEETEEEVQETKL
Bovine	SSRQRSRSNIAALKEETEEEVQETKL
Rabbit	SSKHKSRPQITALKEEAEEEVQGTRL

Table 2. C-terminal sequence of CFTR protein from various species.

3.1 Role of CFTR C-terminus

Patients harbouring a C-terminal truncation of CFTR such as the deletion of the 26 last amino acids (CFTR-S1455X) have a mild CF phenotype. A first study described that a mother and her daughter, both heterozygous for CFTR-S1455X and deletion of exon 14a (del14a) mutations, exhibited no CF phenotype but only an increase in sweat Cl- concentration, while a second daughter homozygous for del14a mutant had a severe CF phenotype (Mickle et al., 1998). A second study described two sisters heterozygous for F508del, the most common CF mutation, and CFTR-S1455X with also no CF phenotype and an elevated sweat Cl- secretion (Salvatore et al., 2005). Those studies suggest that deletion of CFTR C-terminus has no major incidence on the phenotype of patients. The role of CFTR C-terminus was also studied *in vitro* using plasmid constructs where CFTR's PDZ binding motif was deleted (ΔTRL-CFTR). The resulting phenotype of ΔTRL-CFTR in polarized and non-polarized cells is controversial. In type I MDCK cells, Moyer and colleagues have demonstrated that PDZ binding motif is an apical polarization signal and its deletion decreases CFTR activity (Moyer et al., 1999; 2000). On the opposite, several teams have described that deletion of the PDZ binding motif of CFTR has no effect on its apical membrane localization nor its function in numerous cells such as BHK-21, COS-1, type II MDCK, CaCo-2, PANC-1 and primary human airway epithelial cells (Benharouga et al., 2003; Milewski et al., 2005; Ostedgaard et al., 2003). The discrepancy between these studies can be explained by additional sorting motifs (Milewski et al., 2005), but also by the use of MDCK type I cells as the unique polarized cell line by Moyer et al., whereas different non polarized cell models were used by the other groups. Indeed, MDCK type I and II cells exhibit different polarized sorting (Svennevig et al., 1995). Accordingly, CFTR polarized expression would be differentially regulated depending on the type or the origin of the cells. The role in this process of the six PDZ proteins described so far to interact with CFTR is not clearly established, but they indubitably have different functions in CFTR polarized expression.

3.2 Na⁺/H⁺ exchanger regulatory factor family proteins

Na+/H+ Exchanger Regulatory Factor (NHERF) family proteins possess multiple PDZ domains. NHERF1 (also called EBP50 for Ezrin-radixin-moesin Binding Phosphoprotein of 50 kDa), the most studied member of the NHERF family, is the first protein evoked to interact with CFTR through its PDZ domain (Hall et al., 1998; Short et al., 1998; Wang et al., 1998). The NHERF family comprises four members: NHERF1 and NHERF2 (also called E3KARP for Na+/H+ Exchanger 3 Kinase A Regulatory Protein) have two PDZ domains while NHERF3 (also called PDZK1, CAP70 or NaPi CAP-1) and NHERF4 (also called PDZK2, IKEPP or NaPi CAP-2) have 4 PDZ domains (Fig.1). In addition, NHERF1 and NHERF2 have in their C-terminus tail a consensus sequence for ezrin binding, allowing their anchor to the actin cytoskeleton (Reczek et al., 1997).

NHERF1 and NHERF2 have similar functions but their cell expression is generally mutually exclusive *in vivo* (Ingraffea et al., 2002). In human lungs, NHERF1 is expressed in epithelial cells while NHERF2 is expressed in alveolar cells (Ingraffea et al., 2002). However, it seems not to be the case in cell lines. The affinity of CFTR C-terminus for PDZ domains varies across NHERF family members Indeed, CFTR C-terminus tail interacts preferentially with PDZ1 domain of NHERF1 (Wang et al., 1998) but with PDZ2 domain of NHERF2 (Hall et al., 1998; Sun et al., 2000). NHERF1 C-terminus tail interacts with its own PDZ2 domain preventing NHERF1 binding to ezrin. This auto-inhibition of NHERF1 is abolished by PKC phosphorylation (J. Li et al., 2007), which promotes macromolecular complex formation. In addition, both NHERF1 and NHERF2 have been shown to form homo- and heterodimers (Lau & Hall, 2001; Shenolikar et al., 2001).

CFTR C-terminus tail can interact with three out of four PDZ domains of NHERF3 (Wang et al., 2000). To date, only one team has demonstrated an interaction between CFTR and NHERF4 in transfected sf9 insect cells (Hegedüs et al., 2003). On the opposite of NHERF1 and NHERF2, NHERF3 and NHERF4 cannot anchor CFTR to the actin network. However, as NHERF3 is able to bind NHERF1, it can indirectly link CFTR to the cytoskeleton (Lalonde & Bretscher, 2009).

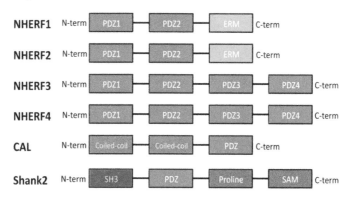

NHERF: Na+/H+ exchanger Regulatory Factor; CAL: CFTR Associated Ligand; ERM: Ezrin-Radixin-Moesin domain; PDZ: Postsynaptic density-95/ Disc large/ Zonula occludens-1; SAM: sterile Alpha Motif; SH3: Src Homology 3 domain; C-term: C-terminal; N-term: N-terminal.

Fig. 1. PDZ domain containing proteins interacting with CFTR C-terminus tail.

3.3 CFTR-associated ligand

CFTR-Associated Ligand (CAL, also called Golgi-associated PDZ and coiled-coil motif containing protein, GOPC, or PDZ Protein Interacting Specifically with TC10, PIST) is a protein of approximately 50 kDa containing a single PDZ domain and two coiled-coil domains (Fig.1). CAL can form homodimers independently of its single PDZ domain but through its N-terminal portion (Cheng et al., 2002; Cushing et al., 2008; Neudauer et al., 2001). CAL is ubiquitously expressed in the Golgi apparatus of human tissues. Although it has no transmembrane domain, CAL is associated with membranes by interacting with resident proteins from the Trans-Golgi network *via* its coiled-coil domain (Cheng et al., 2002). CAL can interact with CFTR C-terminus tail through its PDZ domain as determined by yeast two-hybrid assay and co-immunoprecipiation (Cheng et al., 2002).

3.4 Shank2

Shank2 (also known as Cortactin-binding protein 1, CortBP1; or Proline-rich synapse-associated protein 1, ProSAP1) contains a single PDZ domain and other sites for protein–protein interaction, including an SH3 domain, a long proline-rich region, and a sterile alpha motif (SAM) domain (Fig.1). The SAM domain is able to self-associate to form dimers (Gisler et al., 2001). Shank2 is expressed abundantly in brain as well as in kidney, liver, intestine, and pancreas. In this last tissue, it is localized to the luminal pole in pancreatic duct cells and luminal area of colonic epithelia (Du et al., 1998; Kim et al., 2004; Lee et al., 2007; Lim et al., 1999). Shank2 has been shown to be associated with CFTR through its PDZ domain in the yeast two-hybrid system and in mammalian cells (Kim et al., 2004).

4. PDZ interactions regulate CFTR trafficking

4.1 NHERF family proteins form a subapical network for CFTR plasma membrane docking

NHERF1, NHERF2 and NHERF3 can auto-assemble in a regulated fashion and form a subapical network serving as a cytoskeleton-anchored platform for the docking of multiple regulatory and transmembrane proteins. CFTR binding to this station is PDZ-dependent and results in increased stability at the plasma membrane. Indeed, a CFTR mutant truncated for its C-terminal PDZ interacting motif is highly mobile at the plasma membrane, whereas intact CFTR exhibits a greater immobile fraction or a more confined diffusion (Bates et al., 2006; Haggie et al., 2004; 2006). Moreover, C-terminal truncation of CFTR alters its endocytic/recycling dynamics. While CFTR endocytosis from the apical plasma membrane seems to be unaffected in polarized MDCK type I cells, C-terminal deletion decreases its recycling efficiency (Swiatecka-Urban et al., 2002). Despite the reported decrease in the half-life of ΔTRL-CFTR at the apical plasma membrane, the same group observed that its degradation rate was not accelerated. Albeit this should lead to an intracellular accumulation of ΔTRL-CFTR, it is not the case (Benharouga et al., 2003; Milewski et al., 2005; Ostedgaard et al., 2003), because other trafficking mechanisms may compensate for the recycling defect of ΔTRL-CFTR in order to ensure its observed apical localization. Recently, preliminary results from Bossard et al. (2010) reconcile this discrepancy by reporting a new intracellular trafficking pathway for CFTR polarized sorting. Indeed, apically endocytosed

CFTR is efficiently recycled back to the apical plasma membrane but a significant fraction is constitutively trafficked to the basolateral plasma membrane. This mistargeted pool is transiently localized at the basolateral cell surface, as it is rapidly rerouted to the apical plasma membrane. This transcytotic pathway occurs in various polarized cell lines such as canine kidney (MDCK type II), human airway (CFBE41o⁻) and pig kidney (LLC-PK1) epithelia (Bossard et al., 2010). When comparing wt- and ΔTRL-CFTR dynamics in CFBE epithelia, both proteins exhibit similar half-life and apical surface stability. However, ΔTRL-CFTR undergoes a faster endocytosis from the apical plasma membrane, a slower recycling to the apical membrane and a more intense transcytotic pathway (Fig.2). Those characteristics could compensate for ΔTRL-CFTR recycling defect and explain the comparable half-life and apical stability with its wt counterpart (Bossard et al., 2010). This new insight into CFTR intracellular trafficking uncovers a novel role of PDZ adaptors in protein sorting, and raises further questions about the cause of the mild CF phenotype observed in patients with C-terminally truncated CFTR mutants.

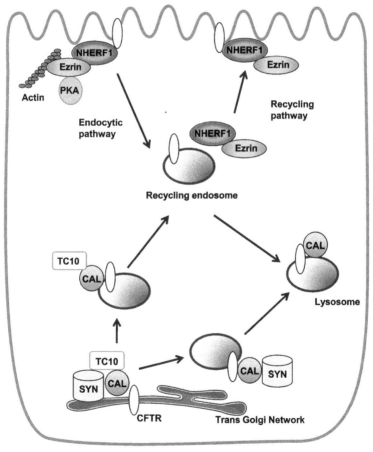

Fig. 2. Regulation of intracellular traffic of CFTR by interaction with several proteins with PDZ domains. SYN: synthaxine 6.

4.2 CAL targets CFTR to lysosomal degradation

PDZ interaction of CAL with CFTR occurs at the endosomal level and targets CFTR to lysosomal degradation (Cheng et al., 2004). This CAL-dependent sorting of CFTR is counteracted by NHERF1 binding (Cheng et al., 2002). Comparable to CFTR, both the beta1-adrenergic receptor and cadherin 23 interact with CAL, leading to their intracellular accumulation and/or degradation (Fig.2); these interactions can be competitively counteracted by binding with other PDZ domain-containing proteins (He et al., 2004; Xu et al., 2010). Likewise, CAL is an intracellular retention partner for the somatostatin receptor subtype 5 and the metabotropic glutamate receptor subtypes 1a (Wente et al., 2005; Zhang et al., 2008).

Accordingly, both inhibition of CAL protein expression and NHERF1 overexpression are efficient in promoting the cell surface expression and function of the most common disease-associated mutant, F508del-CFTR (Bossard et al., 2007; Guerra et al., 2005; Wolde et al., 2007). Interestingly, the conformational and molecular interactions between CFTR and CAL differ from those between CFTR and NHERF1, indicating that PDZ-selective inhibitors can be designed to improve CFTR mutant expression (Amacher et al., 2011; Cushing et al., 2010; Piserchio et al., 2005). CAL/CFTR interaction is modulated by the Rho family small GTPase, TC10. Its activation redistributes CAL to the plasma membrane and reverses CAL-mediated CFTR degradation (Cheng et al., 2005). Thus, CAL can play opposite roles on CFTR trafficking depending on the activation of TC10, which is a molecular switch between the degradation and exocytosis pathways. Moreover, the Q-SNARE [Q-soluble N-ethylmaleimide-sensitive fusion protein (NSF) attachment protein receptor] protein syntaxin 6 interacts with both CAL and CFTR (Charest et al., 2001; Cheng et al., 2010). Syntaxin 6 binds the N-terminal half of CFTR after its interaction with CAL, and this binding mediates CFTR lysosomal degradation (Cheng et al., 2010).

4.3 Do Shank2 and NHERF4 regulate CFTR trafficking?

Only one study reports the modulation of CFTR membrane expression by Shank2. Shank2 overexpression tends to increase CFTR membrane expression and stability (Kim et al., 2004).

Since the first study showing a CFTR/NHERF4 interaction (Hegedüs et al., 2003), no more data were published. This could be explained, in part, by the fact that NHERF4 is not expressed in lungs. Its expression is restricted to the gastrointestinal tract and kidney in mouse (Gisler et al., 2001; Scott et al., 2002; Watanabe et al., 2006) without data in human. In particular, NHERF4 is localized close to or at the apical plasma membrane (Gisler et al., 2001; Scott et al., 2002; Van De Graaf et al., 2006; Watanabe et al., 2006), consistent with CFTR localization.

5. PDZ interactions regulate CFTR function

As a phosphorylation-regulated chloride channel, CFTR physical and functional proximity to kinases and phosphodiesterases has fundamental importance. NHERF1, NHERF2 and NHERF3 have all been reported to link CFTR to PKA. Indeed, NHERF1 and NHERF2 both interact with ezrin, a well known A kinase anchoring protein (AKAP) (Fig.2) (Reczek et al.,

1997; Sun et al., 2000). Likewise, NHERF3 is able to bind the dual-specific A-kinase anchoring protein 2 (D-AKAP2) with higher affinity than NHERF1 (Gisler et al., 2003). Moreover, AKAPs are also anchors for phosphodiesterases (PDE) (Dodge-Kafka et al., 2005; Willoughby et al., 2006), allowing local fine tuning of cAMP concentration for proper regulation of CFTR channel activity. The PDE4D is the most abundant PDE in airway epithelia and forms a cAMP diffusion barrier at the apical confinement where CFTR is localized (Barnes et al., 2005). As Shank2 is associated with PDE4D, thus reducing local cAMP availability, this could explain the observed inhibition of CFTR chloride activity (Lee et al., 2007).

CFTR activation by PKA is potentiated by PKC (Winpenny et al., 1995). As NHERF1 binds the Receptor for Activated C Kinase (RACK1) through PDZ1 interaction, this interaction could anchor PKC epsilon isoform in the vicinity of CFTR and facilitate its activation (Liedtke et al., 2002; 2004).

Besides anchoring cytosolic regulatory proteins, the apical docking station formed by PDZ proteins brings other transmembrane proteins closer to CFTR for reciprocal regulation. Likewise, CFTR and the ENaC display cross-functional regulation (Jiang et al., 2000). This regulation involves NHERF1 that binds the Yes-associated protein 65 (YAP65) through its PDZ2 domain and CFTR C-terminus through PDZ1 (Mohler et al., 1999). YAP65 is an anchoring protein for the cytosolic tyrosine kinase c-Yes, a member of the Src family, which has been reported to inhibit ENaC (Gilmore et al., 2001; Mohler et al., 1999). Furthermore, NHERF1 allows the adrenergic regulation of CFTR by bridging it with the beta2-adrenoceptor at the apical plasma membrane (Naren et al., 2003; Taouil et al., 2003). NHERF2 can form a molecular bond connecting CFTR to the lysophosphatidic acid type 2 receptor or the Na^+/H^+ exchanger isoform 3. The activation of those latter proteins is able to inhibit CFTR chloride current (Bagorda et al., 2002; Favia et al., 2006; C. Li et al., 2005). Moreover, NHERF3 connects CFTR to the cAMP transporter multidrug resistance protein 4 (MRP4), which enhances CFTR function (C. Li et al., 2007).

An additional mechanism for PDZ proteins to regulate CFTR activity is their ability to form CFTR homodimers as detected in the plasma membrane of mammalian cells (Ramjeesingh et al., 2003). The formation of CFTR dimers is triggered by NHERF1, NHERF2 and NHERF3 leading to an increase in CFTR channel activity (Li et al., 2004; J. Li et al., 2005; Wang et al., 2000).

The PDZ protein CAL has not been reported to have direct influence on CFTR chloride current. However, CAL-mediated lysosomal degradation of CFTR indirectly decreases CFTR channel activity by reducing its apical plasma membrane density.

Some studies have reported that annexin A5 (AnxA5) could be involved in the traffic of CFTR. Recently, in oocytes, AnxA5 inhibited CFTR-mediated whole-cell membrane conductance presumably by a mechanism independent of PDZ-binding domain at the C-terminus of CFTR but PKC-dependent and resulted from either endocytosis activation and/or exocytosis block. In contrast, in human cells, co-expression of AnxA5 augmented CFTR whole-cell currents, an effect that was independent of CFTR PDZ-binding domain. Those results suggest that AnxA5 has multiple effects on CFTR, but the effect observed is cell system-dependent (Faria et al., 2011).

6. Are PDZ proteins potential targets for drug therapy in CF?

Because PDZ proteins regulate CFTR membrane expression and/or function, several studies have investigated the potential therapeutic effectiveness of these proteins. To date, only the potential therapeutic role of NHERF1 overexpression or CAL silencing has been investigated.

6.1 NHERF1 overexpression restores F508del-CFTR plasma membrane expression

In 2005, Guerra and colleagues observed that mouse NHERF1 but not NHERF2 overexpression increased F508del-CFTR plasma membrane expression and activity in human bronchial epithelial cell line endogenously expressing F508del-CFTR (CFBE41o-) (Guerra et al., 2005) (Fig.2). Four years later, our team demonstrated in A549 and type II MDCK cells microinjected with F508del-CFTR plasmid that human NHERF1 overexpression restored F508del-CFTR apical plasma membrane expression and chloride channel activity (Bossard et al., 2007). This effect was abolished in the presence of a sense oligonucleotide complementary to NHERF1 mRNA sequence attesting that this mechanism is specific to NHERF1 overexpression (Bossard et al., 2007). Moreover, in type II MDCK cells microinjected with a CFTR double mutant: F508del and K1468X (deletion of the 12 last C-terminus amino acids, thus avoiding PDZ-based interaction), NHERF1 overexpression had no effect on F508del-K1468X-CFTR expression and activity certifying that an interaction between F508del-CFTR and NHERF1 is required (Bossard et al., 2007). Immunostaining experiments confirmed these results by demonstrating a colocalization of F508del-CFTR and NHERF1 at the apical plasma membrane (Bossard et al., 2007). Furthermore, it is important to note that NHERF1 overexpression was not a nonspecific global rescue of ER-retained proteins because it did not restore the plasma membrane expression of an unrelated trafficking defective mutant potassium channel, KCNQ1 [mutant P117L highlighted by Dahimene et al. (2006)] (Bossard et al., 2007).

Thereby, we are currently investigating the effects of NHERF1 overexpression on F508del-CFTR expression and activity *in vivo* by non viral gene transfer using block copolymers in homozygous F508del-CFTR mice (Desigaux et al., 2005).

6.2 CAL silencing restores F508del-CFTR plasma membrane expression

RNA interference targeting endogenous CAL specifically increases cell surface expression of the F508del-CFTR mutant and thus enhances transepithelial chloride currents in polarized CFBE41o- cells overexpressing F508del-CFTR (Wolde et al., 2007) (Fig.3).

Recently, it has been demonstrated that CAL interaction with F508del-CFTR can be avoided by using a blocking peptide, iCAL36 (ANSRWPTSII), which specifically targets CAL but not NHERF1, NHERF2 or NHERF3 PDZ domain (Cushing et al., 2010). The presence of iCAL36 extends F508del-CFTR half-life at the plasma membrane in the human bronchial epithelial cell line CFBE41o- (Cushing et al., 2010) (Fig.3). It is important to mention that this blocking peptide needs a delivery agent to allow its entry into the cells, thereby limiting its potential therapeutic use.

Syntaxin 6 acts at the Trans-Golgi Network where its silencing enhances the protein expression of the rescued, post-ER F508del-CFTR mutant, but not of the non-rescued, ER-trapped F508del-CFTR (Cheng et al., 2010). Thus, impairing CAL interaction with F508del-CFTR or other CFTR mutants as well as the inhibition of CAL/Syntaxin 6 interaction could represent new therapeutic tools for CF (Fig.3).

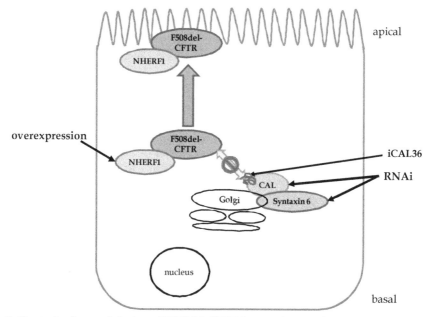

Fig. 3. Strategies for modulation of F508del-CFTR interactions with NHERF1 and CAL to enhance its apical plasma membrane expression.

6.3 Are PDZ interactions a potential drug target for CF treatment?

Since several decades, drug research has focused on finding compounds targeting receptors, ion channels, metabolic transporters and enzymes. More recently, the comprehension of the interrelated omics (genomics, proteomics, transcriptomics, metabonomics, interactomics, signalomics…) suggests that the protein-protein interactions could play a virtually universal role. Among them, PDZ-based interactions are a ubiquitous mechanism to modulate complex cellular processes. Therefore, the inhibition of a single protein-protein interaction should be highly selective in order to avoid undesirable effects.

Besides its conformational-related trafficking defect, the most frequent CFTR mutant, F508del-CFTR, also exhibits an intrinsic functional deficiency, suggesting that its potent rescue to the apical membrane might not be sufficient to restore a healthy phenotype. Consequently, PDZ protein-targeted drugs acting as a corrector treatment should be complemented with a potentiator treatment for effective therapeutic outcome. Moreover, drug or peptide candidates targeting PDZ interaction act exclusively as inhibitors, whereas PDZ interaction reinforcement (e.g. with NHERF1, NHERF2 and NHERF3) would also be suitable for CF treatment. Selective inhibition of interaction between CFTR and PDZ proteins, should likely target CAL and Shank2, which are inhibitors of CFTR expression and/or function. The physical properties of small molecule inhibitors - i.e. cell permeability, good oral bioavailability and high affinity - make them better candidates than peptidic inhibitors (including antibodies) which usually are rapidly degraded and have poor pharmacokinetics. Synthetic inhibitors can target the C-terminus (or sometimes internal)

PDZ motif or the PDZ domain of the PDZ adaptor, rendering either one unavailable for interaction. Taking CFTR as an example target, the inhibitor should avoid CFTR interaction with CAL but not with NHERF1, NHERF2 or NHERF3. This could be accomplished by competitive inhibition (i) if the small molecule inhibitor can block an interaction interface specific to CAL but not to NHERF1, NHERF2 or NHERF3, or (ii) if the affinity of CFTR C-terminus for the small molecule is similar to that for CAL, and lower than that for NHERF1, NHERF2 or NHERF3 which has already been reported (Cushing et al., 2008). It is important that the small molecules that bind CAL to inhibit CAL/CFTR interaction, should not interfere with CAL's other partners in order to prevent any possible adverse effect. In any case, the crystal structure of both interacting partners and especially the geometry of the protein-protein interaction interface can help to rationally design small molecules inhibitors. Moreover, the targeted interaction could only be material in specific organs, tissues, cell types and subcellular compartments, hence complicating the task to achieve targeted drug delivery and selective effects. Although, small molecule inhibitors of PDZ-based interactions are of great interest as research tools for understanding the involvement of these scaffolding proteins in protein trafficking and function, their usefulness as therapeutic agents is still elusive and needs further investigations.

7. Conclusion

In conclusion, PDZ domains containing proteins have a fundamental role in the regulation of CFTR trafficking and chloride channel activity. The modulation of their selective interaction with CFTR using gene therapy and/or drug treatments is an auspicious approach for the treatment of patients harboring CFTR trafficking defect mutations such as F508del, but it remains to be intensively and carefully investigated in order to assess their specificity and possible side effects.

8. Acknowledgment

Our work was supported by the Association "Vaincre la mucoviscidose".

9. References

Altschuler, Y.; Hodson, C. & Milgram, S. L. (2003). The Apical Compartment: Trafficking Pathways, Regulators and Scaffolding Proteins. *Current Opinion in Cell Biology*, 15, 4, pp. 423-429.

Amacher, J. F.; Cushing, P. R.; Weiner, J. A. & Madden, D. R. (2011). Crystallization and Preliminary Diffraction Analysis of the Cal Pdz Domain in Complex with a Selective Peptide Inhibitor. *Acta crystallographica*, 67, Pt 5, pp. 600-603.

Anderson, M. P.; Berger, H. A.; Rich, D. P.; Gregory, R. J.; Smith, A. E. & Welsh, M. J. (1991). Nucleoside Triphosphates Are Required to Open the Cftr Chloride Channel. *Cell*, 67, 4, pp. 775-784.

Bagorda, A.; Guerra, L.; Di Sole, F.; Hemle-Kolb, C.; Cardone, R. A.; Fanelli, T.; Reshkin, S. J.; Gisler, S. M.; Murer, H. & Casavola, V. (2002). Reciprocal Protein Kinase a Regulatory Interactions between Cystic Fibrosis Transmembrane Conductance Regulator and Na+/H+ Exchanger Isoform 3 in a Renal Polarized Epithelial Cell Model. *The Journal of Biological Chemistry*, 277, 24, pp. 21480-21488.

Barasch, J.; Kiss, B.; Prince, A.; Saiman, L.; Gruenert, D. & Al-Awqati, Q. (1991). Defective Acidification of Intracellular Organelles in Cystic Fibrosis. *Nature*, 352, 6330, pp. 70-73.

Barnes, A. P.; Livera, G.; Huang, P.; Sun, C.; O'neal, W. K.; Conti, M.; Stutts, M. J. & Milgram, S. L. (2005). Phosphodiesterase 4d Forms a Camp Diffusion Barrier at the Apical Membrane of the Airway Epithelium. *The Journal of Biological Chemistry*, 280, 9, pp. 7997-8003.

Bates, I. R.; Hebert, B.; Luo, Y.; Liao, J.; Bachir, A. I.; Kolin, D. L.; Wiseman, P. W. & Hanrahan, J. W. (2006). Membrane Lateral Diffusion and Capture of Cftr within Transient Confinement Zones. *Biophysical Journal*, 91, 3, pp. 1046-1058.

Benharouga, M.; Sharma, M.; So, J.; Haardt, M.; Drzymala, L.; Popov, M.; Schwapach, B.; Grinstein, S.; Du, K. & Lukacs, G. L. (2003). The Role of the C Terminus and Na+/H+ Exchanger Regulatory Factor in the Functional Expression of Cystic Fibrosis Transmembrane Conductance Regulator in Nonpolarized Cells and Epithelia. *The Journal of Biological Chemistry*, 278, 24, pp. 22079-22089.

Berger, H. A.; Anderson, M. P.; Gregory, R. J.; Thompson, S.; Howard, P. W.; Maurer, R. A.; Mulligan, R.; Smith, A. E. & Welsh, M. J. (1991). Identification and Regulation of the Cystic Fibrosis Transmembrane Conductance Regulator-Generated Chloride Channel. *The Journal of Clinical Investigation*, 88, 4, pp. 1422-1431.

Bezprozvanny, I. & Maximov, A. (2001). Pdz Domains: More Than Just a Glue. *Proceedings of the National Academy of Sciences of the United States of America*, 98, 3, pp. 787-789.

Bossard, F.; Robay, A.; Toumaniantz, G.; Dahimene, S.; Becq, F.; Merot, J. & Gauthier, C. (2007). Nhe-Rf1 Protein Rescues Deltaf508-Cftr Function. *American Journal of Physiology - Lung Cellular and Molecular Physiology*, 292, 5, pp. L1085-1094.

Bossard, F.; Veit, G.; Borot, F.; Barrière, H. & Lukacs, G. L. (2010). Cellular Mechanism of Cftr Polarized Expression in Epithelia. *Proceedings of 50th annual meeting of the American Society for Cell Biology*, Philadelphia, PA, USA, December 2010. In: *Molecular Biology of the Cell*, 21, pp. 4299.

Charest, A.; Lane, K.; Mcmahon, K. & Housman, D. E. (2001). Association of a Novel Pdz Domain-Containing Peripheral Golgi Protein with the Q-Snare (Q-Soluble N-Ethylmaleimide-Sensitive Fusion Protein (Nsf) Attachment Protein Receptor) Protein Syntaxin 6. *The Journal of Biological Chemistry*, 276, 31, pp. 29456-29465.

Cheng, J.; Moyer, B. D.; Milewski, M. I.; Loffing, J.; Ikeda, M.; Mickle, J. E.; Cutting, G. R.; Li, M.; Stanton, B. A. & Guggino, W. B. (2002). A Golgi-Associated Pdz Domain Protein Modulates Cystic Fibrosis Transmembrane Regulator Plasma Membrane Expression. *The Journal of Biological Chemistry*, 277, 5, pp. 3520-3529.

Cheng, J.; Wang, H. & Guggino, W. B. (2004). Modulation of Mature Cystic Fibrosis Transmembrane Regulator Protein by the Pdz Domain Protein Cal. *The Journal of Biological Chemistry*, 279, 3, pp. 1892-1898.

Cheng, J.; Wang, H. & Guggino, W. B. (2005). Regulation of Cystic Fibrosis Transmembrane Regulator Trafficking and Protein Expression by a Rho Family Small Gtpase Tc10. *The Journal of Biological Chemistry*, 280, 5, pp. 3731-3739.

Cheng, J.; Cebotaru, V.; Cebotaru, L. & Guggino, W. B. (2010). Syntaxin 6 and Cal Mediate the Degradation of the Cystic Fibrosis Transmembrane Conductance Regulator. *Molecular Biology of the Cell*, 21, 7, pp. 1178-1187.

Cheng, S. H.; Gregory, R. J.; Marshall, J.; Paul, S.; Souza, D. W.; White, G. A.; O'riordan, C. R. & Smith, A. E. (1990). Defective Intracellular Transport and Processing of Cftr Is the Molecular Basis of Most Cystic Fibrosis. *Cell*, 63, 4, pp. 827-834.

Cushing, P. R.; Fellows, A.; Villone, D.; BoisgueRin, P. & Madden, D. R. (2008). The Relative Binding Affinities of Pdz Partners for Cftr: A Biochemical Basis for Efficient Endocytic Recycling†. *Biochemistry*, 47, 38, pp. 10084-10098.

Cushing, P. R.; Vouilleme, L.; Pellegrini, M.; Boisguerin, P. & Madden, D. R. (2010). A Stabilizing Influence: Cal Pdz Inhibition Extends the Half-Life of Deltaf508-Cftr. *Angewandte Chemie International Edition in English*, 49, 51, pp. 9907-9911.

Dahimene, S.; Alcolea, S.; Naud, P.; Jourdon, P.; Escande, D.; Brasseur, R.; Thomas, A.; Baro, I. & Merot, J. (2006). The N-Terminal Juxtamembranous Domain of Kcnq1 Is Critical for Channel Surface Expression: Implications in the Romano-Ward Lqt1 Syndrome. *Circulation Research*, 99, 10, pp. 1076-1083.

Dalemans, W.; Hinnrasky, J.; Slos, P.; Dreyer, D.; Fuchey, C.; Pavirani, A. & Puchelle, E. (1992). Immunocytochemical Analysis Reveals Differences between the Subcellular Localization of Normal and Delta Phe508 Recombinant Cystic Fibrosis Transmembrane Conductance Regulator. *Experimental Cell Research*, 201, 1, pp. 235-240.

Desigaux, L.; Gourden, C.; Bello-Roufaï, M.; Richard, P.; Oudrhiri, N.; Lehn, P.; Escande, D.; Pollard, H. & Pitard, B. (2005). Nonionic Amphiphilic Block Copolymers Promote Gene Transfer to the Lung. *Human Gene Therapy*, 16, 7, pp. 821-829.

Dodge-Kafka, K. L.; Soughayer, J.; Pare, G. C.; Carlisle Michel, J. J.; Langeberg, L. K.; Kapiloff, M. S. & Scott, J. D. (2005). The Protein Kinase a Anchoring Protein Makap Coordinates Two Integrated Camp Effector Pathways. *Nature*, 437, 7058, pp. 574-578.

Du, Y.; Weed, S. A.; Xiong, W. C.; Marshall, T. D. & Parsons, J. T. (1998). Identification of a Novel Cortactin Sh3 Domain-Binding Protein and Its Localization to Growth Cones of Cultured Neurons. *Molecular and Cellular Biology*, 18, 10, pp. 5838-5851.

Egan, M.; Flotte, T.; Afione, S.; Solow, R.; Zeitlin, P. L.; Carter, B. J. & Guggino, W. B. (1992). Defective Regulation of Outwardly Rectifying Cl- Channels by Protein Kinase a Corrected by Insertion of Cftr. *Nature*, 358, 6387, pp. 581-584.

Fanning, A. S. & Anderson, J. M. (1999). Protein Modules as Organizers of Membrane Structure. *Current Opinion in Cell Biology*, 11, 4, pp. 432-439.

Faria D., Dahimène S., Alessio L., Scott-Ward T., Schreiber R., Kunzelmann K., Amaral M.D. Effect of Annexin A5 on CFTR: regulated traffic or scaffolding? *Molecular Membrane Biology*, 28(1), pp. 14-29

Favia, M.; Fanelli, T.; Bagorda, A.; Di Sole, F.; Reshkin, S. J.; Suh, P. G.; Guerra, L. & Casavola, V. (2006). Nhe3 Inhibits Pka-Dependent Functional Expression of Cftr by Nherf2 Pdz Interactions. *Biochemical and Biophysical Research Communications*, 347, 2, pp. 452-459.

Fouassier, L.; Yun, C. C.; Fitz, J. G. & Doctor, R. B. (2000). Evidence for Ezrin-Radixin-Moesin-Binding Phosphoprotein 50 (Ebp50) Self-Association through Pdz-Pdz Interactions. *The Journal of Biological Chemistry*, 275, 32, pp. 25039-25045.

Gabriel, S. E.; Clarke, L. L.; Boucher, R. C. & Stutts, M. J. (1993). Cftr and Outward Rectifying Chloride Channels Are Distinct Proteins with a Regulatory Relationship. *Nature*, 363, 6426, pp. 263-268.

Gilmore, E. S.; Stutts, M. J. & Milgram, S. L. (2001). Src Family Kinases Mediate Epithelial Na+ Channel Inhibition by Endothelin. *The Journal of Biological Chemistry*, 276, 45, pp. 42610-42617.

Gisler, S. M.; Stagljar, I.; Traebert, M.; Bacic, D.; Biber, J. R. & Murer, H. (2001). Interaction of the Type Iia Na/Pi Cotransporter with Pdz Proteins. *The Journal of Biological Chemistry*, 276, 12, pp. 9206-9213.

Gisler, S. M.; Madjdpour, C.; Bacic, D.; Pribanic, S.; Taylor, S. S.; Biber, J. & Murer, H. (2003). Pdzk1: Ii. An Anchoring Site for the Pka-Binding Protein D-Akap2 in Renal Proximal Tubular Cells. *Kidney International*, 64, 5, pp. 1746-1754.

Guerra, L.; Fanelli, T.; Favia, M.; Riccardi, S. M.; Busco, G.; Cardone, R. A.; Carrabino, S.; Weinman, E. J.; Reshkin, S. J.; Conese, M. & Casavola, V. (2005). Na+/H+ Exchanger Regulatory Factor Isoform 1 Overexpression Modulates Cystic Fibrosis Transmembrane Conductance Regulator (Cftr) Expression and Activity in Human Airway 16hbe14o- Cells and Rescues Deltaf508 Cftr Functional Expression in Cystic Fibrosis Cells. *The Journal of Biological Chemistry*, 280, 49, pp. 40925-40933.

Haggie, P. M.; Stanton, B. A. & Verkman, A. S. (2004). Increased Diffusional Mobility of Cftr at the Plasma Membrane after Deletion of Its C-Terminal Pdz Binding Motif. *The Journal of biological chemistry*, 279, 7, pp. 5494-5500.

Haggie, P. M.; Kim, J. K.; Lukacs, G. L. & Verkman, A. S. (2006). Tracking of Quantum Dot-Labeled Cftr Shows near Immobilization by C-Terminal Pdz Interactions. *Molecular Biology of the Cell*, 17, 12, pp. 4937-4945.

Hall, R. A.; Ostedgaard, L. S.; Premont, R. T.; Blitzer, J. T.; Rahman, N.; Welsh, M. J. & Lefkowitz, R. J. (1998). A C-Terminal Motif Found in the Beta2-Adrenergic Receptor, P2y1 Receptor and Cystic Fibrosis Transmembrane Conductance Regulator Determines Binding to the Na+/H+ Exchanger Regulatory Factor Family of Pdz Proteins. *Proceedings of the National Academy of Sciences of the United States of America*, 95, 15, pp. 8496-8501.

Harris, B. Z. & Lim, W. A. (2001). Mechanism and Role of Pdz Domains in Signaling Complex Assembly. *Journal of Cell Science*, 114, Pt 18, pp. 3219-3231.

He, J.; Bellini, M.; Xu, J.; Castleberry, A. M. & Hall, R. A. (2004). Interaction with Cystic Fibrosis Transmembrane Conductance Regulator-Associated Ligand (Cal) Inhibits Beta1-Adrenergic Receptor Surface Expression. *The Journal of Biological Chemistry*, 279, 48, pp. 50190-50196.

Hegedüs, T.; Sessler, T.; Scott, R.; Thelin, W.; Bakos, É.; Váradi, A.; Szabó, K.; Homolya, L.; Milgram, S. L. & Sarkadi, B. (2003). C-Terminal Phosphorylation of Mrp2 Modulates Its Interaction with Pdz Proteins. *Biochemical and Biophysical Research Communications*, 302, 3, pp. 454-461.

Hillier, B. J.; Christopherson, K. S.; Prehoda, K. E.; Bredt, D. S. & Lim, W. A. (1999). Unexpected Modes of Pdz Domain Scaffolding Revealed by Structure of Nnos-Syntrophin Complex. *Science*, 284, 5415, pp. 812-815.

Hung, A. Y. & Sheng, M. (2002). Pdz Domains: Structural Modules for Protein Complex Assembly. *The Journal of Biological Chemistry*, 277, 8, pp. 5699-5702.

Ingraffea, J.; Reczek, D. & Bretscher, A. (2002). Distinct Cell Type-Specific Expression of Scaffolding Proteins Ebp50 and E3karp: Ebp50 Is Generally Expressed with Ezrin in Specific Epithelia, Whereas E3karp Is Not. *European Journal of Cell Biology*, 81, 2, pp. 61-68.

Jiang, Q.; Li, J.; Dubroff, R.; Ahn, Y. J.; Foskett, J. K.; Engelhardt, J. & Kleyman, T. R. (2000). Epithelial Sodium Channels Regulate Cystic Fibrosis Transmembrane Conductance Regulator Chloride Channels in Xenopusoocytes. *The Journal of Biological Chemistry*, 275, 18, pp. 13266-13274.

Kerem, B.; Rommens, J. M.; Buchanan, J. A.; Markiewicz, D.; Cox, T. K.; Chakravarti, A.; Buchwald, M. & Tsui, L. C. (1989). Identification of the Cystic Fibrosis Gene: Genetic Analysis. *Science*, 245, 4922, pp. 1073-1080.

Kim, J. Y.; Han, W.; Namkung, W.; Lee, J. H.; Kim, K. H.; Shin, H.; Kim, E. & Lee, M. G. (2004). Inhibitory Regulation of Cystic Fibrosis Transmembrane Conductance Regulator Anion-Transporting Activities by Shank2. *The Journal of Biological Chemistry*, 279, 11, pp. 10389-10396.

Ko, S. B.; Shcheynikov, N.; Choi, J. Y.; Luo, X.; Ishibashi, K.; Thomas, P. J.; Kim, J. Y.; Kim, K. H.; Lee, M. G.; Naruse, S. & Muallem, S. (2002). A Molecular Mechanism for Aberrant Cftr-Dependent Hco(3)(-) Transport in Cystic Fibrosis. *EMBO Journal*, 21, 21, pp. 5662-5672.

Kocher, O.; Comella, N.; Gilchrist, A.; Pal, R.; Tognazzi, K.; Brown, L. F. & Knoll, J. H. (1999). Pdzk1, a Novel Pdz Domain-Containing Protein up-Regulated in Carcinomas and Mapped to Chromosome 1q21, Interacts with Cmoat (Mrp2), the Multidrug Resistance-Associated Protein. *Laboratory Investigation*, 79, 9, pp. 1161-1170.

Kunzelmann, K.; Kiser, G. L.; Schreiber, R. & Riordan, J. R. (1997). Inhibition of Epithelial Na+ Currents by Intracellular Domains of the Cystic Fibrosis Transmembrane Conductance Regulator. *FEBS Letters*, 400, 3, pp. 341-344.

Lalonde, D. P. & Bretscher, A. (2009). The Scaffold Protein Pdzk1 Undergoes a Head-to-Tail Intramolecular Association That Negatively Regulates Its Interaction with Ebp50. *Biochemistry*, 48, 10, pp. 2261-2271.

Lau, A. G. & Hall, R. A. (2001). Oligomerization of Nherf-1 and Nherf-2 Pdz Domains: Differential Regulation by Association with Receptor Carboxyl-Termini and by Phosphorylation. *Biochemistry*, 40, 29, pp. 8572-8580.

Lee, J. H.; Richter, W.; Namkung, W.; Kim, K. H.; Kim, E.; Conti, M. & Lee, M. G. (2007). Dynamic Regulation of Cystic Fibrosis Transmembrane Conductance Regulator by Competitive Interactions of Molecular Adaptors. *The Journal of Biological Chemistry*, 282, 14, pp. 10414-10422.

Li, C.; Roy, K.; Dandridge, K. & Naren, A. P. (2004). Molecular Assembly of Cystic Fibrosis Transmembrane Conductance Regulator in Plasma Membrane. *The Journal of Biological Chemistry*, 279, 23, pp. 24673-24684.

Li, C.; Dandridge, K. S.; Di, A.; Marrs, K. L.; Harris, E. L.; Roy, K.; Jackson, J. S.; Makarova, N. V.; Fujiwara, Y.; Farrar, P. L.; Nelson, D. J.; Tigyi, G. J. & Naren, A. P. (2005). Lysophosphatidic Acid Inhibits Cholera Toxin-Induced Secretory Diarrhea through Cftr-Dependent Protein Interactions. *The Journal of Experimental Medicine*, 202, 7, pp. 975-986.

Li, C.; Krishnamurthy, P. C.; Penmatsa, H.; Marrs, K. L.; Wang, X. Q.; Zaccolo, M.; Jalink, K.; Li, M.; Nelson, D. J.; Schuetz, J. D. & Naren, A. P. (2007). Spatiotemporal Coupling of Camp Transporter to Cftr Chloride Channel Function in the Gut Epithelia. *Cell*, 131, 5, pp. 940-951.

Li, J.; Dai, Z.; Jana, D.; Callaway, D. J. E. & Bu, Z. (2005). Ezrin Controls the Macromolecular Complexes Formed between an Adapter Protein Na+/H+ Exchanger Regulatory

Factor and the Cystic Fibrosis Transmembrane Conductance Regulator. *The Journal of Biological Chemistry*, 280, 45, pp. 37634-37643.

Li, J.; Poulikakos, P. I.; Dai, Z.; Testa, J. R.; Callaway, D. J. & Bu, Z. (2007). Protein Kinase C Phosphorylation Disrupts Na+/H+ Exchanger Regulatory Factor 1 Autoinhibition and Promotes Cystic Fibrosis Transmembrane Conductance Regulator Macromolecular Assembly. *The Journal of Biological Chemistry*, 282, 37, pp. 27086-27099.

Liedtke, C. M.; Yun, C. H. C.; Kyle, N. & Wang, D. (2002). Protein Kinase C(Epsilon)-Dependent Regulation of Cystic Fibrosis Transmembrane Regulator Involves Binding to a Receptor for Activated C Kinase (Rack1) and Rack1 Binding to Na+/H+ Exchange Regulatory Factor. *The Journal of Biological Chemistry*, 277, 25, pp. 22925-22933.

Liedtke, C. M.; Raghuram, V.; Yun, C. C. & Wang, X. (2004). Role of a Pdz1 Domain of Nherf1 in the Binding of Airway Epithelial Rack1 to Nherf1. *American Journal of Physiology - Cell Physiology*, 286, 5, pp. C1037-1044.

Lim, S.; Naisbitt, S.; Yoon, J.; Hwang, J. I.; Suh, P. G.; Sheng, M. & Kim, E. (1999). Characterization of the Shank Family of Synaptic Proteins. Multiple Genes, Alternative Splicing, and Differential Expression in Brain and Development. *The Journal of Biological Chemistry*, 274, 41, pp. 29510-29518.

Lohi, H.; Lamprecht, G.; Markovich, D.; Heil, A.; Kujala, M.; Seidler, U. & Kere, J. (2003). Isoforms of Slc26a6 Mediate Anion Transport and Have Functional Pdz Interaction Domains. *American Journal of Physiology - Cell Physiology*, 284, 3, pp. C769-779.

Loussouarn, G.; Demolombe, S.; Mohammad-Panah, R.; Escande, D. & Baro, I. (1996). Expression of Cftr Controls Camp-Dependent Activation of Epithelial K+ Currents. *American Journal of Physiology*, 271, 5 Pt 1, pp. C1565-1573.

Lukacs, G. L.; Chang, X. B.; Kartner, N.; Rotstein, O. D.; Riordan, J. R. & Grinstein, S. (1992). The Cystic Fibrosis Transmembrane Regulator Is Present and Functional in Endosomes. Role as a Determinant of Endosomal Ph. *The Journal of Biological Chemistry*, 267, 21, pp. 14568-14572.

Mickle, J. E.; Macek, M., Jr.; Fulmer-Smentek, S. B.; Egan, M. M.; Schwiebert, E.; Guggino, W.; Moss, R. & Cutting, G. R. (1998). A Mutation in the Cystic Fibrosis Transmembrane Conductance Regulator Gene Associated with Elevated Sweat Chloride Concentrations in the Absence of Cystic Fibrosis. *Human Molecular Genetics*, 7, 4, pp. 729-735.

Milewski, M. I.; Lopez, A.; Jurkowska, M.; Larusch, J. & Cutting, G. R. (2005). Pdz-Binding Motifs Are Unable to Ensure Correct Polarized Protein Distribution in the Absence of Additional Localization Signals. *FEBS letters*, 579, 2, pp. 483-487.

Mohler, P. J.; Kreda, S. M.; Boucher, R. C.; Sudol, M.; Stutts, M. J. & Milgram, S. L. (1999). Yes-Associated Protein 65 Localizes P62(C-Yes) to the Apical Compartment of Airway Epithelia by Association with Ebp50. *The Journal of Cell Biology*, 147, 4, pp. 879-890.

Moyer, B. D.; Denton, J.; Karlson, K. H.; Reynolds, D.; Wang, S.; Mickle, J. E.; Milewski, M.; Cutting, G. R.; Guggino, W. B.; Li, M. & Stanton, B. A. (1999). A Pdz-Interacting Domain in Cftr Is an Apical Membrane Polarization Signal. *The Journal of Clinical Investigation*, 104, 10, pp. 1353-1361.

Moyer, B. D.; Duhaime, M.; Shaw, C.; Denton, J.; Reynolds, D.; Karlson, K. H.; Pfeiffer, J.; Wang, S.; Mickle, J. E.; Milewski, M.; Cutting, G. R.; Guggino, W. B.; Li, M. & Stanton, B. A. (2000). The Pdz-Interacting Domain of Cystic Fibrosis Transmembrane Conductance Regulator Is Required for Functional Expression in the Apical Plasma Membrane. *The Journal of Biological Chemistry*, 275, 35, pp. 27069-27074.

Naren, A. P.; Cobb, B.; Li, C.; Roy, K.; Nelson, D.; Heda, G. D.; Liao, J.; Kirk, K. L.; Sorscher, E. J.; Hanrahan, J. & Clancy, J. P. (2003). A Macromolecular Complex of Beta 2 Adrenergic Receptor, Cftr, and Ezrin/Radixin/Moesin-Binding Phosphoprotein 50 Is Regulated by Pka. *Proceedings of the National Academy of Sciences of the United States of America*, 100, 1, pp. 342-346.

Neudauer, C. L.; Joberty, G. & Macara, I. G. (2001). Pist: A Novel Pdz/Coiled-Coil Domain Binding Partner for the Rho-Family Gtpase Tc10. *Biochemical and Biophysical Research Communications*, 280, 2, pp. 541-547.

Ostedgaard, L. S.; Randak, C.; Rokhlina, T.; Karp, P.; Vermeer, D.; Ashbourne Excoffon, K. J. & Welsh, M. J. (2003). Effects of C-Terminal Deletions on Cystic Fibrosis Transmembrane Conductance Regulator Function in Cystic Fibrosis Airway Epithelia. *Proceedings of the National Academy of Sciences of the United States of America*, 100, 4, pp. 1937-1942.

Paasche, J. D.; Attramadal, T.; Kristiansen, K.; Oksvold, M. P.; Johansen, H. K.; Huitfeldt, H. S.; Dahl, S. G. & Attramadal, H. (2005). Subtype-Specific Sorting of the Eta Endothelin Receptor by a Novel Endocytic Recycling Signal for G Protein-Coupled Receptors. *Molecular Pharmacology*, 67, 5, pp. 1581-1590.

Pasyk, E. A. & Foskett, J. K. (1995). Mutant (Delta F508) Cystic Fibrosis Transmembrane Conductance Regulator Cl- Channel Is Functional When Retained in Endoplasmic Reticulum of Mammalian Cells. *The Journal of Biological Chemistry*, 270, 21, pp. 12347-12350.

Pietrement, C.; Da Silva, N.; Silberstein, C.; James, M.; Marsolais, M.; Van Hoek, A.; Brown, D.; Pastor-Soler, N.; Ameen, N.; Laprade, R.; Ramesh, V. & Breton, S. (2008). Role of Nherf1, Cystic Fibrosis Transmembrane Conductance Regulator, and Camp in the Regulation of Aquaporin 9. *The Journal of Biological Chemistry*, 283, 5, pp. 2986-2996.

Piserchio, A.; Fellows, A.; Madden, D. R. & Mierke, D. F. (2005). Association of the Cystic Fibrosis Transmembrane Regulator with Cal: Structural Features and Molecular Dynamics. *Biochemistry*, 44, 49, pp. 16158-16166.

Ramjeesingh, M.; Kidd, J. F.; Huan, L. J.; Wang, Y. & Bear, C. E. (2003). Dimeric Cystic Fibrosis Transmembrane Conductance Regulator Exists in the Plasma Membrane. *Biochemical Journal*, 374, 3, pp. 793-797.

Reczek, D.; Berryman, M. & Bretscher, A. (1997). Identification of Ebp50: A Pdz-Containing Phosphoprotein That Associates with Members of the Ezrin-Radixin-Moesin Family. *The Journal of Cell Biology*, 139, 1, pp. 169-179.

Riordan, J. R.; Rommens, J. M.; Kerem, B.; Alon, N.; Rozmahel, R.; Grzelczak, Z.; Zielenski, J.; Lok, S.; Plavsic, N.; Chou, J. L. & Et Al. (1989). Identification of the Cystic Fibrosis Gene: Cloning and Characterization of Complementary DNA. *Science*, 245, 4922, pp. 1066-1073.

Rommens, J. M.; Iannuzzi, M. C.; Kerem, B.; Drumm, M. L.; Melmer, G.; Dean, M.; Rozmahel, R.; Cole, J. L.; Kennedy, D.; Hidaka, N. & Et Al. (1989). Identification of the Cystic Fibrosis Gene: Chromosome Walking and Jumping. *Science*, 245, 4922, pp. 1059-1065.

Salvatore, D.; Tomaiuolo, R.; Vanacore, B.; Elce, A.; Castaldo, G. & Salvatore, F. (2005). Isolated Elevated Sweat Chloride Concentrations in the Presence of the Rare Mutation S1455x: An Extremely Mild Form of Cftr Dysfunction. *American Journal of Medical Genetics*, 133A, 2, pp. 207-208.

Schreiber, R.; Greger, R.; Nitschke, R. & Kunzelmann, K. (1997). Cystic Fibrosis Transmembrane Conductance Regulator Activates Water Conductance in Xenopus Oocytes. *Pflügers Archiv European Journal of Physiology*, 434, 6, pp. 841-847.

Schreiber, R.; Nitschke, R.; Greger, R. & Kunzelmann, K. (1999). The Cystic Fibrosis Transmembrane Conductance Regulator Activates Aquaporin 3 in Airway Epithelial Cells. *The Journal of Biological Chemistry*, 274, 17, pp. 11811-11816.

Scott, R. O.; Thelin, W. R. & Milgram, S. L. (2002). A Novel Pdz Protein Regulates the Activity of Guanylyl Cyclase C, the Heat-Stable Enterotoxin Receptor. *The Journal of Biological Chemistry*, 277, 25, pp. 22934-22941.

Seidler, U.; Singh, A. K.; Cinar, A.; Chen, M.; Hillesheim, J.; Hogema, B. & Riederer, B. (2009). The Role of the Nherf Family of Pdz Scaffolding Proteins in the Regulation of Salt and Water Transport. *Annals of the New York Academy of Sciences*, 1165, pp. 249-260.

Shenolikar, S.; Minkoff, C. M.; Steplock, D. A.; Evangelista, C.; Liu, M. & Weinman, E. J. (2001). N-Terminal Pdz Domain Is Required for Nherf Dimerization. *FEBS letters*, 489, 2-3, pp. 233-236.

Short, D. B.; Trotter, K. W.; Reczek, D.; Kreda, S. M.; Bretscher, A.; Boucher, R. C.; Stutts, M. J. & Milgram, S. L. (1998). An Apical Pdz Protein Anchors the Cystic Fibrosis Transmembrane Conductance Regulator to the Cytoskeleton. *The Journal of Biological Chemistry*, 273, 31, pp. 19797-19801.

Singh, A. K.; Riederer, B.; Krabbenhä¶Ft, A.; Rausch, B.; Bonhagen, J.; Lehmann, U.; De Jonge, H. R.; Donowitz, M.; Yun, C.; Weinman, E. J.; Kocher, O.; Hogema, B. M. & Seidler, U. (2009). Differential Roles of Nherf1, Nherf2, and Pdzk1 in Regulating Cftr-Mediated Intestinal Anion Secretion in Mice. *The Journal of Clinical Investigation*, 119, 3, pp. 540-550.

Slattery, C.; Jenkin, K. A.; Lee, A.; Simcocks, A. C.; Mcainch, A. J.; Poronnik, P. & Hryciw, D. H. (2011). Na+-H+ Exchanger Regulatory Factor 1 (Nherf1) Pdz Scaffold Binds an Internal Binding Site in the Scavenger Receptor Megalin. *Cellular Physiology and Biochemistry*, 27, 2, pp. 171-178.

Stutts, M.; Canessa, C.; Olsen, J.; Hamrick, M.; Cohn, J.; Rossier, B. & Boucher, R. (1995). Cftr as a Camp-Dependent Regulator of Sodium Channels. *Science*, 269, 5225, pp. 847-850.

Sun, F.; Hug, M. J.; Lewarchik, C. M.; Yun, C. H.; Bradbury, N. A. & Frizzell, R. A. (2000). E3karp Mediates the Association of Ezrin and Protein Kinase a with the Cystic Fibrosis Transmembrane Conductance Regulator in Airway Cells. *The Journal of Biological Chemistry*, 275, 38, pp. 29539-29546.

Svennevig, K.; Prydz, K. & Kolset, S. O. (1995). Proteoglycans in Polarized Epithelial Madin-Darby Canine Kidney Cells. *Biochemical Journal*, 311 (Pt 3), pp. 881-888.

Swiatecka-Urban, A.; Duhaime, M.; Coutermarsh, B.; Karlson, K. H.; Collawn, J.; Milewski, M.; Cutting, G. R.; Guggino, W. B.; Langford, G. & Stanton, B. A. (2002). Pdz Domain

Interaction Controls the Endocytic Recycling of the Cystic Fibrosis Transmembrane Conductance Regulator. *The Journal of Biological Chemistry*, 277, 42, pp. 40099-40105.

Tabcharani, J. A.; Chang, X. B.; Riordan, J. R. & Hanrahan, J. W. (1991). Phosphorylation-Regulated Cl- Channel in Cho Cells Stably Expressing the Cystic Fibrosis Gene. *Nature*, 352, 6336, pp. 628-631.

Taouil, K.; Hinnrasky, J.; Hologne, C.; Corlieu, P.; Klossek, J.-M. & Puchelle, E. (2003). Stimulation of Î²2-Adrenergic Receptor Increases Cystic Fibrosis Transmembrane Conductance Regulator Expression in Human Airway Epithelial Cells through a Camp/Protein Kinase a-Independent Pathway. *The Journal of Biological Chemistry*, 278, 19, pp. 17320-17327.

Van De Graaf, S.; Hoenderop, J.; Van Der Kemp, A.; Gisler, S. & Bindels, R. (2006). Interaction of the Epithelial Ca≪Sup≫2+≪/Sup≫ Channels Trpv5 and Trpv6 with the Intestine- and Kidney-Enriched Pdz Protein Nherf4. *Pflügers Archiv European Journal of Physiology*, 452, 4, pp. 407-417.

Wang, S.; Raab, R. W.; Schatz, P. J.; Guggino, W. B. & Li, M. (1998). Peptide Binding Consensus of the Nhe-Rf-Pdz1 Domain Matches the C-Terminal Sequence of Cystic Fibrosis Transmembrane Conductance Regulator (Cftr). *FEBS letters*, 427, 1, pp. 103-108.

Wang, S.; Yue, H.; Derin, R. B.; Guggino, W. B. & Li, M. (2000). Accessory Protein Facilitated Cftr-Cftr Interaction, a Molecular Mechanism to Potentiate the Chloride Channel Activity. *Cell*, 103, 1, pp. 169-179.

Watanabe, C.; Kato, Y.; Sugiura, T.; Kubo, Y.; Wakayama, T.; Iseki, S. & Tsuji, A. (2006). Pdz Adaptor Protein Pdzk2 Stimulates Transport Activity of Organic Cation/Carnitine Transporter Octn2 by Modulating Cell Surface Expression. *Drug Metabolism and Disposition*, 34, 11, pp. 1927-1934.

Wei, L.; Vankeerberghen, A.; Cuppens, H.; Eggermont, J.; Cassiman, J. J.; Droogmans, G. & Nilius, B. (1999). Interaction between Calcium-Activated Chloride Channels and the Cystic Fibrosis Transmembrane Conductance Regulator. *Pflügers Archiv European Journal of Physiology*, 438, 5, pp. 635-641.

Welsh, M. J.; Tsui, L. C.; Boat, T. M. & Beaudet, A. L. (1995). Cystic Fibrosis, In: *The Metabolic and Molecular Bases of Inherited Disease.*, Scriver, C. R., Beaudet, A. L., Sly, W. S. & Valle, D., pp. 3799-3876, McGraw-Hill, New-York, NY.

Wente, W.; Stroh, T.; Beaudet, A.; Richter, D. & Kreienkamp, H.-J. R. (2005). Interactions with Pdz Domain Proteins Pist/Gopc and Pdzk1 Regulate Intracellular Sorting of the Somatostatin Receptor Subtype 5. *The Journal of Biological Chemistry*, 280, 37, pp. 32419-32425.

Willoughby, D.; Wong, W.; Schaack, J.; Scott, J. D. & Cooper, D. M. F. (2006). An Anchored Pka and Pde4 Complex Regulates Subplasmalemmal Camp Dynamics. *EMBO Journal*, 25, 10, pp. 2051-2061.

Winpenny, J. P.; Mcalroy, H. L.; Gray, M. A. & Argent, B. E. (1995). Protein Kinase C Regulates the Magnitude and Stability of Cftr Currents in Pancreatic Duct Cells. *American Journal of Physiology - Cell Physiology*, 268, 4, pp. C823-C828.

Wolde, M.; Fellows, A.; Cheng, J.; Kivenson, A.; Coutermarsh, B.; Talebian, L.; Karlson, K.; Piserchio, A.; Mierke, D. F.; Stanton, B. A.; Guggino, W. B. & Madden, D. R. (2007). Targeting Cal as a Negative Regulator of Deltaf508-Cftr Cell-Surface Expression: An Rna Interference and Structure-Based Mutagenetic Approach. *The Journal of Biological Chemistry*, 282, 11, pp. 8099-8109.

Xu, Z.; Oshima, K. & Heller, S. (2010). Pist Regulates the Intracellular Trafficking and Plasma Membrane Expression of Cadherin 23. *BMC cell biology*, 11, pp. 80.

Yoo, D.; Flagg, T. P.; Olsen, O.; Raghuram, V.; Foskett, J. K. & Welling, P. A. (2004). Assembly and Trafficking of a Multiprotein Romk (Kir 1.1) Channel Complex by Pdz Interactions. *The Journal of Biological Chemistry*, 279, 8, pp. 6863-6873.

Zhang, J.; Cheng, S.; Xiong, Y.; Ma, Y.; Luo, D.; Jeromin, A.; Zhang, H. & He, J. (2008). A Novel Association of Mglur1a with the Pdz Scaffold Protein Cal Modulates Receptor Activity. *FEBS Letters*, 582, 30, pp. 4117-4124.

Zhang W., Penmatsa H., Ren A., Punchihewa C., Lemoff A., Yan B., Fujii N., Naren A.P. (2011). Functional regulation of cystic fibrosis transmembrane conductance regulator-containing macromolecular complexes: a small-molecule inhibitor approach. *Biochemical Journal*, 435(2), pp. 451-62.

3

Pharmacological Potential of PDE5 Inhibitors for the Treatment of Cystic Fibrosis

Bob Lubamba, Barbara Dhooghe, Sabrina Noël and Teresinha Leal
Louvain Centre for Toxicology and Applied Pharmacology,
Université Catholique de Louvain, Brussels,
Belgium

1. Introduction

Recent basic research has aroused great interest in the therapeutic potential of phosphodiesterase type 5 (PDE5) inhibitors, such as sildenafil, vardenafil and taladafil, for the treatment of cystic fibrosis (CF). CF is the most common, life-threatening, recessively inherited disease in Caucasian populations. An estimated 1 in 2,500 Caucasian live births are affected and approximately 80,000 people in the world are diagnosed with CF. Due to mutation in the CF transmembrane conductance regulator (*CFTR*) gene [1,2], which encodes the main chloride channel expressed in epithelia, CF causes abnormal mucociliary clearance mainly in the lungs, leading to a vicious cycle of obstruction/infection/inflammation that progressively and irreversibly damages the lung tissue and architecture. Although many organs are affected in CF, pulmonary disease is the major cause of morbidity and mortality [3,4]. Despite more than two decades of intensive investigation of the genetics [1,2], pathophysiology and clinical phenotypes of CF [3,4], there is still no cure for CF. As a matter of fact, therapies have been limited to alleviating clinical manifestations. Although life expectancy and quality of life have progressively improved, CF continues to inflict major burdens and to shorten lives.

The most common disease allele, p.Phe508del (F508del), corresponding to deletion of a single phenylalanine residue at position 508 of a single polypeptide chain of 1480 amino acids, interferes with CFTR function because the mutant protein does not efficiently fold into the native protein structure. Although the mutant F508del is correctly translated, it is held back in the endoplasmic reticulum; the misfolded protein is directed towards proteosomal degradation and fails to reach the apical membrane of many epithelial cells [5]. An effective candidate drug to treat F508del-CF patients should be able to correct the localization of CFTR protein by increasing its expression at the apical membrane of epithelial cells. Indeed, it has been recognized that rescuing F508del-CFTR to the plasma membrane is followed by an improved efflux of chloride ions across the epithelium related to some residual channel activity of the mutant protein [6]. Therefore, finding a compound that promotes CFTR channel activity would be of great benefit. Searching for such compounds, we and others have demonstrated the potential of PDE5 inhibitors for the treatment of CF. Indeed, basic studies have provided evidence that PDE5 inhibitors, already in clinical use for the treatment of erectile dysfunction and/or of pulmonary arterial hypertension, rescue F508del-CFTR trafficking [7,8] and improve its channel activity [9,10].

PDE are enzymes that regulate the intracellular levels of the second messengers, such as cyclic AMP and GMP, by controlling their rate of degradation. The enzymes catalyze the hydrolysis of the 3' cyclic phosphate bonds of adenosine (Figure 1) and/or guanosine 3'5' cyclic monophosphate.

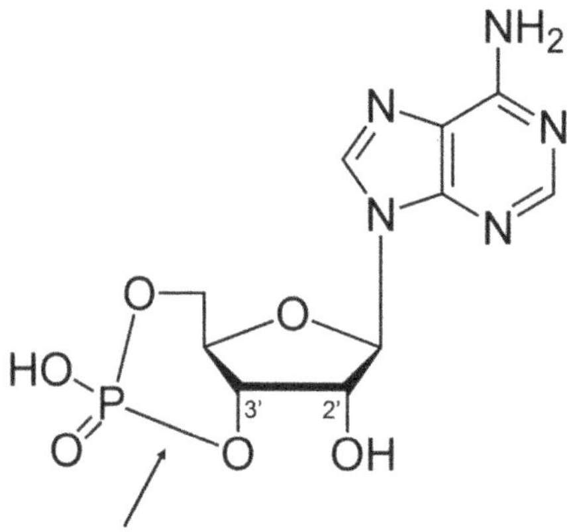

Fig. 1. **Structure of cyclic AMP.** Arrow indicates the site of hydrolyses by phosphodiesterases: the 3' cyclic phosphate bond.

Many of the early studies on cyclic nucleotides were directed toward understanding PDE activity since at that time it was much easier to measure PDE activity than either cAMP or cGMP themselves or the enzymes that catalyzed their synthesis. More recently, it became clear that there were likely to be multiple isoforms of PDEs with different kinetic and regulatory properties. They are characterized by their specificity and sensitivity to calcium-calmodulin and by their affinity for cAMP or cGMP [11]. PDEs were classified on the basis of their amino acid sequences, substrate specificities, pharmacological properties and tissue distributions.

2. Cyclic nucleotide phosphodiesterases

2.1 Isoforms of phosphodiesterases

It is now very clear that any single cell type can express several different PDE isoforms and also that the nature and localization of these PDEs are likely to be major regulators of the local concentrations of cAMP or cGMP in the cell. Eleven cyclic PDE families with varying selectivities for cAMP and/or cGMP have been identified in mammalian tissues [12-16] (Table 1).

PDEs are therefore important regulators of diverse biochemical mechanisms mediated by cAMP and /or cGMP. Despite this heterogeneity, there is a surprising degree of homology within their catalytic domains; however, slight structural differences in these domains determine whether a PDE is cAMP-specific (PDE4, PDE7, PDE8), cGMPspecific (PDE5, PDE6, PDE9) or has dual substrate specificity (PDE1, PDE2, PDE3, PDE10, PDE11) [17-18].

PDE isoenzyme	Substrate	Km (µM) cAMP	Km (µM) GMP	Tissue expression	Specific inhibitors
1	Ca^{2+}/calmodulin stimulated	80	3	Heart, brain, lung, smooth muscle, T lymphocytes, sperm	KS505a, bepril, Vinpocetine, Flunarizine and Amiodarone
2	cGMP-stimulated	30	10	Adrenal gland, heart, lung, liver, platelets	EHNA, BAY 60-7550, Oxindole and PDP
3	cGMP-inhibited cAMP-selective	0.4	0.3	Heart, lung, liver, platelets, Kidney, T lymphocytes, adipocytes, inflammatory cells	Cilostamide, Enoxamone, Milrinone, Siguazodan
4	cAMP-specific	4		Sertoli cells, kidney, brain, liver, lung, inflammatory cells	Rolipram, Roflumilast, Cilomilast, Drotaverine, ibudilast
5	cGMP-specific	150	1	Lung, platelets, vascular, smooth muscle	Sildenafil, Vardenafil, Tadalafil, Zaprinast
6	cGMP-specific		60	Photoreceptor	Dipyridamole
7	cAMP-specific, high-affinity	700	15	Skeletal muscle, heart, kidney, Brain, pancreas, T lymphocytes	BRL-50481, BC30
8	cAMP-selective	0.06		Testes, eye, liver, skeletal muscle, Heart, kidney, ovary, brain, T lymphocytes	PF-04957325
9	cGMP-specific	230	0.2	Kidney, liver, lung, brain	BAY 73-6691
10	cGMP-sensitive, cAMP-selective	0.2	13	Testes, brain	None
11	cGMP-sensitive, dual specificity	0.7	0.6	Skeletal muscle, prostate, kidney, liver, pituitary, testes and salivary glands	None

Table 1. Phosphodiesterase families and specific inhibitors

PDE1s are calcium dependent activators or regulators: they have been shown to activate cyclic nucleotide PDE in a calcium-dependent manner. PDE1s are present in many tissues and are abundant mainly in the central nervous system, heart, skeletal muscle and kidney [19-21].

PDE2 metabolizes both cGMP and cAMP although its affinity for cGMP is slightly higher than for cAMP [22]. High PDE2 activity can be found in heart [23] and brain. Lower expression of PDE2 was found in lung, placenta, liver, skeletal muscle, kidney and pancreas [24].

PDE3s are characterized by their high affinity and their ability to metabolize both cAMP and cGMP. They are also distinguished by their ability to be activated by several phosphorylation pathways including the PKA and PI3K/PKB pathways. PDE3s are moderately expressed in platelets as well as in vascular smooth muscle [25] and oocytes.

PDE4s have a higher affinity for cAMP, they are expressed in inflammatory cells such as T cells, B cells, eosinophils, neutrophils, airway epithelial cells and endothelial cells [26-28], cardiovascular tissues and smooth muscles. Differential expression of PDE4s can be modulated by inflammatory factors and expressed in lung macrophages from patients with chronic obstructive pulmonary disease (COPD).

PDE5 has a higher affinity for cGMP and was identified, isolated and characterized in rat platelets [29,30] and rat lung [31,32]. PDE5 is widely expressed in pulmonary vascular smooth muscle of pulmonary arteries and veins, bronchial blood vessels and airway smooth muscle [33]. Recent data show that PDE5 may modulate pulmonary arterial pressure induced by cardiac hypertrophy and fibrosis ([34].

PDE6s are phosphodiesterases characterized by their affinity for cGMP and are expressed in the photoreceptor outer segments of the mammalian retina, in which they mediate transduction of the light signal into an electrical response [35].

PDE7 are characterized by their high affinity and selectivity for cAMP as substrate. PDE7 protein expression is largest in T cell lines, blood T cells, epithelial cell lines, airway and vascular smooth muscle cells, lung fibroblasts and eosinophils and in neutrophils [36].

PDE8s are cAMP specific and have a very high affinity for cAMP as a substrate. PDE8s are distributed in various human tissues and are abundant in testis [37-40]. Functionally, PDE8s have been reported to be involved in regulation of T-cell activation [41], chemotaxis of activated lymphocytes [42], modulation of testosterone production in Leydig cells [43], and possibly potentiation of biphasic insulin response to glucose [44].

PDE9 is one of the more recently discovered PDE families. It is perhaps most notable as the PDE family having the highest affinity for cGMP. Further, compared with other cGMP-specific PDEs, PDE9 apparently lacks the non catalytic cGMP-binding domain, which is present in PDE5, PDE6, and also PDE2. The mRNA encoding PDE9 is well expressed in many examined human tissues, including spleen, small intestine, and brain [45,46].

PDE10 was isolated and characterized as a dual-substrate gene family in 1999 from mouse [47] as well as from human fetal lung [48] and fetal brain [49]. This PDE family was recently shown to be associated to the progressive neurodegenerative Huntington's disease (HD) since PDE10 mRNA decreases prior to the onset of motor symptoms in transgenic HD mice expressing exon 1 of the human Huntington gene [50].

PDE11 are characterized by their high affinity for both cAMP and cGMP, although kinetic characteristics for the variants are different [51-53]. PDE 11 mRNA occurs at higher levels in skeletal muscle, prostate, kidney, liver, pituitary and salivary glands, and testis.

3. PDE inhibitors as pharmacological tools in the treatment of diseases

The principle that inhibition of PDE activity could be a valid therapeutic tool is now well accepted. It is commonly accepted that concentrations of cAMP and cGMP in most cells are typically <1 to 10μM [54]. This means that a competitive inhibitor would not need to compete with very high levels of endogenous substrate in order to be effective.

The history of the PDE starts with the work of Henry Hyde Salter in 1887. It has been shown that caffeine has a bronchodilatator effect and that it was a non selective inhibitor of PDE activity. The caffeine and other xanthines have been used as therapeutic agents in respiratory diseases [55].

Inhibition of cyclic nucleotide PDEs allow cAMP/cGMP concentrations to increase within cells. Therefore, inhibition of PDE is a useful way of causing a variety of cellular effects and can influence various physiological mechanisms. Many PDE inhibitors are recognized as pharmacological agents. In fact, some compounds such as theophylline have been used as drugs in medical practice long before they were identified as PDE inhibitors. Currently, both non selective and selective PDE inhibitors are explored as therapeutic agents.

3.1 Non selective PDE inhibitors

Non selective inhibitors of the PDE such as theophylline, caffeine and papaverin have been used for more than 70 years in the western world for treatment of various diseases [56-59] and were identified as PDE inhibitors, i.e. as compounds that specifically inhibit the activity of PDE and not of other phosphohydrolases. During the last 10 years, a better understanding of physiological roles, cellular expression, specific inhibitors of the PDE isoforms, as well as of their clinical indications has been acquired. These non selective PDE inhibitors inhibit PDE competitively with low affinity and do not discriminate between PDE isozymes; both cAMP and cGMP–PDE activities are inhibited. Theophylline and other methylxantines are potent antagonists of adenosine receptors [60]. Theophylline had been prescribed for the first time in 1937 for the treatment of asthma; it is also perceived to be an orally active anti-inflammatory agent for use in asthma or COPD [57,61]. Paraxanthine, the primary metabolite of caffeine, acts through the ryanodine receptor to elevate intracellular calcium concentration and increases viability of neuronal cells in culture [62]. 3-isobutyl-1-methylxanthine (IBMX) was synthesized by Wells et al (1975), it has a much higher affinity for PDEs and at low concentrations, it preferentially inhibits cGMP-PDE over cAMP-PDE [63].

3.2 Selective PDE inhibitors

3.2.1 Inhibitors without therapeutic action

PDE2 is involved in a variety of physiological processes. The availability of PDE selective inhibitors has greatly facilitated the elucidation of PDE2 function in various tissues. One of the first specific inhibitors for PDE2 was erythro 9-(2 hydroxy-3-nonyl) adenine (EHNA) which potentiates the effects of NMDA (N-methyl-D-aspartate) activated receptors in cGMP, but has no effect on cAMP concentration [64]. EHNA is also a potent inhibitor of adenosine deaminase (ADA); it exerts a concentration dependent inhibition of the cGMP-stimulated PDE2 but does not inhibit other PDEs [65]. The strong expression of PDE2 in neurons of the hippocampus and cortex [66] suggests that this enzyme may control intraneuronal second messenger concentrations in these areas. Bayer (Germany) has developed a selective PDE2 inhibitor, the Bay 60-7550, which enhances long-term potentiation of synaptic transmission without altering basal synaptic transmission. BAY 60-7550 can improve memory functions by enhancing neural plasticity [67,68].

3.2.2 Inhibitors with therapeutic action

Some selective PDE inhibitors act directly on the catalytic site of PDE1s, such as vinpocetine. This PDE inhibitor has been used in memory loss [69] and in treating detrusor instabilities and urgency incontinence [70]. PDE inhibitor can improve neural plasticity or restore this function in different neurological conditions [71,72]. Vinpocetine treatment was also shown to revert the effects of early alcohol exposure in learning performance in the water maze [73]. It was recently demonstrated that vinpocetine has a strong anti-inflammatory effect [74]. This new action of vinpocetine, combined with its potential to enhance neuronal plasticity suggest that this drug may have beneficial effects in conditions such as Alzheimer and Parkinson diseases where inflammation and poor neuronal plasticity are present [75].

There are a relatively large number of PDE3 selective inhibitors including milrinone, cilostamide and cilostazol, which were identified as potential therapeutic tools in cardiovascular disease and asthma. Inhibition of PDE3 activity increase L-type Ca^{2+} currents in cardiomyocytes isolated from human, rat and frog heart, an effect that contributes to the positive inotropic effects of these inhibitors [76]. Milrinone has an inotropic and vasodilator effect for "wet and cold" heart failure [77], a case of heart failure with congestion and hypoperfusion [78]. It has been reported that the combination of inhaled and intravenous milrinone could be an effective treatment of secondary pulmonary hypertension in high-risk cardiac valve surgery patients [79].

PDE4 inhibitors have been developed for the treatment of asthma and COPD, diseases characterised by inflammatory and immune responses [80]. Rolipram is a highly selective first generation PDE4 inhibitor that has been used for many years as a research tool to investigate the role of PDE4. Several studies have shown that rolipram inhibits neutrophilic and eosinophilic inflammation [81]; it proved to be an effective antidepressant, but side effects such as nausea and gastro-intestinal disturbance terminated its clinical development [82]. Roflumilast was beneficial, as assessed by improvement in lung function, even when added to a long acting β_2 agonist or a long acting inhaled antimuscarinic [83].

The use of inhibitors of PDE5 (sildenafil (Viagra; Pfizer Inc, US), vardenafil (Levitra; GlaxoSmithKline, UK) and tadalafil (Cialis; Eli Lilly, US)) in the treatment of male erectile dysfunction is the first commercial success for PDE inhibitors. Sildenafil (under the tradename Revatio) and tadalafil (under the tradename Adcirca) have also been approved for the treatment of pulmonary arterial hypertension (PAH). PDE5 is a cGMP-specific phosphodiesterase encoded by a single gene. Recent data show that PDE5 may modulate pressure-induced cardiac hypertrophy and fibrosis [34]. Although sildenafil has an acceptable degree of selectivity, increased specificity for PDE5, particularly over PDE1 and PDE6 will reduce or eliminate the incidence of visual disturbances associated with the flushing and headaches that are observed with sildenafil [84]. In the case of all the other PDE5 inhibitors that have been described in the peer-reviewed literature, improvements in selectivity were determined empirically, and compounds were optimized on the basis of structure- activity explorations of the chemical series in question. PDE5 is abundantly expressed in lung tissue and appears to be up regulated in PAH [85,86]. PDE5 is involved in endothelial dysfunction by inactivating cGMP, the second messenger of the nitric oxide (NO) pathway in the pulmonary vasculature [85-87]. It has been reported that sildenafil and vardenafil raise hippocampal cGMP levels and improve memory in aged rats [88] and mice [89].

The PDE7 family is composed of two genes coding for high-affinity, rolipram-insensitive, cAMP-specific enzymes. The presence of high concentrations of PDE7 mRNA in the human striatum and dentate gyrus suggests that selective inhibitors could be used to increase cAMP concentration in these areas without some of the side effects associated with PDE4 inhibition [40,90,91]. Several distinct PDE7 inhibitors have been reported [92,93]; however, their effects on central nervous system (CNS) function have yet to be described. It has been shown that selective inhibition of PDE7 or dual PDE4/7 inhibition may provide a novel therapeutic approach for the treatment of chronic lymphocytic leukemia (CLL) by enhancing killing and increasing specificity for CLL cells [94].

The company Pfizer reported on a small molecule called PF-04957325 that selectively inhibits PDE8 with an *in vitro* IC50 of 0.7nM against PDE8A, of 0.2nM against PDE8B, and >1.5µM against all other PDE isoforms [95]. PDE8-selective inhibitors might be used to correct adrenal insufficiency, and a PDE8 activator might be used to treat Cushing's syndrome [96].

4. Pharmacological potential of PDE inhibitors for the treatment of cystic fibrosis

As an important second messenger signaling molecule, cAMP controls a wide variety of eukaryotic and prokaryotic responses to extracellular cues [97]. For cAMP-dependent signaling pathways to be effective, the intracellular cAMP concentration is tightly controlled at the level of both of synthesis and degradation. CF is characterized by defective cAMP-dependent chloride conductance in epithelial cells and is caused by a defect in the targeting of the chloride channel CFTR.

4.1 Non selective PDE inhibitors

Non specific inhibitors of the PDE such as IBMX, theophylline and DPMX (7-methyl-1,3 dipropyl xanthine) have been shown to activate normal and mutated CFTR chloride channels in epithelia [98]. It is well known that the methylxanthines, found naturally in tea, coffee and cocoa, stimulate the central nervous system, relax bronchial smooth muscle, and stimulate cardiac muscle. These purine derivatives function as adenosine receptor antagonists and as PDE inhibitors. Due to impact on the cAMP pathway and activity at low concentrations, studies have been done looking at their effect on the cAMP activated CFTR channel. The PDE inhibitor, IBMX also functions as an adenosine receptor antagonist. It has been reported that IBMX increases the CFTR chloride current in Xenopus oocytes expressing the F508del-CFTR [99]. In 1993, when studying CF nasal bronchial epithelial tissues with F508del-CFTR, Grubb et al. found that IBMX (5 mM) associated to forskolin (0.01 mM) did not stimulate chloride efflux *in vitro* [100]. Haws et al. studied the effect of IBMX and 8-cyclopentyl-1,3-dipropylxanthine (CPX), another non specific PDE and an A1 adenosine receptor antagonist, on stably transfected cells with F508del-CFTR [101]. In this study, both IBMX (5 mM) and CPX potentiated the effect of forskolin on CFTR-mediated efflux of ^{125}I by 2.5-fold. There was a 7-fold increase in cAMP levels associated with IBMX treatment, but not CPX treatment. A potentiation by IBMX of prostaglandin E (PGE2)-induced HCO_3^- secretion has been reported in the rat duodenum *in vivo* [102,103].

4.2 Selective PDE inhibitors

PDE inhibitors increase cAMP by inhibiting one or more enzymes involved in cAMP degradation. Cyclic AMP-activated PKA mediates phosphorylation of CFTR and increases the open probability of the CFTR channel. Drugs in this class include amrinone and milrinone. These drugs also cause vasodilation, which may be beneficial for the CF airways. In 1991, Drumm et al. showed that inhibiting PDE had a larger effect on CFTR activation than have adenylate cyclase stimulants [99]. Using airway epithelial cell lines expressing wild-type CFTR, Calu-3 and 16HBE cells, it has been found that, at 100µM concentrations, PDE 3 inhibitors (milrinone, amrinone) without adenylate cyclase activators, stimulate chloride efflux 13.7-fold [104]. They found no effect on chloride efflux by IBMX, a non specific PDE, by rolipram, a PDE4 inhibitor or by dipyridamole, a PDE5 inhibitor. The increase of channel efflux by the type 3 PDE inhibitor was not associated with a significant rise in cAMP concentrations but it was inhibited by protein kinase A inhibitors (H-8 and Rp-cAMPS), suggesting that it might work through a more distal signal. Kelley et al. also looked at endogenous CFTR in transformed nasal polyp tissue of patients homozygous for F508del (CF-T43) [105]. They found that, when administered in the presence of a β-agonist (isoproterenol) and protein kinase A activator, milrinone and amrinone, at 100µM concentrations, increased chloride efflux by 19-61% from baseline. Mice homozygous for F508del Cftr were administered with a combination of milrinone (100 µM) and forskolin (10 µM) [106]. This combination of drugs resulted in an increased magnitude of the murine nasal potential difference (PD). The implications of this study are exciting; but the effect has not been confirmed by others [107].

It has been shown that CFTR has a major role in the regulation of duodenal HCO_3^- secretion [108]. Furthermore, O'Grady et al. [109] showed that both PDE1 and PDE3 are involved in the activation of CFTR in T84 cells and human colonic epithelial cells. In 2007, Hayashi M et al. [110] suggested that PDE1 and PDE3 are involved in the regulation of duodenal HCO_3^- secretion and that the response to PGE2 is associated with both PDE1 and PDE3, while the response to NO is mainly modulated by PDE1 [110]. McPherson et al. showed that a selective cyclic nucleotide PDE5 inhibitor partially corrected defective L-adrenergic stimulation of mucin secretion in CFTR antibody-inhibited submandibular cells. The PDE5 inhibitor did not increase cAMP levels, nor did it potentiate isoproterenol-induced cAMP rise [111]. Of note, Dormer et al. (2005) demonstrated that the PDE5 inhibitor sildenafil (Viagra) also acts as a pharmacological chaperone. Because sildenafil is approved for clinical use, they speculated that their data might speed up the development of new therapies for CF [7].

5. The clinical pharmacokinetics of PDE5 inhibitors

Lung tissue is a rich source of PDE, including PDE5, the major function of which is acceleration of the decay of cGMP [112].

5.1 Sildenafil

Sildenafil citrate was the first selective PDE5 inhibitor approved for the treatment of erectile dysfunction. Sildenafil, however, is only approximately 10-fold as potent for PDE5 as for PDE6, which is found in the photoreceptors of the human retina. This lower selectivity toward PDE6 is presumed to be the cause for color vision abnormalities observed with high doses or plasma levels of sildenafil.

Sildenafil is relatively lipophilic with a weakly basic center in the piperazine tertiary amine, resulting in only partial ionization at physiological pH. Following oral administration, sildenafil is rapidly absorbed, reaching peak plasma concentrations within 1 hour (range, 0.5-2 hours). The first-order absorption rate constant was estimated as 2.6 hours^{-1} based on population pharmacokinetic data in patients with erectile dysfunction [113]. Administration of sildenafil after a high-fat meal caused reductions in the rate of absorption and extent of systemic exposure. The time-to-peak (t_{max}) was delayed by approximately 1 hour, and maximum concentration (C_{max}) was reduced by 29%. The systemic exposure of sildenafil after a high-fat meal was reduced by 11% [114].

Sildenafil is highly bound to plasma proteins, and the protein binding is independent of drug concentrations. After intravenous administration, the mean steady-state volume of distribution of sildenafil is 105 L, which substantially exceeds the total volume of body water (approximately 42 L), indicating distribution into tissues and possibly binding to extravascular proteins. Sildenafil is extensively metabolized, without unchanged sildenafil being detected in either urine or feces. After an oral dose, metabolites are predominantly excreted into the feces (73%-88%) and to a lesser extent into the urine (6%-15%) [115]. Plasma concentrations of sildenafil was reported to decline biexponentially, with a mean terminal half-life of 3 to 5 hours, independent of the route of administration [114]. Sildenafil is primarily metabolized by the cytochrome P-450 (CYP) isoenzyme CYP3A4 and to a lesser extent CYP2C9 [116]. Sildenafil is extensively metabolized, with more than 12 metabolites identified.

The principal routes of metabolism are N-demethylation, oxidation, and aliphatic hydroxylation [115]. Plasma concentrations of N-demethylation are approximately 40% that of sildenafil, so that the metabolite accounts for approximately 20% of the pharmacological effects of sildenafil. The metabolite profile is qualitatively similar after intravenous and oral administration, but higher concentrations of N-desmethyl sildenafil after oral administration indicate the important role of first-pass metabolism in the metabolite formation.

5.2 Vardenafil

Vardenafil hydrochloride was the first second generation PDE5 inhibitor approved for the treatment of erectile dysfunction. Vardenafil has a high selectivity for the inhibition of PDE5 compared with the other known phosphodiesterases [117,118]. Unlike sildenafil and tadalafil, vardenafil was developed from the outset specifically to treat erectile dysfunction.

Vardenafil is rapidly absorbed, with plasma concentrations being detected in all subjects within 8 to 15 minutes after oral administration.

Peak plasma concentrations were observed 0.25 to 3 hours after administration, with a median of 0.7 hours for the 20 and 40 mg dose level, and slightly later, with 0.9 hours for the 10 mg dose level [117,119]. The absolute bioavailability of vardenafil was described as approximately 15%. Vardenafil pharmacokinetics is largely unaffected by food containing moderate amounts of fat. Minimal changes (<15%) in mean vardenafil C_{max} and no change in median t_{max} were observed when vardenafil was administered with a moderate-fat evening meal compared to dosing on an empty stomach. When 20mg oral vardenafil was administered immediately after consumption of a high-fat breakfast, the mean C_{max} was 18% lower and the median t_{max} was delayed by 1 hour.

Based on *in vitro* investigations in human plasma, approximately 93% to 95% of the drug is bound to plasma proteins, approximately 80% to albumin, and 11% to α1-acid glycoprotein [120]. It was also demonstrated that the binding to plasma proteins was fully reversible in all the tested species and was concentration independent. The major metabolite of vardenafil has similar protein-binding properties as the parent drug, with a bound fraction of 93% to 95%. The volume of distribution estimate for vardenafil after intravenous administration is relatively high, 208 L, implying extensive drug distribution into tissues.

Vardenafil is extensively metabolized, with more than 14 metabolites identified. The major metabolite, M1, and 2 minor metabolites, M4 and M5, as well as their respective glucuronides, are all a result of the degradation of vardenafil's piperazine ring. M1 is N-desethyl vardenafil, M4 is reduced by a 2-carbon fragment of the piperazine ring of vardenafil, and M5 is the N-desethyl derivative of M4. Metabolism is predominantly mediated by CYP3A4 and to a smaller extent by CYP3A5 and CYP2C isoforms. All 3 metabolites have pharmacologic activity. The major circulating metabolite, M1, has 28% of vardenafil's potency for PDE5 inhibition, while M4 and M5 possess 5.6% and 4.9%, respectively [120].

5.3 Tadalafil

Tadalafil is a selective and potent inhibitor of PDE5 with an IC50 of 0.94 nM. It exhibits high selectivity toward PDE5 compared to other PDEs. Tadalafil is structurally different from both sildenafil and vardenafil, and the different structures are reflected in distinct differences in the clinical pharmacology profiles of these drugs [121]. Like sildenafil, tadalafil was developed initially for use in cardiovascular disease and was subsequently used for the treatment of erectile dysfunction [122]. Tadalafil was the last of the 3 PDE5 inhibitors approved for erectile dysfunction.

Tadalafil is rapidly absorbed after oral administration with a median time to reach peak plasma concentration of 2 hours (range, 0.5-6 hours) [118,121]. Absolute bioavailability of tadalafil following oral dosing has not been reported, but at least 36% of the dose is absorbed from an oral solution. The time course of oral absorption could successfully be modeled by a rapid first-order process. Population estimates of the first-order absorption rate constant from phase II and phase III studies are 1.75 and 1.86 hours[-1], respectively [123]. The absorption and pharmacodynamic properties of tadalafil are not affected by either food or alcohol, and thus the drug can be administered without regard for food or alcohol consumption [124]. Smoking and body mass index had a weak effect on the pharmacokinetics of tadalafil. It has been reported that the clinical response to tadalafil may be evident as early as 16 minutes and may persist for up to 24 to 36 hours post dose [124,125]

Tadalafil has an apparent volume of distribution of 60 to 70 L, with an interindividual variability of 40% to 50%. This indicates that tadalafil is distributed into tissues. Plasma protein binding was reported as 94%, with α1-acid glycoprotein and albumin as principal binding proteins. A population pharmacokinetic analysis in patients taking tadalafil suggests a body weight dependency of the volume of distribution at steady state.

Tadalafil is excreted primarily as inactive metabolites, mainly in the feces and to a lesser extent in urine. The mean elimination half-life for tadalafil was 17.5 hours, and the mean apparent oral clearance was 2.5 L/h in healthy subjects [126]. The nearly exclusive elimination via hepatic metabolism and the relatively low value for oral clearance indicate that tadalafil has a low intrinsic clearance with regard to hepatic metabolism and can be classified as a drug with low hepatic extraction ratio.

Tadalafil is primarily metabolized by CYP3A4 to a catechol metabolite, which further undergoes extensive methylation and glucuronidation to form methylcatechol and methylcatechol glucuronide metabolites. This was confirmed by interaction studies with rifampin as potent CYP3A inducer and

ketoconazole as a potent CYP3A inhibitor. The main circulating metabolite in plasma is methylcatechol glucuronide, which has a $\geq$ 10 000-fold less affinity for PDE5 than the analogue drug, tadalafil, and is thus expected to be clinically inactive at observed metabolite concentrations [126]. Several other inactive metabolites have also been identified in plasma, urine, or feces.

5.4 Comparison of PDE5 inhibitors

Although the 3 currently available PDE5 inhibitors, sildenafil, vardenafil, and tadalafil, have all shown to be effective in the treatment of erectile dysfunction, there are distinct differences between the compounds regarding their selectivity and specificity for PDE inhibition with consequences especially for the safety profile but also biopharmaceutic and pharmacokinetic disparities that largely affect the efficacy profile of these compounds. Sildenafil and vardenafil are very similar in terms of their chemical structure, whereas tadalafil with a methyldione structure differs markedly from sildenafil and vardenafil (Figure 2). These chemical similarities and differences are also reflected in similarities and dissimilarities of their clinical pharmacokinetics.

All 3 PDE5 inhibitors are rapidly absorbed after oral administration, with peak concentrations reached slightly earlier for vardenafil compared to sildenafil and tadalafil. Although no clear concentration-effect relationships have been established for any of the 3 PDE5 inhibitors, rapid absorption is considered an essential for a rapid onset of efficacy. Administration of a high-fat meal had no significant effect on the rate and extent of absorption of tadalafil but decreased the rate of absorption for sildenafil and vardenafil. All 3 drugs are lipophilic and have a volume of distribution larger than the volume of total body water, indicating tissue uptake and binding. Furthermore, all 3 compounds are highly protein bound, with free plasma concentration fractions of only 4% to 6%.

The major route of elimination for all PDE5 inhibitors is hepatic metabolism, with renal excretion of unchanged drug accounting for 1% or less of the elimination pathways. Based on their relatively high systemic clearance after intravenous administration, sildenafil and vardenafil can be classified as non restrictively cleared drugs with intermediate to high hepatic extraction ratio. The relatively comparable distribution volumes together with the substantial differences in systemic clearance among the PDE5 inhibitors result in distinct differences of the elimination half-life, 3 to 5 hours for sildenafil and vardenafil compared to 17.5 hours for tadalafil. Tadalafil, however, has been detected in plasma even 5 days after oral administration due to its long half-life. This suggests the possibility of accumulation if taken regularly and in short intervals, which may result in an increased risk of side effects with the excessive use of this PDE5 inhibitor.

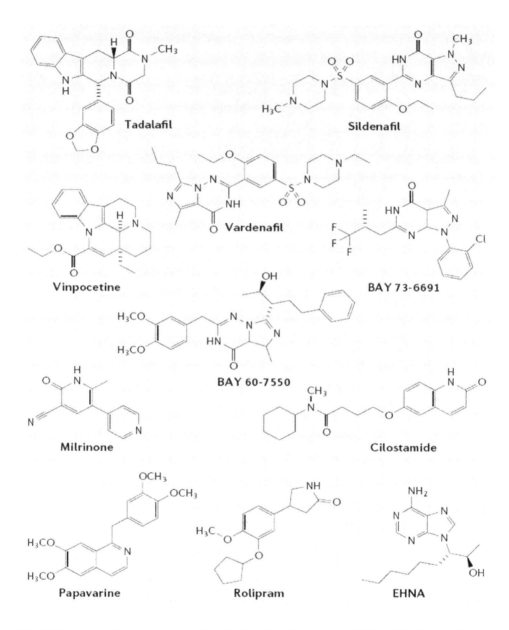

Fig. 2. Structures of selected examples of phosphodiesterase inhibitors. The figure shows various selective phosphodiesterase (PDE) inhibitors mentioned in this chapter. Of these, the PDE5 inhibitors sildenafil, vardenafil and tadalafil have been approved for treatment of erectile dysfunction. Sildenafil and vardenafil have also recently been approved as a treatment for pulmonary hypertension.

6. Administration of PDE5 inhibitors at clinical doses activates defective chloride transport in CF

At present, many efforts are focused on CFTR pharmacotherapy which corrects the abnormal protein pharmacologically by various approaches such as the direct correction of stop codon mutations, CFTR channel activation, or correction of CFTR trafficking defects.

High-throughput screening (HTS) has been used to identify molecules that increase F508del-CFTR activity [127,129]. Such molecules have been categorized according to whether they alleviate the folding/cellular processing defect (correctors) or increase the responsiveness of F508del-CFTR channels already present in the membrane to cAMP activation (potentiators). Sildenafil has also been shown to correct F508del-CFTR processing when used at high micromolar concentrations [7].

To test the hypothesis that PDE5 inhibitors (sildenafil, vardenafil and taladafil) are able to restore transepithelial ion transport abnormalities of the F508del-CFTR protein, we have conducted experimental studies [9,10] in CF mice homozygous for the F508del mutation [130] and in their corresponding wild-type homozygous normal mice. The F508del-Cftr mouse model has been chosen because F508del is the most common and one of the most severe CF mutation and because the mouse model recapitulates, at different levels, the human disease. Epithelia of the F508del-CF mouse model are characterized by defective electrolyte transport, and *Pseudomonas aeruginosa* lipopolysaccharide (LPS) exposure mimics several aspects of CF airway epithelial inflammation such as increased pro-inflammatory cytokines, most notably interleukin (IL)-8, IL-6, and Tumor Necrosis Factor (TNF)-α, and neutrophil infiltrate cells.

In our protocols, CFTR function has been assessed *in vivo* by measuring the transepithelial nasal PD, a delicate technique that has been increasingly used as an index of therapeutic efficacy in novel fundamental therapies, either in animal models [9,10,131] or in CF patients [132]. Our results provide clear evidence that intraperitoneal injection of PDE5 inhibitors (Figure 3), at clinical doses, to F508del-CF mice interact with CFTR, propping open the mutant protein to allow a normal flow of chloride ions across the epithelium of nasal mucosa, thereby completely restoring the decreased or even abolished CFTR-dependent chloride transport [9]. In F508del mice, but not in *Cftr* knockout mice, the chloride conductance, evaluated by perfusing the nasal mucosa with a chloride-free solution in the presence of amiloride and with forskolin, is corrected 1 h after sildenafil administration. A more prolonged effect, persisting for at least 24 h, is observed with vardenafil. Moreover, vardenafil, but not sildenafil, is able to stimulate chloride transport associated with normal wild-type Cftr protein [9]. The forskolin response is increased after treatment with sildenafil or vardenafil in wild-type and in F508del mutant animals. In F508del mice, the chloride conductance in the presence of 200 µM DIDS (4-4'-diisothiocyanostilbene-2,2'-disulphonic acid), an inhibitor of alternative chloride channels, was much higher after sildenafil injection than following placebo treatment (Figure 4). No effect on the sodium conductance was detected in any group of animals. Altogether, these data provide preclinical evidence that sildenafil and vardenafil stimulate, by a direct and not a by-pass effect, chloride transport activity of F508del-CFTR protein.

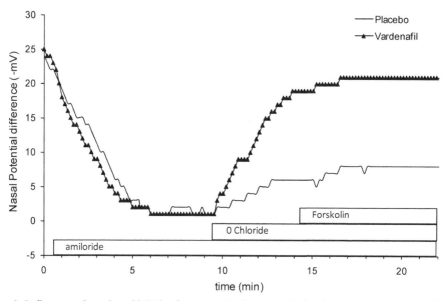

Fig. 3. Influence of vardenafil (24h after a single therapeutic dose) on ion transport evaluated by the nasal potential difference (PD) in F508del-CF mice. Chloride conductance in response to perfusion of the nasal mucosa with a solution without chloride and to forskolin is dramatically increased as compared to placebo-treated CF mice.

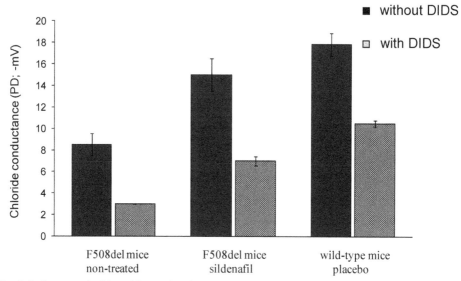

Fig. 4. Influence of sildenafil on Cftr -dependent chloride conductance evaluated by the nasal potential difference (PD) in the presence or the absence of DIDS, an inhibitor of alternative chloride conductance. Increased DIDS-insensitive conductance after sildenafil treatment reflects activation of Cftr function.

More recently, using a nebulizer setup specifically developed for mice (Figure 5), we have demonstrated that administration of PDE5 inhibitors through a single inhalation exposure is able to locally activate Cftr protein and correct the basic defects in CF [10] and that the effect lasts for at least 8 h (Figure 6). Our data have identified the inhalational route as a potential therapy for PDE5 inhibitors in CF. Consistent with our results, it has recently been demonstrated that the inhalation route of administration for vardenafil is associated with an acceptable safety profile. Apart from brief coughing on inspiration, no clinically significant changes in blood pressure or heart rate and no serious adverse events were recorded [133]. Inhalation drug therapy has several potential advantages over oral and intravenous routes, including rapid onset of pharmacological action, minimized systemic adverse effects and reduced effective drug doses compared to the same drug delivered orally [134]; this greatly highlights the impact of our work for translational science.

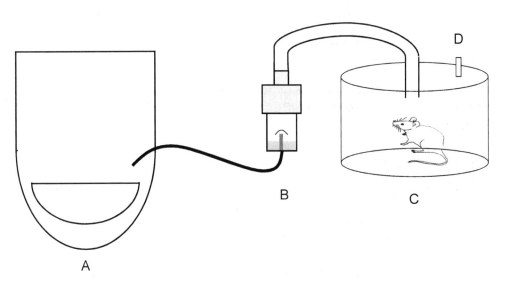

Fig. 5. Schematic representation of the whole-body immersion inhalation chamber setup we developed for a single mouse. (A) compressor, (B) nebulizer, (C) inhalation chamber with (D) expiratory gate.

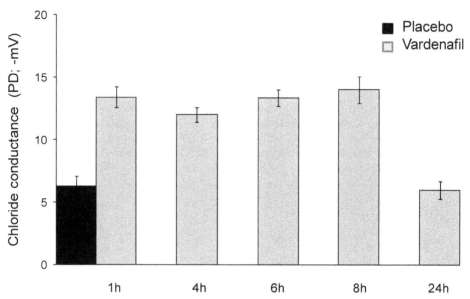

Fig. 6. Duration of the correcting effect of inhaled vardenafil on chloride conductance, evaluated by nasal potential difference (PD) in F508del-CF mice 1, 4, 6, 8 and 24h after a single nebulisation with placebo or with vardenafil. The correcting effect of vardenafil lasts at least 8 h after inhalation.

7. Intraperitoneal administration of PDE5 inhibitors administration at clinical doses attenuates exaggerated inflammatory responses in CF in vivo conditions

Another important goal of mutation-specific CF treatment is attenuation of exaggerated lung inflammatory responses [134-137]. As lung inflammation plays a major role in morbi-mortality in CF, identifying a therapeutic strategy that combines ability to correct the basic ion transport defect and to reduce dysregulated inflammatory responses is very exciting and promising. It has been reported that sildenafil reduces neutrophil lung infiltration in murine airways infected with *P. aeruginosa* [138]. In addition, toxicological studies have shown that sildenafil pretreatment attenuates acrolein-triggered airway inflammation associated with mucin overproduction [139].

More recently, we have found that vardenafil, selected as a representative PDE5 inhibitor for its longer-lasting Cftr activating effect, modulates the vicious circle of lung inflammation and attenuates the expression of pro-inflammatory cytokines and chemokines and cell infiltrates in the bronchoalveolar lavage (BAL) of CF and wild-type mice [140] Our data indicate that intraperitoneal administration of a single pharmacological dose (0.14 mg/kg body weight) of vardenafil is followed by a reducing response in cell infiltrate and in the biosynthesis of several biomarkers of the inflammatory response. Most notably, levels of CCL-2 (chemokine C-C motif ligand), a cytokine playing a key role in the contribution of macrophages in the inflammatory response [136], are significantly reduced in the BAL fluid after vardenafil treatment, particularly in CF animals (Figure 7).

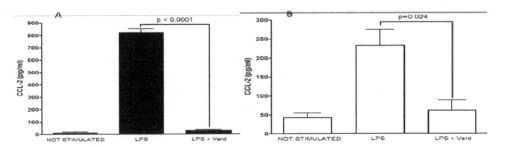

Fig. 7. Anti-inflammatory effect of *in vivo* treatment, by intraperitoneal injection, of a single therapeutic dose of vardenafil (vard) to F508del-CF (A) and wild-type (B) mice on the lipopolyssaccharide (LPS of *P. aeruginosa*) induced inflammatory response. Biosynthesis of CCL-2 is significantly reduced in the bronchoalveolar lavage (BAL) of vardenafil-treated CF and non-CF animals.

The mechanism of action of vardenafil as an anti-inflammatory agent in CF as well as the target-effector cells involved in these responses are under investigation by our group. Altogether, our data indicate that PDE5 inhibitors have a strong therapeutic potential for treating CF. A clinical trial aimed at investigating the safety and efficacy of sildenafil in CF lung disease is listed on www.clinicaltrials.gov (NCT00659529).

8. Conclusions

There is still no cure for CF. The CF patient may benefit from today's privileged strategy which consists on targeting a pharmacological mutation-specific treatment. Currently candidate molecules suitable for CFTR pharmacotherapy are either being sought after or under investigation. Based on the high prevalence of *F508del-CFTR* mutation – more than two-thirds of patients with CF carry at least one copy of the allele -, strategies to rescue the functional status of the mutated protein will benefit most of the CF population. As PDE5 inhibitors such as sildenafil, vardenafil and tadalafil are able to correct transepithelial ion transport abnormalities and to limit exaggerated inflammatory responses related to the presence of F508del-CF protein, the drugs are promising compounds for fundamental pharmacotherapy in CF. Since the drugs are in clinical use, therapeutic approaches to address F508del-CFTR defects by PDE5 inhibitors could be considered as a 'low-hanging fruit' strategy in the drug discovery tree. The fact that such compounds have been approved for other therapeutic indications could speed up their development as CF therapeutics, as compared to other agents that are under investigation only for CF therapy and for which further exploratory studies are needed before being streamed towards clinical testing.

In summary, CFTR correction with PDE5 inhibitors is a promising therapeutic approach based on functional correction of F508del-CFTR activity and on a possible anti-inflammatory action in F508del mice. The effects of these compounds on other CF mutation classes remain to be assessed.

9. Acknowledgements

TL is an associate researcher with the Fonds de la Recherche Scientifique Médicale (FRSM). BL is a PhD fellow with the Fonds Spéciaux de Recherche (FSR; Université catholique de Louvain). SN is a postdoctoral fellow with the FSR and Marie Curie Actions of the European Commission. We thank Gregory Reychler for his assistance in the development of the inhalation chamber setup. Supported by grants of the French CF Association (Vaincre la Mucoviscidose), the FRSM, FSR and the Foundation St Luc (St Luc University Hospital and Université catholique de Louvain).

10. References

[1] Kerem B, Rommens JM, Buchanan JA, Markiewicz D, Cox TK, Chakravarti A, Buchwald M, Tsui LC (1989) Identification of the cystic fibrosis gene: Genetic analysis. *Science* 245:1073-1080.

[2] Riordan JR, Rommens JM, Kerem B, Alon N, Rozmahel R, Grzelczak Z, Zielenski J, Lok S, Plavsic N, Chou JL, et al (1989). Identification of the cystic fibrosis gene: Cloning and characterization of complementary DNA. *Science* 245:1066-1073.

[3] Rowe SM, Miller S, Sorscher EJ (2005) Cystic fibrosis. *N Engl J Med* 352:1992-2001.

[4] Davis PB (2006) Cystic fibrosis since 1938. *Am J Respir Crit Care Med* 173:475-482.

[5] Lukacs GL, Mohamed A, Kartner N, Chang XB, Riordan JR, Grinstein S (1994). Conformational maturation of CFTR but not its mutant counterpart (Delta F508) occurs in the endoplasmic reticulum and requires atp. *EMBO J* 13:6076-6086.

[6] Amaral MD (2004) CFTR and chaperones: processing and degradation. *J Mol Neurosci* 23:41-8.

[7] Dormer RL, Harris CM, Clark Z, Pereira MM, Doull IJ, Norez C, Becq F, McPherson MA (2005) Sildenafil (Viagra) corrects DeltaF508-CFTR location in nasal epithelial cells from patients with cystic fibrosis. *Thorax* 60:55-59.

[8] Robert R, Carlile GW, Pavel C, Liu N, Anjos SM, Liao J, Luo Y, Zhang D, Thomas DY, Hanrahan JW (2008) Structural analog of sildenafil identified as a novel corrector of the F508del-CFTR trafficking defect. *Mol Pharmacol* 73:478-489.

[9] Lubamba B, Lecourt H, Lebacq J, Lebecque P, De Jonge H, Wallemacq P, Leal T (2008). Preclinical evidence that sildenafil and vardenafil activate chloride transport in cystic fibrosis. *Am J Respir Crit Care Med* 177:506-515.

[10] Lubamba B, Lebacq J, Reychler G, Marbaix E, Wallemacq P, Lebecque P, Leal T (2011) Inhaled phosphodiesterase type 5 inhibitors restore chloride transport in cystic fibrosis mice. *Eur Respir J* 37:72-78.

[11] Beavo JA, Rogers NL, Crofford OB, Hardman JG, Sutherland EW, Newman EV (1970) Effects of xanthine derivatives on lipolysis and on adenosine 3',5'-monophosphate phosphodiesterase activity. *Mol Pharmacol* 6:597-603.

[12] Cheung WY (1970) Cyclic nucleotide phosphodiesterase. *Adv Biochemical Psychopharmacol* 3:51-65.

[13] Conti M (2000) Phosphodiesterases and cyclic nucleotide signaling in endocrine cells. *Mol Endocrinol* 14:1317-1327.

[14] Soderling SH, Beavo JA (2000) Regulation of cAMP and cGMP signaling: new phosphodiesterases and new functions. *Curr Opin Cell Biol* 12:174-179

[15] Francis SH, Turko IV, Corbin JD (2001) Cyclic nucleotide phosphodiesterases: relating structure and function. *Prog Nucleic Acid Res Mol Biol* 65:1-52.

[16] Mehats C, Andersen CB, Filopanti M, Jin SL, Conti M (2002) Cyclic nucleotide phosphodiesterases and their role in endocrine cell signaling. *Trends Endocrinol Metabol* 13:29-35.

[17] Xu RX, Rocque WJ, Lambert MH, Vanderwall DE, Luther MA, Nolte RT (2004) Crystal structures of the catalytic domain of phosphodiesterase 4B complexed with AMP, 8-Br-AMP, and rolipram. *J Mol Biol* 337:355-365.

[18] Zhang HT, Zhao Y, Huang Y, Dorairaj NR, Chandler LJ, O'Donnell JM (2004) Inhibition of the phosphodiesterase 4 (PDE4) enzyme reverses memory deficits produced by infusion of the MEK inhibitor U0126 into the CA1 subregion of the rat hippocampus. *Neuropsychopharmacology* 29:1432-1439.

[19] Yan C, Zhao AZ, Bentley JK, Loughney K, Ferguson K, Beavo JA (1995) Molecular cloning and characterization of a calmodulin-dependent phosphodiesterase enriched in olfactory sensory neurons. *Proc Natl Acad Sci USA* 92:9677-9681.

[20] Loughney K, Martins TJ, Harris EA, Sadhu K, Hicks JB, Sonnenburg WK, Beavo JA, Ferguson K (1996) Isolation and characterization of cDNAs corresponding to two human calcium, calmodulin-regulated, 3',5'-cyclic nucleotide phosphodiesterases. *J Biol Chem* 271:796-806.

[21] Yu SM, Hung LM, Lin CC (1997) cGMP-elevating agents suppress proliferation of vascular smooth muscle cells by inhibiting the activation of epidermal growth factor signaling pathway. *Circulation* 95:1269-1277.

[22] Rosman GJ, Martins TJ, Sonnenburg WK, Beavo JA, Ferguson K, Loughney K (1997) Isolation and characterization of human cDNAs encoding a cGMP-stimulated 3',5'-cyclic nucleotide phosphodiesterase. *Gene* 191:89-95.

[23] Rivet-Bastide M, Vandecasteele G, Hatem S, Verde I, Benardeau A, Mercadier JJ, Fischmeister R (1997) cGMP-stimulated cyclic nucleotide phosphodiesterase regulates the basal calcium current in human atrial myocytes. *J Clin Invest* 99:2710-2718.

[24] Sadhu K, Hensley K, Florio VA, Wolda SL (1999) Differential expression of the cyclic GMP-stimulated phosphodiesterase PDE2A in human venous and capillary endothelial cells. *J Histochem Cytochem* 47:895-906.

[25] Palmer D, Maurice DH (2000) Dual expression and differential regulation of phosphodiesterase 3A and phosphodiesterase 3B in human vascular smooth muscle: implications for phosphodiesterase 3 inhibition in human cardiovascular tissues. *Mol Pharmacol* 58:247-252.

[26] Tenor H, Hatzelmann A, Kupferschmidt R, Stanciu L, Djukanovic R, Schudt C, Wendel A, Church MK, Shute JK (1995) Cyclic nucleotide phosphodiesterase isoenzyme activities in human alveolar macrophages. *Clin Exp Allergy* 25:625-633.

[27] Tenor H, Hatzelmann A, Wendel A, Schudt C (1995) Identification of phosphodiesterase IV activity and its cyclic adenosine monophosphate-dependent up-regulation in a human keratinocyte cell line (HaCaT). *J Invest Dermatol* 105:70-74.

[28] Tenor H, Staniciu L, Schudt C, Hatzelmann A, Wendel A, Djukanovic R, Church MK, Shute JK (1995) Cyclic nucleotide phosphodiesterases from purified human CD4+ and CD8+ T lymphocytes. *Clin Exp Allergy* 25:616-624.

[29] Hamet P, Coquil JF (1978) Cyclic GMP binding and cyclic GMP phosphodiesterase in rat platelets. *J Cyclic Nucleotide Res* 4:281-290.

[30] Coquil JF, Franks DJ, Wells JN, Dupuis M, Hamet P (1980) Characteristics of a new binding protein distinct from the kinase for guanosine 3':5'-monophosphate in rat platelets. *Biochim Biophys Acta* 631:148-165.

[31] Francis SH, Corbin JD (1988) Purification of cGMP-binding protein phosphodiesterase from rat lung. *Meth Enzymol* 159:722-729.

[32] Francis SH, Lincoln TM, Corbin JD (1980) Characterization of a novel cGMP binding protein from rat lung. *J Biol Chem* 255:620-626.

[33] Sebkhi A, Strange JW, Phillips SC, Wharton J, Wilkins MR (2003) Phosphodiesterase type 5 as a target for the treatment of hypoxia-induced pulmonary hypertension. *Circulation* 107:3230-3235.

[34] Takimoto E, Belardi D, Tocchetti CG, Vahebi S, Cormaci G, Ketner EA, Moens AL, Champion HC, Kass DA (2007) Compartmentalization of cardiac beta-adrenergic inotropy modulation by phosphodiesterase type 5. *Circulation* 115:2159-2167.

[35] Zhang X, Feng Q, Cote RH (2005) Efficacy and selectivity of phosphodiesterase-targeted drugs in inhibiting photoreceptor phosphodiesterase (PDE6) in retinal photoreceptors. *Invest Ophthalmol Vis Sci* 46:3060-3066.

[36] Smith SJ, Brookes-Fazakerley S, Donnelly LE, Barnes PJ, Barnette MS, Giembycz MA (2003) Ubiquitous expression of phosphodiesterase 7A in human proinflammatory and immune cells. *Am J Physiol* 284:L279-289.

[37] Wang P, Wu P, Egan RW, Billah MM (2001) Human phosphodiesterase 8A splice variants: cloning, gene organization, and tissue distribution. *Gene* 280:183-194.

[38] Hayashi M, Kita K, Ohashi Y, Aihara E, Takeuchi K (2007) Phosphodiesterase isozymes involved in regulation of HCO3- secretion in isolated mouse duodenum in vitro. *Biochem Pharmacol* 74:1507-1513.

[39] Kobayashi T, Gamanuma M, Sasaki T, Yamashita Y, Yuasa K, Kotera J, Omori K (2003) Molecular comparison of rat cyclic nucleotide phosphodiesterase 8 family: unique expression of PDE8B in rat brain. *Gene* 319:21-31.

[40] Perez-Torres S, Cortes R, Tolnay M, Probst A, Palacios JM, Mengod G (2003) Alterations on phosphodiesterase type 7 and 8 isozyme mRNA expression in Alzheimer's disease brains examined by in situ hybridization. *Exp Neurol* 182:322-334.

[41] Glavas NA, Ostenson C, Schaefer JB, Vasta V, Beavo JA (2001) T cell activation up-regulates cyclic nucleotide phosphodiesterases 8A1 and 7A3. *Proc Natl Acad Sci USA* 98:6319-6324.

[42] Dong H, Osmanova V, Epstein PM, Brocke S (2006) Phosphodiesterase 8 (PDE8) regulates chemotaxis of activated lymphocytes. *Biochem Biophys Res Commun* 345:713-719.

[43] Vasta V, Shimizu-Albergine M, Beavo JA (2006) Modulation of Leydig cell function by cyclic nucleotide phosphodiesterase 8A. *Proc Natl Acad Sci USA* 103:19925-19930.

[44] Dov A, Abramovitch E, Warwar N, Nesher R (2008) Diminished phosphodiesterase-8B potentiates biphasic insulin response to glucose. *Endocrinology* 149:741-748.

[45] Soderling SH, Bayuga SJ, Beavo JA (1998) Cloning and characterization of a cAMP-specific cyclic nucleotide phosphodiesterase. *Proc Natl Acad Sci USA* 95:8991-8996.

[46] Soderling SH, Bayuga SJ, Beavo JA (1998) Identification and characterization of a novel family of cyclic nucleotide phosphodiesterases. *J Biol Chem* 273:15553-15558.

[47] Soderling SH, Bayuga SJ, Beavo JA (1999) Isolation and characterization of a dual-substrate phosphodiesterase gene family: PDE10A. *Proc Natl Acad Sci USA* 96:7071-7076.

[48] Fujishige K, Kotera J, Michibata H, Yuasa K, Takebayashi S, Okumura K, Omori K (1999) Cloning and characterization of a novel human phosphodiesterase that hydrolyzes both cAMP and cGMP (PDE10A). *J Biol Chem* 274:18438-18445.

[49] Loughney K, Snyder PB, Uher L, Rosman GJ, Ferguson K, Florio VA (1999) Isolation and characterization of PDE10A, a novel human 3', 5'-cyclic nucleotide phosphodiesterase. *Gene* 234:109-117.

[50] Hebb AL, Robertson HA, Denovan-Wright EM (2004) Striatal phosphodiesterase mRNA and protein levels are reduced in Huntington's disease transgenic mice prior to the onset of motor symptoms. *Neuroscience* 123:967-981.

[51] Fawcett L, Baxendale R, Stacey P, McGrouther C, Harrow I, Soderling S, Hetman J, Beavo JA, Phillips SC (2000) Molecular cloning and characterization of a distinct human phosphodiesterase gene family: PDE11A. *Proc Natl Acad Sci USA* 97:3702-3707.

[52] Hetman JM, Soderling SH, Glavas NA, Beavo JA (2000) Cloning and characterization of PDE7B, a cAMP-specific phosphodiesterase. *Proc Natl Acad Sci USA* 97:472-476.

[53] Weeks JL 2nd, Zoraghi R, Francis SH, Corbin JD (2007) N-Terminal domain of phosphodiesterase-11A4 (PDE11A4) decreases affinity of the catalytic site for substrates and tadalafil, and is involved in oligomerization. *Biochemistry* 46:10353-10364.

[54] Bender AT, Beavo JA (2006) Cyclic nucleotide phosphodiesterases: molecular regulation to clinical use. *Pharmacol Rev* 58:488-520.

[55] Bhatt-Mehta V, Schumacher RE. Treatment of apnea of prematurity. Paediatr Drugs 2003;5:195-210.

[56] Barnes PJ (2003) Theophylline: new perspectives for an old drug. *Am J Respir Crit Care Med* 167:813-818.

[57] Barnes PJ (2003) Therapy of chronic obstructive pulmonary disease. *Pharmacol Ther* 97:87-94.

[58] Barnes PJ (200) Theophylline in chronic obstructive pulmonary disease: new horizons. *Proc Am Thorac Soc* 2:334-339.

[59] Barnes PJ, Stockley RA (2005) COPD: current therapeutic interventions and future approaches. *Eur Respir J* 25:1084-1106.

[60] Muller CE, Jacobson KA (2011) Xanthines as adenosine receptor antagonists. *Handb Exp Pharmacol*:151-199.

[61] Sullivan M, Egerton M, Shakur Y, Marquardsen A, Houslay MD (1994) Molecular cloning and expression, in both COS-1 cells and S. cerevisiae, of a human cytosolic type-IVA, cyclic AMP specific phosphodiesterase (hPDE-IVA-h6.1). *Cell Signal* 6:793-812.

[62] Guerreiro S, Toulorge D, Hirsch E, Marien M, Sokoloff P, Michel PP (2008) Paraxanthine, the primary metabolite of caffeine, provides protection against dopaminergic cell death via stimulation of ryanodine receptor channels. *Mol Pharmacol* 74:980-989.

[63] Wells JN, Wu YJ, Baird CE, Hardman JG (1975) Phosphodiesterases from porcine coronary arteries: inhibition of separated forms by xanthines, papaverine, and cyclic nucleotides. *Mol Pharmacol* 11:775-783.

[64] Suvarna NU, O'Donnell JM (2002) Hydrolysis of N-methyl-D-aspartate receptor-stimulated cAMP and cGMP by PDE4 and PDE2 phosphodiesterases in primary neuronal cultures of rat cerebral cortex and hippocampus. *J Pharmacol Exp Ther* 302:249-256.

[65] Podzuweit T, Nennstiel P, Muller A (1995) Isozyme selective inhibition of cGMP-stimulated cyclic nucleotide phosphodiesterases by erythro-9-(2-hydroxy-3-nonyl) adenine. *Cell Signal* 7:733-738.

[66] Repaske DR, Swinnen JV, Jin SL, Van Wyk JJ, Conti M (1992) A polymerase chain reaction strategy to identify and clone cyclic nucleotide phosphodiesterase cDNAs. Molecular cloning of the cDNA encoding the 63-kDa calmodulin-dependent phosphodiesterase. *J Biol Chem* 267:18683-18688.

[67] Boess FG, Hendrix M, van der Staay FJ, Erb C, Schreiber R, van Staveren W, de Vente J, Prickaerts J, Blokland A, Koenig G (2004) Inhibition of phosphodiesterase 2 increases neuronal cGMP, synaptic plasticity and memory performance. *Neuropharmacology* 47:1081-1092.

[68] Rutten K, Van Donkelaar EL, Ferrington L, Blokland A, Bollen E, Steinbusch HW, Kelly PA, Prickaerts JH (2009) Phosphodiesterase inhibitors enhance object memory independent of cerebral blood flow and glucose utilization in rats. *Neuropsychopharmacology* 34:1914-1925.

[69] Reed TM, Repaske DR, Snyder GL, Greengard P, Vorhees CV (2002) Phosphodiesterase 1B knock-out mice exhibit exaggerated locomotor hyperactivity and DARPP-32 phosphorylation in response to dopamine agonists and display impaired spatial learning. *J Neurosci* 22:5188-5197.

[70] Truss MC, Stief CG, Uckert S, Becker AJ, Wefer J, Schultheiss D, Jonas U (2001) Phosphodiesterase 1 inhibition in the treatment of lower urinary tract dysfunction: from bench to bedside. *World J Urol* 19:344-350.

[71] Medina AE, Krahe TE, Ramoa AS (2006) Restoration of neuronal plasticity by a phosphodiesterase type 1 inhibitor in a model of fetal alcohol exposure. *J Neurosci* 26:1057-1060.

[72] Menniti FS, Faraci WS, Schmidt CJ (2006) Phosphodiesterases in the CNS: targets for drug development. *Nat Rev Drug Discov* 5:660-670.

[73] Filgueiras CC, Krahe TE, Medina AE (2010) Phosphodiesterase type 1 inhibition improves learning in rats exposed to alcohol during the third trimester equivalent of human gestation. *Neurosci Lett* 473:202-207.

[74] Jeon KI, Xu X, Aizawa T, Lim JH, Jono H, Kwon DS, Abe J, Berk BC, Li JD, Yan C (2010) Vinpocetine inhibits NF-kappaB-dependent inflammation via an IKK-dependent but PDE-independent mechanism. *Proc Natl Acad Sci USA* 107:9795-9800.

[75] Medina AE (2010) Vinpocetine as a potent antiinflammatory agent. *Proc Natl Acad Sci USA* 107:9921-9922.

[76] Vandecasteele G, Verde I, Rucker-Martin C, Donzeau-Gouge P, Fischmeister R (2001) Cyclic GMP regulation of the L-type Ca(2+) channel current in human atrial myocytes. *J Physiol* 533:329-340.

[77] Shin DD, Brandimarte F, De Luca L, Sabbah HN, Fonarow GC, Filippatos G, Komajda M, Gheorghiade M (2007) Review of current and investigational pharmacologic agents for acute heart failure syndromes. *Am J Cardiol* 99:4A-23A.

[78] Nohria A, Tsang SW, Fang JC, Lewis EF, Jarcho JA, Mudge GH, Stevenson LW (2003) Clinical assessment identifies hemodynamic profiles that predict outcomes in patients admitted with heart failure. *J Am Coll Cardiol* 41:1797-1804.

[79] Carev M, Bulat C, Karanovic N, Lojpur M, Jercic A, Nenadic D, Marovih Z, Husedzinovic I, Letica D (2010) Combined usage of inhaled and intravenous milrinone in pulmonary hypertension after heart valve surgery. *Coll Antropol* 34:1113-1117.

[80] Essayan DM (2001) Cyclic nucleotide phosphodiesterases. *J Allergy Clin Immunol* 108:671-680.

[81] Toward TJ, Smith N, Broadley KJ (2004) Effect of phosphodiesterase-5 inhibitor, sildenafil (Viagra), in animal models of airways disease. *Am J Respir Crit Care Med* 169:227-234.

[82] Scott AI, Perini AF, Shering PA, Whalley LJ (1991) In-patient major depression: is rolipram as effective as amitriptyline? *Eur J Clin Pharmacol* 40:127-129.

[83] O'Byrne PM, Gauvreau G (2009) Phosphodiesterase-4 inhibition in COPD. *Lancet* 374:665-667.

[84] Ghofrani HA, Osterloh IH, Grimminger F (2006) Sildenafil: from angina to erectile dysfunction to pulmonary hypertension and beyond. *Nature Rev Drug Discov* 5:689-702.

[85] Corbin JD, Beasley A, Blount MA, Francis SH (2005) High lung PDE5: a strong basis for treating pulmonary hypertension with PDE5 inhibitors. *Biochem Biophys Res Commun* 334:930-938.

[86] Wharton J, Strange JW, Moller GM, Growcott EJ, Ren X, Franklyn AP, Phillips SC, Wilkins MR (2005) Antiproliferative effects of phosphodiesterase type 5 inhibition in human pulmonary artery cells. *Am J Respir Crit Care Med* 172:105-113.

[87] Moncada S, Martin JF (1993) Evolution of nitric oxide. *Lancet* 341:1511.

[88] Prickaerts J, van Staveren WC, Sik A, Markerink-van Ittersum M, Niewohner U, van der Staay FJ, Blokland A, de Vente J (2002) Effects of two selective phosphodiesterase type 5 inhibitors, sildenafil and vardenafil, on object recognition memory and hippocampal cyclic GMP levels in the rat. *Neuroscience* 113:351-361.

[89] Baratti CM, Boccia MM (1999) Effects of sildenafil on long-term retention of an inhibitory avoidance response in mice. *Behav Pharmacol* 10:731-737.

[90] Gardner C, Robas N, Cawkill D, Fidock M (2000) Cloning and characterization of the human and mouse PDE7B, a novel cAMP-specific cyclic nucleotide phosphodiesterase. *Biochem Biophys Res Commun* 272:186-192.

[91] Sasaki T, Kotera J, Yuasa K, Omori K (2000) Identification of human PDE7B, a cAMP-specific phosphodiesterase. *Biochem Biophys Res Commun* 271:575-583.

[92] Pitts WJ, Vaccaro W, Huynh T, Leftheris K, Roberge JY, Barbosa J, Guo J, Brown B, Watson A, Donaldson K, Starling GC, Kiener PA, Poss MA, Dodd JH, Barrish JC (2004) Identification of purine inhibitors of phosphodiesterase 7 (PDE7). *Bioorg Med Chem Lett* 14:2955-2958.

[93] Vergne F, Bernardelli P, Lorthiois E, Pham N, Proust E, Oliveira C, Mafroud AK, Royer F, Wrigglesworth R, Schellhaas J, Barvian M, Moreau F, Idrissi M, Tertre A, Bertin B, Coupe M, Berna P, Soulard P (2004) Discovery of thiadiazoles as a novel structural class of potent and selective PDE7 inhibitors. Part 1: design, synthesis and structure-activity relationship studies. *Bioorg Med Chem Lett* 14:4607-4613.

[94] Zhang L, Murray F, Zahno A, Kanter JR, Chou D, Suda R, Fenlon M, Rassenti L, Cottam H, Kipps TJ, Insel PA (2008) Cyclic nucleotide phosphodiesterase profiling reveals increased expression of phosphodiesterase 7B in chronic lymphocytic leukemia. *Proc Natl Acad Sci USA* 105:19532-19537.

[95] Vang AG, Ben-Sasson SZ, Dong H, Kream B, DeNinno MP, Claffey MM, Housley W, Clark RB, Epstein PM, Brocke S (2010) PDE8 regulates rapid Teff cell adhesion and proliferation independent of ICER. *PLoS One* 5:e12011.

[96] Tsai LC, Shimizu-Albergine M, Beavo JA (2011) The high affinity cAMP-specific phosphodiesterase 8B (PDE8B) controls steroidogenesis in the mouse adrenal gland. *Mol Pharmacol* 79:639-648.

[97] Antoni FA (2000) Molecular diversity of cyclic AMP signalling. *Front Neuroendocrinol* 21:103-132.

[98] Chappe V, Mettey Y, Vierfond JM, Hanrahan JW, Gola M, Verrier B, Becq F (1998) Structural basis for specificity and potency of xanthine derivatives as activators of the CFTR chloride channel. *Br J Pharmacol* 123:683-693.

[99] Drumm ML, Wilkinson DJ, Smit LS, Worrell RT, Strong TV, Frizzell RA, Dawson DC, Collins FS (1991) Chloride conductance expressed by delta F508 and other mutant CFTRs in Xenopus oocytes. *Science* 254:1797-1799.

[100] Grubb B, Lazarowski E, Knowles M, Boucher R (1993) Isobutylmethylxanthine fails to stimulate chloride secretion in cystic fibrosis airway epithelia. *Am J Respir Cell Mol Biol* 8:454-460.

[101] Haws CM, Nepomuceno IB, Krouse ME, Wakelee H, Law T, Xia Y, Nguyen H, Wine JJ (1996) Delta F508-CFTR channels: kinetics, activation by forskolin, and potentiation by xanthines. *Am J Physiol* 270:C1544-1555.

[102] Takeuchi K, Yagi K, Kato S, Ukawa H (1997) Roles of prostaglandin E-receptor subtypes in gastric and duodenal bicarbonate secretion in rats. *Gastroenterology* 113:1553-1559.

[103] Aoi M, Aihara E, Nakashima M, Takeuchi K (2004) Participation of prostaglandin E receptor EP4 subtype in duodenal bicarbonate secretion in rats. *Am J Physiol Gastrointest Liver Physiol* 287:G96-103.

[104] Kelley TJ, Al-Nakkash L, Drumm ML (1995) CFTR-mediated chloride permeability is regulated by type III phosphodiesterases in airway epithelial cells. *Am J Respir Cell Mol Biol* 13:657-664.

[105] Kelley TJ, Al-Nakkash L, Cotton CU, Drumm ML (1996) Activation of endogenous deltaF508 cystic fibrosis transmembrane conductance regulator by phosphodiesterase inhibition. *J Clin Invest* 98:513-520.

[106] Kelley TJ, Thomas K, Milgram LJ, Drumm ML (1997) In vivo activation of the cystic fibrosis transmembrane conductance regulator mutant deltaF508 in murine nasal epithelium. *Proc Natl Acad Sci USA* 94:2604-2608.

[107] Smith SN, Middleton PG, Chadwick S, Jaffe A, Bush KA, Rolleston S, Farley R, Delaney SJ, Wainwright B, Geddes DM, Alton EW (1999) The in vivo effects of milrinone on the airways of cystic fibrosis mice and human subjects. *Am J Respir Cell Mol Biol* 20:129-134.

[108] Hogan DL, Crombie DL, Isenberg JI, Svendsen P, Schaffalitzky de Muckadell OB, Ainsworth MA (1997) CFTR mediates cAMP- and Ca2+-activated duodenal epithelial HCO3- secretion. *Am J Physiol* 272:G872-878.

[109] O'Grady SM, Jiang X, Maniak PJ, Birmachu W, Scribner LR, Bulbulian B, Gullikson GW (2002) Cyclic AMP-dependent Cl secretion is regulated by multiple phosphodiesterase subtypes in human colonic epithelial cells. *J Membr Biol* 185:137-144.

[110] Hayashi M, Kita K, Ohashi Y, Aihara E, Takeuchi K (2007) Phosphodiesterase isozymes involved in regulation of HCO3- secretion in isolated mouse duodenum in vitro. *Biochem Pharmacol* 74:1507-1513.

[111] McPherson MA, Pereira MM, Lloyd Mills C, Murray KJ, Dormer RL (1999) A cyclic nucleotide PDE5 inhibitor corrects defective mucin secretion in submandibular

cells containing antibody directed against the cystic fibrosis transmembrane conductance regulator protein. *FEBS Lett* 464:48-52.

[112] Ahn HS, Foster M, Cable M, Pitts BJ, Sybertz EJ (1991) Ca/CaM-stimulated and cGMP-specific phosphodiesterases in vascular and non-vascular tissues. *Adv Exp Med Biol* 308:191-197.

[113] Milligan PA, Marshall SF, Karlsson MO (2002) A population pharmacokinetic analysis of sildenafil citrate in patients with erectile dysfunction. *Br J Clin Pharmacol* 53 Suppl 1:45S-52S.

[114] Nichols DJ, Muirhead GJ, Harness JA (2002) Pharmacokinetics of sildenafil after single oral doses in healthy male subjects: absolute bioavailability, food effects and dose proportionality. *Br J Clin Pharmacol* 53 Suppl 1:5S-12S.

[115] Muirhead GJ, Rance DJ, Walker DK, Wastall P (2002) Comparative human pharmacokinetics and metabolism of single-dose oral and intravenous sildenafil. *Br J Clin Pharmacol* 53 Suppl 1:13S-20S.

[116] Burgess G, Hoogkamer H, Collings L, Dingemanse J (2008) Mutual pharmacokinetic interactions between steady-state bosentan and sildenafil. *Eur J Clin Pharmacol* 64:43-50.

[117] Klotz T, Sachse R, Heidrich A, Jockenhovel F, Rohde G, Wensing G, Horstmann R, Engelmann R (2001) Vardenafil increases penile rigidity and tumescence in erectile dysfunction patients: a RigiScan and pharmacokinetic study. *World J Urol* 19:32-39.

[118] Gresser U, Gleiter CH (2002) Erectile dysfunction: comparison of efficacy and side effects of the PDE-5 inhibitors sildenafil, vardenafil and tadalafil--review of the literature. *Eur J Med Res* 7:435-446.

[119] Stark S, Sachse R, Liedl T, Hensen J, Rohde G, Wensing G, Horstmann R, Schrott KM (2001) Vardenafil increases penile rigidity and tumescence in men with erectile dysfunction after a single oral dose. *Eur Urol* 40:181-188; discussion 189-190.

[120] Ormrod D, Easthope SE, Figgitt DP (2002) Vardenafil. *Drugs Aging* 19:217-227.

[121] Eardley I, Cartledge J (2002) Tadalafil (Cialis) for men with erectile dysfunction. *Int J Clin Pract* 56:300-304.

[122] Bella AJ, Brock GB (2003) Tadalafil in the treatment of erectile dysfunction. *Curr Urol Rep* 4:472-478.

[123] Staab A, Tillmann C, Forgue ST, Mackie A, Allerheiligen SR, Rapado J, Troconiz IF (2004) Population dose-response model for tadalafil in the treatment of male erectile dysfunction. *Pharm Res* 21:1463-1470.

[124] Brock GB (2003) Tadalafil: a new agent for erectile dysfunction. *Can J Urol* 10 Suppl 1:17-22.

[125] Porst H, Padma-Nathan H, Giuliano F, Anglin G, Varanese L, Rosen R (2003) Efficacy of tadalafil for the treatment of erectile dysfunction at 24 and 36 hours after dosing: a randomized controlled trial. *Urology* 62:121-125; discussion 125-126.

[126] Curran M, Keating G (2003) Tadalafil. *Drugs* 63:2203-2212; discussion 2213-2214.

[127] Pedemonte N, Lukacs GL, Du K, Caci E, Zegarra-Moran O, Galietta LJ, Verkman AS (2005) Small-molecule correctors of defective DeltaF508-CFTR cellular processing identified by high-throughput screening. *J Clin Invest* 115:2564-2571.

[128] Van Goor F, Straley KS, Cao D, Gonzalez J, Hadida S, Hazlewood A, Joubran J, Knapp T, Makings LR, Miller M, Neuberger T, Olson E, Panchenko V, Rader J, Singh A, Stack JH, Tung R, Grootenhuis PD, Negulescu P (2006) Rescue of DeltaF508-CFTR trafficking and gating in human cystic fibrosis airway primary cultures by small molecules. *Am J Physiol Lung Cell Mol Physiol* 290:L1117-1130.

[129] Carlile GW, Robert R, Zhang D, Teske KA, Luo Y, Hanrahan JW, Thomas DY (2007) Correctors of protein trafficking defects identified by a novel high-throughput screening assay. *Chem Biochem* 8:1012-1020.

[130] van Doorninck JH, French PJ, Verbeek E, Peters RH, Morreau H, Bijman J, Scholte BJ (1995) A mouse model for the cystic fibrosis delta F508 mutation. *EMBO J* 14:4403-4411.

[131] Lubamba B, Lebacq J, Lebecque P, Vanbever R, Leonard A, Wallemacq P, Leal T (2009) Airway delivery of low dose miglustat normalizes nasal potential differenece in F508del cystic fibrosis mice. *Am J Respir Crit Care Med* 179:1022-8.

[132] Sermet-Gaudelus I, De Boeck K, Casimir GJ, Vermeulen F, Leal T, Mogenet A, Roussel D, Fritsch J, Constantine S, Reha A, Hirawat S, Miller NL, Ajayi T, Elfring GL, Miller L (2010) Ataluren (PTC124) Induces CFTR Protein Expression and Activity in Children with Nonsense Mutation Cystic Fibrosis. *Am J Respir Crit Care Med* 182:1262-72.

[133] Berry B, Altman P, Rowe J, Vaisman T (2009) Comparison of pharmacokinetics of vardenafil administered using an ultrasonic nebulizer for inhalation versus a single 10-mg oral tablet. *J Sex Med* July 28 [Epub ahead of print].

[134] Dalby R, Suman J (2003) Inhalation therapy: technological milestones in asthma treatment. *Adv Drug Deliv Rev* 55: 779–791.

[135] Legssyer R, Huaux F, Lebacq J, Delos M, Marbaix E, Lebecque P, Lison D, Scholte BJ, Wallemacq P, Leal T (206) Azithromycin reduces spontaneous and induced inflammation in delta F508 cystic fibrosis mice. *Respir Res* 7:134.

[136] Meyer M, Huaux F, Gavilanes X, van den Brûle S, Lebecque P, Lo Re S, Lison D, Scholte B, Wallemacq P, Leal T (2009) Azithromycin reduces exaggerated cytokine production by M1 alveolar macrophages in cystic fibrosis. *Am J Respir Cell Mol Biol* 41:590-602.

[137] Gavilanes X, Huaux F, Meyer M, Lebecque P, Marbaix E, Lison D, Scholte B, Wallemacq P, Leal T (2009) Azithromycin fails to reduce increased expression of neutrophil-related cytokines in primary-cultured epithelial cells from cystic fibrosis mice. *J Cyst Fibros* 8:203-210.

[138] Poschet JF, Timmins GS, Taylor-Cousar JL, Ornatowski W, Fazio J, Perkett E, Wilson KR, Yu HD, de Jonge HR, Deretic V (2007) Pharmacological modulation of cGMP levels by phosphodiesterase 5 inhibitors as a therapeutic strategy for treatment of respiratory pathology in cystic fibrosis. *Am J Physiol Lung Cell Mol Physiol* 293:L712-719.

[139] Wang Y, Loo TW, Bartlett MC, Clarke DM (2007) Correctors promote maturation of cystic fibrosis transmembrane conductance regulator (CFTR)-processing mutants by binding to the protein. *J Biol Chem* 282:33247-33251.

[140] Lubamba BA, Panin N, Wauthier S, Huaux F, Lison D, Lebecque P, Wallemacq P, Leal T (2010) Anti-inflammatory effect of vardenafil in CF lung disease. *Ped Pulmonol* 45(S33):308-309.

4

VIP as a Corrector of CFTR Trafficking and Membrane Stability

Valerie Chappe[1] and Sami I. Said[2]
[1]Dalhousie University,
[2]SUNY-Stony Brook University
[1]Canada,
[2]USA

1. Introduction

Cystic Fibrosis (CF) is a fatal autosomal recessive disease characterized by abnormal ion transport across epithelia, viscous mucus secretions, chronic bacterial infections, and inflammation in the airways that result from misprocessed or nonfunctional CFTR (Cystic Fibrosis Transmembrane conductance Regulator) chloride channels, normally located at the apical membrane of epithelial cells in exocrine tissues. CFTR activity is regulated by the Vasoactive Intestinal Peptide (VIP), a neuropeptide with potent anti-inflammatory, bronchodilatory and immunomodulatory functions. In airway sub-mucosal glands and other exocrine tissues, VIP is the major physiological activator for CFTR-dependent secretions, which contribute to local innate defense. When CFTR is defective or absent from the apical membrane of epithelial cells, due to mutations in the CFTR gene, airway glands no longer secrete in response to VIP stimulation and synergy with acetylcholine is lost. Although it is thought that VIP receptors are not altered in CF epithelial tissues, early studies have demonstrated that innervations by VIP-containing nerve fibers of the skin sweat glands, nasal and intestinal mucosa of CF patients is almost absent compared to healthy individuals, suggesting that absence of VIP stimulation could play a central role in the development of CF pathology.

Our group has recently demonstrated that VIP regulates CFTR membrane stability via activation of the $VPAC_1$ receptor and the $G_{\alpha i/q}$ signaling cascade in a PKCε-dependent manner. We also found that prolonged VIP exposure can rescue trafficking to the cell membrane and function of ΔF508-CFTR channels; the most commonly found mutation in CF. Our most recent *in vivo* studies using VIP knock-out (KO) mice provides clear evidence of the importance of VIP in maintaining healthy exocrine tissues, and the molecular link, between the absence of VIP stimulation and the development of a CF-like phenotype. We also observed a corrective effect with exogenous VIP administration, which restored normal trafficking and stabilized functional CFTR channels at the apical membrane of epithelial cells of the lung and small intestine (Fig. 1&2).

This mini-review summarizes recent and past findings on the role VIP in CFTR regulation and how it relates to the development of CF.

2. VIP historical background: Discovery as a vasodilator peptide in lung and intestine and rediscovery as a neuropeptide

First discovered as a smooth-muscle-relaxant, vasodilator peptide in the lung (Said, 1969), VIP was soon thereafter isolated from porcine intestine (Said and Mutt, 1970), chemically characterized (Mutt and Said, 1974), and synthesized (Bodanszky et al, 1973).

A 28 amino-acid residue peptide, VIP is structurally related to several other peptides, said to make up a "family," including pituitary adenylate cyclase-activating peptides (PACAP) 27 & 38, secretin, glucagon, helodermin, sauvagine, urotensin I, and gastric inhibitory peptide (glucose-dependent insulinotropic peptide) (Said, 2006).

With the aid of specific radioimmunoassay and immunofluorescence techniques, VIP immunoreactivity was detected in normal tissues and organs outside of the gastrointestinal tract, and found at high concentrations, as well as in certain neurogenic and endocrine tumors associated with excessive VIP secretion and high plasma levels (Said and Faloona, 1975). Eventually, the peptide was "rediscovered" in normal brain and peripheral nerves (Said and Rosenberg, 1976), and its true identity was recognized as a neuropeptide with neurotransmitter or neuromodulator properties. VIP is now considered to have physiologic regulatory influences on multiple organ systems, to be involved in the pathogenesis of several human disorders, and to have potential therapeutic benefit in a variety of disorders (Said, 1991b).

3. Role of VIP in exocrine secretion

As a neuropeptide, VIP was found to richly innervate all exocrine glands, including the pancreas, sweat, salivary, lachrymal, bronchial, and intestinal glands. Investigators learned that VIP worked in unison with cholinergic nerves, serving primarily to promote blood flow, and together with acetylcholine, to regulate and coordinate exocrine function (Lundberg et al, 1980). Evidence was accumulating that VIP, acting via receptors on these glands (Heinz-Erian et al, 1986), stimulated water and chloride transport across intestinal and tracheobronchial mucosa, HCO_3^- secretion by pancreatic acini, and promoted the movement of water and chloride across other epithelial surfaces (Heinz-Erian et al, 1985).

4. Is there a link to CF?

The above observations suggested that VIP exerted a regulatory influence on exocrine function, that appeared to run opposite to the observed defects in CF. With my associates (Said & colleagues), therefore, we postulated that the exocrine abnormalities of CF might be caused by a deficiency of VIP innervation. Accordingly, we examined the presence, distribution, and density of VIP-immunoreactive nerves supplying the sweat glands of normal subjects and CF patients. We selected sweat glands because: a) they express one of the cardinal functional abnormalities of the disease; b) unlike other exocrine organs involved in the disease, such as the lungs, sweat glands remain free of infection or morphologic changes; and c) they are easily accessible through skin biopsy (Heinz-Erian et al, 1985).

4.1 Deficient VIP – Containing nerves in CF exocrine tissues

Normal skin showed a rich network of VIP-immunoreactive nerves around secretory sweat gland acini, and a moderate innervation of the reabsorptive ducts. Individual VIP-positive nerve fibers were closely associated with basement membrane of both acini and duct cells. VIP innervation in CF samples, by contrast, was either absent or minimal both in the acini and in the ducts (Heinz-Erian *et al*, 1985).

Other than the skin, VIPergic neurons are also present in other sites of important CF manifestation such as the mucosa of the small intestinal, the pancreas and the respiratory epithelium. As observed in the skin, a deficiency, specifically in VIP-immunoreactive nerves, was observed in the nasal and intestinal mucosa of CF patients (Wattchow *et al*, 1988) while other types of nerve fibers were still present. The loss of VIP-immunoreactive nerve fibers was not however generalized and normal innervation was observed in intestinal muscles.

These findings, later confirmed by other investigators (Savage *et al*, 1990), raised the questions: 1) Is the decreased VIP innervation of CF glands and ducts causally related to the chloride ion abnormality in CF? and 2) what is the role of VIP, if any, in the pathogenesis, or correction, of CF pathology? Both questions remained unanswered for many years to follow.

4.2 Changes in CF submucosal glands

In response to VIP stimulation, normal human submucosal glands, in which CFTR is highly expressed, secrete low level of mucus which participates in the airways innate defense noteworthy by enabling mucociliary clearance (Wine, 2007). In CF glands, however, mucous secretion in response to VIP or cAMP elevation is altered (Joo *et al*, 2002). Mucus becomes more acidic (Song *et al*, 2006) and more viscous (Jayaraman *et al*, 2001) compared to normal. The same dysfunction is observed in CFTR-KO mice (Ianowski *et al*, 2007). VIP and cholinergic agonists synergistically induce mucous secretion from healthy human and pig glands but this synergy is absent in CF tissues (Choi *et al*, 2007). However, the secretion of large amounts of mucus in response to acute stimulation, primarily under the vagal pathway[1], and cholinergic stimulation are still present although altered (Wine, 2007).

5. Recent confirmation of a link, from studies of VIP and VIP-KO mice

We have recently used VIP knockout C57/Bl6 mice to demonstrate *in vivo* the central role of VIP in CFTR regulation and exocrine epithelial tissue integrity. These mice have been proven to be a very good model for airways diseases such as bronchial asthma (Szema *et al*, 2006; Hamidi *et al*, 2006; Said, 2009). They display airways inflammation and hyper-responsiveness to methacholine. They also present moderate pulmonary hypertension, right ventricular hypertrophy, and thickened pulmonary arteries (Said et al, 2007). We have used H&E staining for pathological assessment of the lung, small intestine and pancreas (Fig. 1). Interestingly, changes observed resembled those seen in CF. VIP-KO intestinal tissues had a significant increase in goblet and inflammatory cells. In the lung, we observed lymphocyte aggregation, increased airway secretion, alveolar thickening and edema. The pancreas presented increased secretion and increased infiltration with inflammatory cells surrounding ducts. These pathological changes could be reversed, closed to a wild-type phenotype, by VIP treatment consisting of intra-peritoneal injections of VIP (15µg) every other day for 3 weeks (Fig. 1) (Alcolado, 2010).

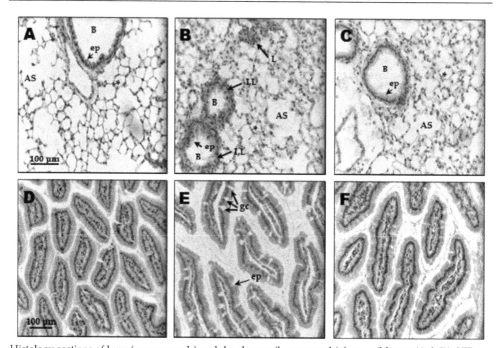

Histology sections of lung (upper panels) and duodenum (lower panels) from wild-type (**A** & **D**), VIP-KO (**B** & **E**) and VIP-KO treated (**C** & **F**) mice. Samples were embedded in paraffin before sectioning. 5 µm thick sections were mounted onto microscopy slides before hematoxylin and eosin (H & E) staining. Images were taken with a light microscope at 20X magnification. Compared to normal tissue, VIP-KO lungs show signs of inflammation (I) and lymphocyte aggregation (dark blue staining), thickening of the mucosa around bronchiolar space, thickening of the alveolar walls and the presence of inflammatory cells. The bronchiolar epithelium (ep) is also damaged. All these pathological signs are reversed to normal after VIP treatment (**C**). In the duodenum, transversal sections show increased amount of goblet cells and epithelium damage in the upper villi of VIP-KO mice tissues. As for the lung, these pathological signs are reversed by VIP treatment.
AS= alveolar sac, B = bronchioles, ep=epithelium, gc = goblet cells, I = inflammation, L = lymphocytes aggregation, * alveoli.

Fig. 1. VIP-KO mice lung and duodenum present pathological signs reversible by VIP treatment (adapted from Alcolado, 2010).

VIP binds to class II seven transmembrane spanning domain G protein-coupled receptors (GPCR) on the basolateral membrane of epithelial cells (Laburthe *et al*, 2007, 2002; Dickson *et al*, 2006; Chastre *et al*, 1989). VIP can bind to 3 receptors: $VPAC_1$, $VPAC_2$ and PAC_1. The highest affinity is for $VPAC_1$ ($EC_{50} < 0.1nM$) followed by $VPAC_2$ ($EC_{50} = 10$ nM) and very little affinity for PAC_1 ($EC_{50} \sim 40$ nM). The PAC_1 receptor has a much greater affinity for Pituitary Adenylate Cyclase-Activating Polypeptide ($EC_{50} \sim 0.2$ nM) (Dickson and Finlayson, 2009). Other members of this peptide family, such as secretin and helodermin, can also bind to VPAC receptors although with much lower affinity than VIP (Laburthe *et al*, 2007) . Although VIP innervating fibres were found to be absent from CF intestinal mucosa (Wattchow *et al*, 1988), a study on CF foetuses revealed the presence of VIP receptors with unaltered pharmacology in the small intestine (Chastre *et al*, 1989).

In the VIP-KO mice model, we confirmed the expression of $VPAC_1$, $VPAC_2$ and PAC_1 by RT-PCR. Immunoblotting of lung and duodenum tissue lysates revealed unchanged PAC_1 expression in VIP-KO mice tissues compared to wild-type (WT), whereas VPAC 1 and 2 were found to be more abundant in VIP-KO tissues. These 2 receptors expression level remained up-regulated after VIP treatment (Conrad, 2011). CFTR localization was examined by immunostaining followed by confocal microscopy (Fig. 2). WT tissues showed CFTR predominantly at the apical membrane of epithelial cells in contrast to VIP-KO tissues, where CFTR distribution was mainly observed intracellularly. No changes in CFTR protein abundance or maturation were observed in immunoblots. Interestingly, VIP treatment restored strong CFTR membrane localization (Fig. 2), confirming the important role of VIP chronic exposure to maintain CFTR channels at the membrane, where it can exert its function, and for exocrine epithelial tissues integrity. Inflammation and damage observed in VIP-KO tissues can be attributed, at least in part, to the lack of CFTR-dependent secretions which ultimately depend on VIP stimulation both for acute and long-term regulation of CFTR function. These observations provide evidence of the molecular link between early observations of deficient VIP-containing fibers innervation of epithelial layers of exocrine organs in CF tissues and the absence of CFTR-dependent secretions.

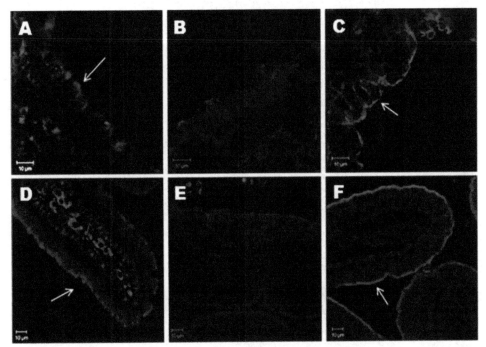

Paraffin embedded tissues (lung: upper panels, duodenum: lower panels) were sliced into 5 μm sections and mounted onto microscopy slides before immunostaining with the monoclonal anti-CFTR antibody MAB1660 (1:100). Arrows indicate apical CFTR signal. A & D: wild-type, B & E: VIP-KO, C & F: VIP-KO treated mice.

Fig. 2. CFTR localization at the apical membrane of epithelial cells is lost in VIP-KO tissues and restored by VIP treatment (adapted from Alcolado, 2010).

6. Molecular role of VIP in CFTR regulation

6.1 Regulation of CFTR activation by VIP acute stimulation

CFTR is activated mainly by protein kinase A (PKA)-dependent phosphorylation, with protein kinase C (PKC) stimulation playing an enhancing and permissive role to subsequent responsiveness to PKA (Chappe *et al*, 2008; Jia *et al*, 1997), in part through direct phosphorylation of conserved consensus sequences in CFTR Regulatory (R) domain (Chappe *et al*, 2003; Chappe *et al*, 2004). Hormones and neurotransmitters, such as VIP, which raise cellular cyclic AMP level, can stimulate acute CFTR channel activity. VIP is the most abundant peptide in the airways and the $VPAC_1$ receptor has been shown to stimulate CFTR-dependent chloride secretion upon VIP binding through activation of both PKA- and PKC-dependent signaling pathways in airway submucosal glands epithelial cell line Calu-3 (Chappe *et al*, 2008; Derand *et al*, 2004). Although class II GPCR are generally coupled to $G_{\alpha s}$[2] and adenylate cyclase activation to increase intracellular cAMP content, numerous reports have demonstrated that VIP receptors can couple to alternate G proteins and elicit signaling cascades cross-talk involving $G_{\alpha i/q}$[2], PKC and calcium release on top of the conventional $G_{\alpha s}$ and cAMP cascade (Derand *et al*, 2004; Bewley *et al*, 2006; Chappe *et al*, 2008; Sreedharan *et al*, 1994; Xia *et al*, 1996; Shreeve *et al*, 2000; Rafferty *et al*, 2009) (Fig. 3).

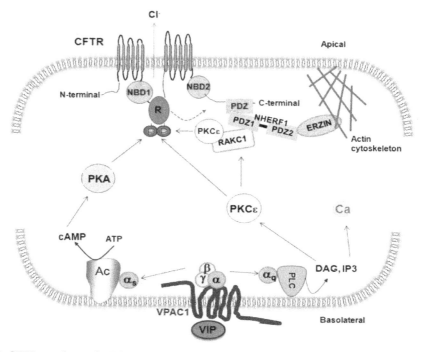

Fig. 3. CFTR regulation by VIP.

After binding to the $VPAC_1$ receptor, on the basolateral membrane, VIP induces the activation of both PKA and PKC signalling cascades. On the right end side of this cartoon is displayed the PKCε cascade of activation, as observed in our experiments and by others. The $G\alpha_q$ protein activates phospholipase C (PLC) which produces inositol tri-phosphate (IP3) and diacylglycerol (DAG). IP3 induces calcium release whereas DAG stimulates PKCε. PKCε can directly phosphorylate membrane CFTR on specific sites in the Regulatory domain. The activated PKCε also binds to the receptor for active kinase C (RAKC1) and translocate to the plasma membrane where RAKC1 binds to the PDZ domain 1 of NHERF1 (Na+/H+ Exchanger Regulatory Factor-1). This complex interacts with CFTR C-terminal, on a PDZ motif, and to ERZIN which anchors the whole complex to the actin cytoskeleton. This regulation maintains CFTR at the membrane and reduces its endocytosis. The co-localization of PKCε and CFTR is thought to maintain CFTR phosphorylation which contributes to its activation. We observed that the phosphorylated R domain relocates from its initial position, close to the Nucleotide Binding domains (NBD), to a new position with increased binding strength. We hypothesize here that re-binding of the phosphorylated R domain will further increase CFTR stability at the membrane through interaction with the PKCε-RAKC1-NHERF1 complex. In parallel (see left side), the VPAC$_1$ receptor can activate the PKA signalling cascade by associating with the Gα$_s$ protein which activates Adenylyl cyclase (Ac) to produce intracellular cAMP. This second messenger stimulates PKA. Direct phosphorylation of the CFTR R domain by PKA activates the channel gating. CFTR gating is further enhanced by PKC phosphorylation.

6.2 Role of VIP in CFTR membrane insertion and stability

Control of CFTR recycling is an important mechanism for the regulation of CFTR-dependent secretions. Adapters and proteins involved in CFTR endocytosis have been studied in detail (Ameen et al, 2007; Okiyoneda and Lukacs, 2007), but its regulation by physiological agonists is far less well understood and seems to be cell-type specific. Although CFTR function as a chloride channel requires apical membrane localization to participate in the regulation of exocrine secretions, it is mostly present in recycling endosomes, forming an important submembranar pool of mature proteins (Bradbury et al, 1994; Bradbury and Bridges, 1994; Webster et al, 1994). CFTR has a relatively long half-life: 16-24 hrs and a rapid turnover, although variable among cell lines: 2-16% per minute (Chappe et al, 2008; Lukacs et al, 1993; Swiatecka-Urban et al, 2005). CFTR is internalized by clathrin coated vesicles due to the presence of a dileucine and tyrosine endocytotic signals in its C-terminal. The tyrosine based motif interacts with the clathrin adapter complex AP-2 to enter into clathrin coated pits. CFTR also interacts with actin-binding proteins like myosin VI and to N-SWAP to recycle back to the plasma membrane via recycling endosomes (Okiyoneda and Lukacs, 2007; Swiatecka-Urban et al, 2004; Ganeshan et al, 2006). Conflicting results exist regarding the role of cAMP or other second messengers in CFTR recycling probably due to disparity in epithelial cells studied or the use of over-expressing systems which might saturate the normal pathway for CFTR trafficking. Both PKA and PKC-dependent mechanisms have been reported.

6.2.1 In intact tissues

Spiny dogfish shark (*Squalus acanthias*) rectal glands highly regulate salt secretion upon hormonal signals. These glands express a CFTR ortholog with 72% identity to the human CFTR. Acute VIP stimulation of these glands produces an increase in CFTR-mediated chloride secretions. Immunofluorescence labeling also revealed a redistribution of CFTR from intracellular to apical membrane localization following VIP stimulation (Lehrich et al, 1998).

In rats, a subpopulation of epithelial cells found in the small intestinal villi was identified as CFTR High Expresser cells (CHE) (Ameen *et al*, 1995). In response to VIP stimulation, CFTR present in sub-apical vesicular pool redistributed to the apical membrane but returned to the intracellular pool after removal of VIP (Ameen *et al*, 1999; Ameen *et al*, 2000).

6.2.2 In cell lines

Our lab has established that prolonged VIP stimulation of polarized airway epithelial cells stabilizes CFTR at the cell surface by reducing its internalization rate by more than 50%. The consequence of this regulation is an increase in CFTR-mediated chloride secretion. This was demonstrated initially in Calu-3 cells, a widely used model for submucosal gland serous cells, which express $VPAC_1$ receptors on their basolateral membrane and wild-type CFTR at the apical surface. Analysis of surface proteins by biotinylation and streptavidin extraction methods, revealed a large increase in apical CFTR after VIP exposure which was significant after 10 min and maximal within 2 hrs of VIP treatment. No changes in total CFTR or the proportion of fully glycosylated CFTR were measured in any tested condition, confirming that the VIP regulation was on mature CFTR recycling and did not affect its trafficking. Interestingly, the signaling cascade involved in this mechanism was $VPAC_1$ and $G_{\alpha i}$ mediated and involved the activation of PKC (Chappe *et al*, 2008). Direct activation of PKC by phorbol esters could mimic VIP effect with more than 2 fold increase in apical CFTR after 2 hrs of treatment. Functional evidence of increased membrane CFTR density after PKC stimulation were also reported in the human colon cell line HT29 together with increased mucus secretion (Bajnath *et al*, 1995). Contrary to previous observations in intestinal epithelial cells (Ameen *et al*, 2003; Bradbury and Bridges, 1992), raising intracellular cAMP by forskolin had no effect on the amount of CFTR at the apical membrane of Calu-3 cells. It is thus evident that VIP effect on CFTR membrane insertion is coupled to different signaling pathways in airways and intestinal cells, with the latter having more complex regulation possibly depending on the cellular model considered.

6.2.3 Rescue of ΔF508-CFTR maturation and membrane stability

The most common mutation in CF is the deletion of a phenylalanine residue at position 508 (ΔF508) that causes improper folding of the CFTR protein, resulting in its retention in the endoplasmic reticulum and proteosomal degradation of the majority of the newly synthesized CFTR proteins (Cheng *et al*, 1990; Kartner *et al*, 1992; Penque *et al*, 2000). However, part of the ΔF508-CFTR protein can still mature and reach the cell membrane where it retains some chloride channel function (Bronsveld *et al*, 2000; Penque *et al*, 2000; Kopito, 1999). Many efforts on CF research are devoted to attempt to rescue ΔF508-CFTR defective trafficking to restore normal epithelial function. Interestingly, ΔF508-CFTR retains some chloride channel activity when rescued from degradation by low temperature, chemical chaperones or other correctors. However, the half-life of the mutant protein is considerably shorter than that of the wild-type CFTR, mainly due to instability at the apical membrane (Lukacs *et al*, 1993; Denning *et al*, 1992; Dormer *et al*, 2001; Sharma *et al*, 2001).

We have investigated the potential rescue and stability at the cell membrane of ΔF508-CFTR by VIP treatment in the human nasal epithelial cells JME/CF15, derived from a ΔF508 homozygous patient (Jefferson *et al*, 1990). Immunostaining experiments with specific anti-

CFTR antibodies, followed by confocal microscopy confirmed intracellular localization of ΔF508-CFTR under control conditions, at 37°C, whereas membrane localization was observed in cells cultured at 27°C for 48hrs (Rafferty *et al*, 2009). The important finding of this study was that when JME/CF15 cells, maintained at physiological temperature (37°C), were treated with VIP (300 nM) for 1 or 2 hrs, mature ΔF508-CFTR proteins were observed in western blot experiments and immunostaining confirmed localization at the cell membrane. Functional assays confirmed the presence of CFTR-dependent chloride secretion after VIP treatment at 37°C. In these nasal cells, which express the VPAC$_1$ receptor, we found that VIP-dependent rescue of ΔF508-CFTR trafficking was mediated by the PKA-dependent signaling cascade (Fig. 4). We also found that ΔF508-CFTR membrane insertion obtained at low temperature could be enhanced by prolonged VIP treatment (1 to 2 hrs) which induced a large increase in ΔF508-CFTR function. As previously observed for wild-type CFTR, this regulation involved the $G_{\alpha q}$ and PKC signaling cascade but not the $G_{\alpha s}$ - PKA cascade (Fig. 4).

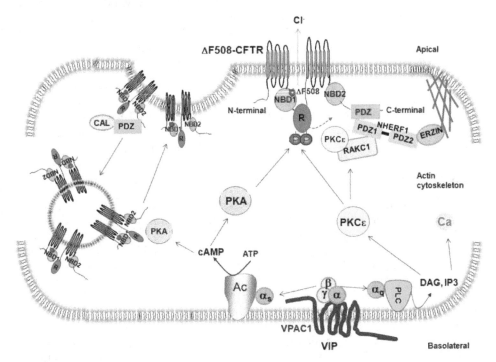

Fig. 4. Regulation of ΔF508-CFTR by VIP.

After binding to the VPAC$_1$ receptor, on the basolateral membrane, VIP induces the activation of both PKA and PKC signalling cascades. On the right side of this cartoon is displayed the PKCε cascade of activation, as observed in our experiments and by others. The $G_{\alpha q}$ protein activates phospholipase C (PLC) which produces inositol tri-phosphate (IP3) and diacylglycerol (DAG). IP3 induces calcium release whereas DAG stimulates PKCε. PKCε can directly phosphorylate membrane CFTR on specific sites in the Regulatory domain. The activated PKCε also binds to the receptor for active kinase C (RAKC1) and translocates to the plasma membrane where RAKC1 binds to the PDZ domain 1 of NHERF1. This complex interacts with CFTR C-terminal, on a PDZ motif, and to ERZIN which anchors the whole complex to the actin cytoskeleton. This regulation maintains CFTR at the membrane and reduces its endocytosis. The co-localization of PKCε and CFTR is thought to maintain CFTR phosphorylation which contributes to its activation. We observed that the phosphorylated R domain relocates from its initial position, close to the Nucleotide Binding domains (NBD), to a new unidentified position with increased binding strenght. We hypothesize here that re-binding of the phosphorylated R domain will further increase CFTR stability at the membrane through interaction with the PKCε-RAKC1-NHERF1 complex. In parallel (see left side), the VPAC$_1$ receptor can activate the PKA signalling cascade by associating with the Gα$_s$ protein which activates Adenylyl cyclase (Ac) to produce intracellular cAMP. This second messenger stimulates PKA. Direct phosphorylation of the CFTR R domain by PKA activates the channel and is further enhanced by PKC phosphorylation. We also observed that the activated PKA contributes to ΔF508-CFTR trafficking and insertion to the plasma membrane. We hypothesize that PKA effect counteracts the action of the CFTR Associated Ligand (CAL) which had been shown to bind to CFTR C-terminal PDZ motif, and compete with NHERF1, to retain CFTR in endosomes and target ΔF508-CFTR to lysosomal degradation.

Evidence from airway cells thus demonstrates that VIP mechanism of regulation of CFTR activity involves both PKA and PKC signaling in a synergistic manner to rescue defective trafficking of mutant CFTR, activate CFTR gating through direct phosphorylation of its regulatory domain, and most importantly, stabilize CFTR channels at the cell surface by reducing their internalization rate, thus optimizing CFTR-dependent secretions.

6.2.4 Role of PKCε

In both recombinant and native systems, we have investigated the role of PKC on VIP-dependent CFTR membrane stability. PKC isoforms comprise calcium-dependent (α, β$_1$, β$_2$, γ) and calcium-independent novel isoforms (δ, ε, η, θ). All necessitate diacyl glycerol to be activated (Reyland, 2009; Dempsey et al, 2000; Gallegos and Newton, 2008). With specific inhibitors and siRNA treatments we found that only PKCε, a novel calcium-independent isoform, mediated VIP-dependent increase in CFTR membrane stability in the JME/CF15 epithelial nasal cells and also in the recombinant BHK cells stably expressing wild-type or ΔF508-CFTR (Alcolado et al, 2011). This is not surprising as PKCε was previously reported to co-localize with CFTR at the apical membrane of airway epithelial cells and to play a permissive role on CFTR-dependent chloride secretion (Liedtke and Cole, 1998; Liedtke et al, 2001; Liedtke et al, 2002). The C-terminal of CFTR interacts with either CAL or NHERF1. These two scaffolding proteins regulate CFTR membrane density in an opposite manner. While CAL, which is mostly found in the trans-golgi network, promotes CFTR targeting to lysosomal degradation, NHERF1, which is localized at the cell apical membrane, rather participate in maintaining CFTR at the membrane by tethering it to the actin cytoskeleton (Cheng, J., 2002, 2004). Structural studies indicate that CAL and NEHRF1 might compete for the same binding site in CFTR C-terminal, and their differential interaction with CFTR is thought to regulate the steady-state level of mature CFTR present at the apical membrane of epithelial cells (Ladias ,

2003; Wolde, 2007). Part of this regulation involves activated PKCε which binds to RACK1 and translocates to the plasma membrane. RACK1 interacts directly with NHERF1 by PDZ domain interaction at the apical membrane of epithelial cells. It is hypothesized that the complex composed of PKCε – RACK1-NHERF1 interacts with CFTR to regulate its membrane stability (Fig. 3 & 4).

7. Conclusions

Although VIP binding to the VPAC$_2$ receptor plays an important role in the relaxation of smooth muscles and is a matter of intense study for respiratory diseases such as bronchial asthma (Hamidi et al, 2006; Alessandrini et al, 1993; Groneberg et al, 2001; Groneberg et al, 2006; Jaeger et al, 1996; Onoue et al, 2004; Said, 1991a), our recent studies have highlighted the important role of the VPAC$_1$ receptor and differential activation of the PKA or PKC signalling pathways in airway epithelial cells to regulate CFTR-dependent secretions. In vivo data set VIP, or its analogs, as a potential candidate for the treatment of CF as it corrects many features of this disease including the molecular basis. Further investigation of VIP potential to rescue exocrine epithelial secretions should be conducted to uncover the large potential of this peptide in the treatment of respiratory diseases, which are the third cause of hospitalization and death in North America.

8. Footnotes

1. Airway defense in response to acute stress such as intense exercise is under the control of the vagal nerve pathway (see Kubin, 2006 and Wine, 2007 for review).
2. G proteins are composed of 3 subunits: α, β and γ. They mediate signaling cascades initiated by ligand binding to membrane receptors of the G protein coupled receptors (GPCR) family. Once activated, the α subunit dissociates from βγ and translocates to a target effector: cellular enzymes and ion channels. The α subunits, which mediate most of the known signals, comprise 4 different types which will initiate specific signaling cascades: α_s, α_q, α_i, $\alpha_{12/13}$. The α_s subunit's effector is the adenylyl cylcase and it initiates the cAMP signaling cascade. The α_q subunit rather activates phospolipase C and initiates the calcium and PKC signaling cascades (for review see Musnier, 2010).

9. Acknowledgments

The authors thank all lab members and collaborators involved in this research: Nicole Alcolado, Dustin Conrad, Frederic Chappe, Dr.Younes Anini, Dr. Zaholin Xu. We also thank Cystic Fibrosis Canada, Nova Scotia Health Research Foundation, Canadian Institutes of Health Research, Canadian Foundation for Innovation, The National Science and Engineering Research Council of Canada and The National Institutes of Health for funding.

10. References

Alcolado N, Conrad DJ, Rafferty S, Chappe FG, Chappe VM. (2011). VIP-dependent increase in F508del-CFTR membrane localization is mediated by PKCε. Am J Physiol Cell Physiol ; 301(1): C56-65.

Alcolado N. (2010). Regulation of CFTR membrane localization by Vasoactive Intestinal Peptide (VIP). *Dalhousie University, Master of Science-Physiology* .

Alessandrini F, Thakkar M, Foda HD, Said SI, Lodi R, Pakbaz H, et al. (1993). Vasoactive intestinal peptide enhances lung preservation. *Transplantation* 56, 964-73.

Ameen N, Silvis M, Bradbury NA. (2007). Endocytic trafficking of CFTR in health and disease. *J Cyst Fibros* 6, 1-14.

Ameen NA, Ardito T, Kashgarian M, Marino CR. (1995). A unique subset of rat and human intestinal villus cells express the cystic fibrosis transmembrane conductance regulator. *Gastroenterology* 108, 1016-23.

Ameen NA, Marino C, Salas PJ. (2003). cAMP-dependent exocytosis and vesicle traffic regulate CFTR and fluid transport in rat jejunum in vivo. *Am J Physiol Cell Physiol* 284, C429-38.

Ameen NA, Martensson B, Bourguinon L, Marino C, Isenberg J, McLaughlin GE. (1999). CFTR channel insertion to the apical surface in rat duodenal villus epithelial cells is upregulated by VIP in vivo. *J Cell Sci* 112 (Pt 6), 887-94.

Ameen NA, van Donselaar E, Posthuma G, de Jonge H, McLaughlin G, Geuze HJ, et al. (2000). Subcellular distribution of CFTR in rat intestine supports a physiologic role for CFTR regulation by vesicle traffic. *Histochem Cell Biol* 114, 219-28.

Bajnath RB, Dekker K, De Jonge HR, Groot JA. (1995). Chloride secretion induced by phorbol dibutyrate and forskolin in the human colonic carcinoma cell line HT-29Cl.19A is regulated by different mechanisms. *Pflugers Arch* 430, 705-12.

Bewley MS, Pena JT, Plesch FN, Decker SE, Weber GJ, Forrest JN,Jr. (2006). Shark rectal gland vasoactive intestinal peptide receptor: Cloning, functional expression, and regulation of CFTR chloride channels. *Am J Physiol Regul Integr Comp Physiol* 291, R1157-64.

Bodanszky M, Klausner YS, Said SI. (1973). Biological activities of synthetic peptides corresponding to fragments of and to the entire sequence of the vasoactive intestinal peptide. *Proc Natl Acad Sci U S A* 70, 382-4.

Bradbury NA. (1999). Intracellular CFTR: Localization and function. *Physiol Rev* 79, S175-91.

Bradbury NA, Bridges RJ. (1994). Role of membrane trafficking in plasma membrane solute transport. *Am J Physiol* 267, C1-24.

Bradbury NA, Bridges RJ. (1992). Endocytosis is regulated by protein kinase A, but not protein kinase C in a secretory epithelial cell line. *Biochem Biophys Res Commun* 184, 1173-80.

Bradbury NA, Cohn JA, Venglarik CJ, Bridges RJ. (1994). Biochemical and biophysical identification of cystic fibrosis transmembrane conductance regulator chloride channels as components of endocytic clathrin-coated vesicles. *J Biol Chem* 269, 8296-302.

Bronsveld I, Mekus F, Bijman J, Ballmann M, Greipel J, Hundrieser J, et al. (2000). Residual chloride secretion in intestinal tissue of deltaF508 homozygous twins and siblings with cystic fibrosis. the european CF twin and sibling study consortium. *Gastroenterology* 119, 32-40.

Chappe FG, Loewen ME, Hanrahan JW, Chappe VM. (2008). VIP increases CFTR levels in the apical membrane of calu-3 cells through a PKC-dependent mechanism. *J Pharmacol Exp Ther* 327, 226-38.

Chappe V, Hinkson DA, Howell LD, Evagelidis A, Liao J, Chang XB, et al. (2004). Stimulatory and inhibitory protein kinase C consensus sequences regulate the cystic fibrosis transmembrane conductance regulator. *Proc Natl Acad Sci U S A* 101, 390-5.

Chappe V, Hinkson DA, Zhu T, Chang XB, Riordan JR, Hanrahan JW. (2003). Phosphorylation of protein kinase C sites in NBD1 and the R domain control CFTR channel activation by PKA. *J Physiol* 548, 39-52.

Chastre E, Bawab W, Faure C, Emami S, Muller F, Boue A, et al. (1989). Vasoactive intestinal peptide and its receptors in fetuses with cystic fibrosis. *Am J Physiol* 257, G561-9.

Cheng J, Moyer BD, Milewski M, Loffing J, Ikeda M, Mickle JE, et al. (2002). A golgi-associated PDZ domain protein modulates cystic fibrosis transmembrane regulator plasma membrane expression. *J Biol Chem* 277, 3520-9.

Cheng J, Wang H, Guggino WB. (2004). Modulation of mature cystic fibrosis transmembrane regulator protein by the PDZ domain protein CAL. *J Biol Chem* 279, 1892-8.

Cheng SH, Gregory RJ, Marshall J, Paul S, Souza DW, White GA, et al. (1990). Defective intracellular transport and processing of CFTR is the molecular basis of most cystic fibrosis. *Cell* 63, 827-34.

Choi JY, Joo NS, Krouse ME, Wu JV, Robbins RC, Ianowski JP, et al. (2007). Synergistic airway gland mucus secretion in response to vasoactive intestinal peptide and carbachol is lost in cystic fibrosis. *J Clin Invest* 117, 3118-27.

Conrad DJ. (2011). Increased VIP receptors expression mediates CFTR membrane localization in response to VIP treatment in VIP knockout mice. *Dalhousie University, Master of Science-Physiology* .

Denning GM, Anderson MP, Amara JF, Marshall J, Smith AE, Welsh MJ. (1992). Processing of mutant cystic fibrosis transmembrane conductance regulator is temperature-sensitive. *Nature* 358, 761-4.

Derand R, Montoni A, Bulteau-Pignoux L, Janet T, Moreau B, Muller JM, et al. (2004). Activation of VPAC1 receptors by VIP and PACAP-27 in human bronchial epithelial cells induces CFTR-dependent chloride secretion. *Br J Pharmacol* 141, 698-708.

Dickson L, Aramori I, McCulloch J, Sharkey J, Finlayson K. (2006). A systematic comparison of intracellular cyclic AMP and calcium signalling highlights complexities in human VPAC/PAC receptor pharmacology. *Neuropharmacology* 51, 1086-98.

Dickson L, Finlayson K. (2009). VPAC and PAC receptors: From ligands to function. *Pharmacol Ther* 121, 294-316.

Dormer RL, Derand R, McNeilly CM, Mettey Y, Bulteau-Pignoux L, Metaye T, et al. (2001). Correction of delF508-CFTR activity with benzo(c)quinolizinium compounds through facilitation of its processing in cystic fibrosis airway cells. *J Cell Sci* 114, 4073-81.

Ganeshan R, Nowotarski K, Di A, Nelson DJ, Kirk KL. (2006). CFTR surface expression and chloride currents are decreased by inhibitors of N-WASP and actin polymerization. *Biochim Biophys Acta* ; DOI: S0167-4889(06)00313-2 [pii]; 10.1016/j.bbamcr.2006.09.031 [doi].

Groneberg DA, Hartmann P, Dinh QT, Fischer A. (2001). Expression and distribution of vasoactive intestinal polypeptide receptor VPAC(2) mRNA in human airways. *Lab Invest* 81, 749-55.

Groneberg DA, Rabe KF, Fischer A. (2006). Novel concepts of neuropeptide-based drug therapy: Vasoactive intestinal polypeptide and its receptors. *Eur J Pharmacol* 533, 182-94.

Groneberg DA, Springer J, Fischer A. (2001). Vasoactive intestinal polypeptide as mediator of asthma. *Pulm Pharmacol Ther* 14, 391-401.

Hamidi SA, Szema AM, Lyubsky S, Dickman KG, Degene A, Mathew SM, et al. (2006). Clues to VIP function from knockout mice. *Ann N Y Acad Sci* 1070, 5-9.

Heinz-Erian P, Dey RD, Flux M, Said SI. (1985). Deficient vasoactive intestinal peptide innervation in the sweat glands of cystic fibrosis patients. *Science* 229, 1407-8.

Heinz-Erian P, Paul S, Said SI. (1986). Receptors for vasoactive intestinal peptide on isolated human sweat glands. *Peptides* 7 Suppl 1, 151-4.

Ianowski JP, Choi JY, Wine JJ, Hanrahan JW. (2007). Mucus secretion by single tracheal submucosal glands from normal and cystic fibrosis transmembrane conductance regulator knockout mice. *J Physiol* 580, 301-14.

Jaeger E, Bauer S, Joyce MW, Foda HD, Berisha HI, Said SI. (1996). Structure-activity studies on VIP: IV. the synthetic agonist helodermin-fragment-(1-28)-amide is a potent VIP-agonist with prolonged duration of tracheal relaxant activity. *Ann N Y Acad Sci* 805, 499-504.

Jayaraman S, Joo NS, Reitz B, Wine JJ, Verkman AS. (2001). Submucosal gland secretions in airways from cystic fibrosis patients have normal [na(+)] and pH but elevated viscosity. *Proc Natl Acad Sci U S A* 98, 8119-23.

Jefferson DM, Valentich JD, Marini FC, Grubman SA, Iannuzzi MC, Dorkin HL, et al. (1990). Expression of normal and cystic fibrosis phenotypes by continuous airway epithelial cell lines. *Am J Physiol* 259, L496-505.

Jia Y, Mathews CJ, Hanrahan JW. (1997). Phosphorylation by protein kinase C is required for acute activation of cystic fibrosis transmembrane conductance regulator by protein kinase A. *J Biol Chem* 272, 4978-84.

Joo NS, Irokawa T, Wu JV, Robbins RC, Whyte RI, Wine JJ. (2002). Absent secretion to vasoactive intestinal peptide in cystic fibrosis airway glands. *J Biol Chem* 277, 50710-5.

Kartner N, Augustinas O, Jensen TJ, Naismith AL, Riordan JR. (1992). Mislocalization of delta F508 CFTR in cystic fibrosis sweat gland. *Nat Genet* 1, 321-7.

Kopito RR. (1999). Biosynthesis and degradation of CFTR. *Physiol Rev* 79, S167-73.

Kubin L, Alheid GF, Zuperku EJ, McCrimmon DR. (2006). Central pathways of pulmonary and lower airway vagal afferents. *J Appl Physiol* 101, 618-27.

Laburthe M, Couvineau A, Marie JC. (2002). VPAC receptors for VIP and PACAP. *Receptors Channels* 8, 137-53.

Laburthe M, Couvineau A, Tan V. (2007). Class II G protein-coupled receptors for VIP and PACAP: Structure, models of activation and pharmacology. *Peptides* 28, 1631-9.

Ladias JA. (2003). Structural insights into the CFTR-NHERF interaction. *J Membr Biol* 192, 79-88.

Lehrich RW, Aller SG, Webster P, Marino CR, Forrest JN,Jr. (1998). Vasoactive intestinal peptide, forskolin, and genistein increase apical CFTR trafficking in the rectal gland of the spiny dogfish, squalus acanthias. acute regulation of CFTR trafficking in an intact epithelium. *J Clin Invest* 101, 737-45.

Liedtke CM, Cole TS. Antisense oligonucleotide to PKC-epsilon alters cAMP-dependent stimulation of CFTR in calu-3 cells. Am J Physiol. 1998 Nov;275(5 Pt 1):C1357-64.

Liedtke CM, Cody D, Cole TS. Differential regulation of Cl- transport proteins by PKC in Calu-3 cells. Am J Physiol Lung Cell Mol Physiol. 2001 Apr;280(4):L739-47.

Liedtke CM, Yun CH, Kyle N, Wang D. Protein kinase C epsilon-dependent regulation of cystic fibrosis transmembrane regulator involves binding to a receptor for activated C kinase (RACK1) and RACK1 binding to Na+/H+ exchange regulatory factor. J Biol Chem. 2002 Jun 21;277(25):22925-33.

Lukacs GL, Chang XB, Bear C, Kartner N, Mohamed A, Riordan JR, et al. (1993). The delta F508 mutation decreases the stability of cystic fibrosis transmembrane conductance regulator in the plasma membrane. determination of functional half-lives on transfected cells. J Biol Chem 268, 21592-8.

Lundberg JM, Anggard A, Fahrenkrug J, Hokfelt T, Mutt V. (1980). Vasoactive intestinal polypeptide in cholinergic neurons of exocrine glands: Functional significance of coexisting transmitters for vasodilation and secretion. Proc Natl Acad Sci U S A 77, 1651-5.

Musnier A, Blanchot B, Reiter E, Crepieux P. (2010). GPCR signalling to the translation machinery. Cell Signal 22, 707-16.

Mutt V, Said SI. (1974). Structure of the porcine vasoactive intestinal octacosapeptide. the amino-acid sequence. use of kallikrein in its determination. Eur J Biochem 42, 581-9.

Okiyoneda T, Lukacs GL. (2007). Cell surface dynamics of CFTR: The ins and outs. Biochim Biophys Acta 1773, 476-9.

Onoue S, Endo K, Ohmori Y, Yamada S, Kimura R, Yajima T, et al. (2004). Long-acting analogue of vasoactive intestinal peptide, [R15, 20, 21, L17]-VIP-GRR (IK312532), protects rat alveolar L2 cells from the cytotoxicity of cigarette smoke. Regul Pept 123, 193-9.

Penque D, Mendes F, Beck S, Farinha C, Pacheco P, Nogueira P, et al. (2000). Cystic fibrosis F508del patients have apically localized CFTR in a reduced number of airway cells. Lab Invest 80, 857-68.

Rafferty S, Alcolado N, Norez C, Chappe F, Pelzer S, Becq F, et al. (2009). Rescue of functional F508del-CFTR by VIP in the human nasal epithelial cell line JME/CF15. J Pharmacol Exp Ther 331(1), 2-13.

Said SI. (2006). Vasoactive intestinal peptide. In Encyclopedia of Respiratory Medicine, ed. Laurent GJ SS. pp. 517-520. Elsevier.

Said SI, Hamidi SA, Dickman KG, Szema AM, Lyubsky S, Lin RZ etal. (2007). Moderate Pulmonary Arterial Hypertension in Male Mice Lacking the Vasoactive Intestinal Peptide Gene. Ciculation 115:1260-1268

Said SI. (1969). A peptide fraction from lung tissue with prolonged peripheral vasodilator activity. Scandinavian journal of clinical laboratory investigation.Supplement 107, 51-6.

Said SI. (2009). Animal models of airway hyperresponsiveness. Eur Respir J 33, 217-8.

Said SI. (1991a). Vasoactive intestinal polypeptide (VIP) in asthma. Ann N Y Acad Sci 629, 305-18.

Said SI. (1991b). Vasoactive intestinal polypeptide biologic role in health and disease. Trends Endocrinol Metab 2, 107-12.

Said SI, Faloona GR. (1975). Elevated plasma and tissue levels of vasoactive intestinal polypeptide in the watery-diarrhea syndrome due to pancreatic, bronchogenic and other tumors. N Engl J Med 293, 155-60.

Said SI, Mutt V. (1970). Polypeptide with broad biological activity: Isolation from small intestine. *Science* 169, 1217-8.

Said SI, Rosenberg RN. (1976). Vasoactive intestinal polypeptide: Abundant immunoreactivity in neural cell lines and normal nervous tissue. *Science* 192, 907-8.

Savage MV, Brengelmann GL, Buchan AM, Freund PR. (1990). Cystic fibrosis, vasoactive intestinal polypeptide, and active cutaneous vasodilation. *J Appl Physiol* 69, 2149-54.

Sharma M, Benharouga M, Hu W, Lukacs GL. (2001). Conformational and temperature-sensitive stability defects of the delta F508 cystic fibrosis transmembrane conductance regulator in post-endoplasmic reticulum compartments. *J Biol Chem* 276, 8942-50.

Shreeve SM, Sreedharan SP, Hacker MP, Gannon DE, Morgan MJ. (2000). VIP activates G(s) and G(i3) in rat alveolar macrophages and G(s) in HEK293 cells transfected with the human VPAC(1) receptor. *Biochem Biophys Res Commun* 272, 922-8.

Song Y, Salinas D, Nielson DW, Verkman AS. (2006). Hyperacidity of secreted fluid from submucosal glands in early cystic fibrosis. *Am J Physiol Cell Physiol* 290, C741-9.

Sreedharan SP, Patel DR, Xia M, Ichikawa S, Goetzl EJ. (1994). Human vasoactive intestinal peptide1 receptors expressed by stable transfectants couple to two distinct signaling pathways. *Biochem Biophys Res Commun* 203, 141-8.

Swiatecka-Urban A, Boyd C, Coutermarsh B, Karlson KH, Barnaby R, Aschenbrenner L, et al. (2004). Myosin VI regulates endocytosis of the cystic fibrosis transmembrane conductance regulator. *J Biol Chem* 279, 38025-31.

Swiatecka-Urban A, Brown A, Moreau-Marquis S, Renuka J, Coutermarsh B, Barnaby R, et al. (2005). The short apical membrane half-life of rescued {delta}F508-cystic fibrosis transmembrane conductance regulator (CFTR) results from accelerated endocytosis of {delta}F508-CFTR in polarized human airway epithelial cells. *J Biol Chem* 280, 36762-72.

Szema AM, Hamidi SA, Lyubsky S, Dickman KG, Mathew S, Abdel-Razek T, et al. (2006). Mice lacking the VIP gene show airway hyperresponsiveness and airway inflammation, partially reversible by VIP. *Am J Physiol Lung Cell Mol Physiol* 291, L880-6.

Wattchow DA, Furness JB, Costa M. (1988). Distribution and coexistence of peptides in nerve fibers of the external muscle of the human gastrointestinal tract. *Gastroenterology* 95, 32-41.

Webster P, Vanacore L, Nairn AC, Marino CR. (1994). Subcellular localization of CFTR to endosomes in a ductal epithelium. *Am J Physiol* 267, C340-8.

Wine JJ. (2007). Parasympathetic control of airway submucosal glands: Central reflexes and the airway intrinsic nervous system. *Auton Neurosci* 133, 35-54.

Wolde M, Fellows A, Cheng J, Kivenson A, Coutermarsh B, Talebian L, Karlson,K.; Piserchio,A.; Mierke,D.F.; Stanton,B.A.; Guggino,W.B.; Madden,D.R. (2007). Targeting CAL as a negative regulator of DeltaF508-CFTR cell-surface expression: An RNA interference and structure-based mutagenetic approach. *J Biol Chem* 282, 8099-109.

Xia M, Sreedharan SP, Goetzl EJ. (1996). Predominant expression of type II vasoactive intestinal peptide receptors by human T lymphoblastoma cells: Transduction of both Ca2+ and cyclic AMP signals. *J Clin Immunol* 16, 21-30.

5

Improving Cell Surface Functional Expression of ΔF508 CFTR: A Quest for Therapeutic Targets

Yifei Fan, Yeshavanth K. Banasavadi-Siddegowda and Xiaodong Wang
University of Toledo College of Medicine
USA

1. Introduction

Cystic fibrosis (CF) is largely a protein misfolding disease. The deletion of a phenylalanine at residue 508 (ΔF508) in the cystic fibrosis transmembrane conductance regulator (CFTR) accounts for 70% of all disease-causing alleles and is present in at least one copy in 90% of CF patients (Kerem et al., 1989). The ΔF508 mutation impairs the conformational maturation of nascent CFTR (Lukacs et al., 1994), and arrests it in an early folding intermediate (Zhang et al., 1998). As a result, the mutant CFTR is retained in the endoplasmic reticulum (ER) (Cheng et al., 1990) in a chaperone-bound state (Yang et al., 1993), The ER-accumulated mutant CFTR fails to efficiently couple to the coatomer complex II (COPII) ER export machinery (Wang et al., 2004), and is degraded by the ubiquitin proteasome system through the ER-associated degradation (ERAD) pathway (Jensen et al., 1995; Ward et al., 1995), leading to loss of CFTR function at the cell surface.

The folding defect of ΔF508 CFTR appears kinetic in nature (Qu et al., 1997). A small fraction of ΔF508 CFTR is able to exit the ER but the escaped mutant protein is not stable at the cell periphery and is rapidly cleared through lysosomal degradation (Lukacs et al., 1993). This second defect further reduces the cell surface localization of this mutant CFTR. Aside from localization defect, the ΔF508 mutation also impairs the channel gating of CFTR, leading to reduced open probability (Dalemans et al., 1991). The threefold defect of ΔF508 CFTR stems from its defective conformation, and impairs the CFTR functional expression at the cell surface, leading to severe clinical phenotype. Given the autosomal recessive inheritance of the disease, improving plasma membrane functional expression of ΔF508 CFTR will benefit the vast majority of CF patients (Gelman & Kopito, 2002).

Numerous research efforts have been made to improve ΔF508 CFTR cell surface functional expression, including elevating its expression, reducing its degradation, enhancing the efficiency of its maturation, increasing its post-ER stability and improving its channel gating. Restoring ΔF508 CFTR conformation will potentially improve its ER folding, its cell surface stability and its channel gating, leading to efficient ΔF508 CFTR rescue. In this chapter, multiple approaches for ΔF508 CFTR rescue will be reviewed, and their advantages as well as limitations will be discussed.

2. Overview of CFTR biogenesis, quality control and exocytic trafficking

CFTR is a member of the ATP-binding cassette (ABC) transporter family, and is composed of two homologous modules each containing a membrane spanning domain (MSD) followed by a nucleotide-binding domain (NBD) (Riordan et al., 1989) (Fig. 1). CFTR is unique in that it has an unstructured regulatory (R) domain inserted between the two homologous modules (Fig. 1). CFTR has two N-linked glycosylation sites on the fourth extracellular loop (Fig. 1). In the ER, the newly synthesized CFTR acquires core-glycosylation at these two sites. Upon transport to the Golgi, the core-glycosylation is processed into the Golgi-specific complex glycosylation, leading to an up-shift in its apparent molecular weight. This difference in processing provides an important means of discriminating the ER-localized, immature CFTR (band B) and the Golgi-processed, mature form (band C). At the steady state, the majority of CFTR is in its mature form. As ΔF508 CFTR is unable to exit the ER, it largely exists in band B. All the major functional domains of CFTR reside on the cytoplasmic side of membrane. Therefore, chaperone-mediated folding events in the cytoplasm play an important role in CFTR maturation and quality control (Yang et al., 1993; Loo et al., 1998; Meacham et al., 1999; Wang et al., 2006).

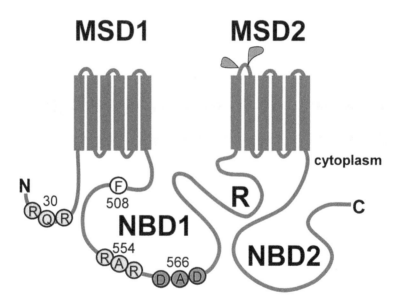

Fig. 1. Domain structure and putative sorting signals of CFTR.

2.1 CFTR de novo folding in the ER

CFTR is synthesized on the ER membrane. Domain folding occurs largely co-translationally (Kleizen et al., 2005). However, further conformational maturation is necessary to form a fully assembled molecule competent for passing the ER quality control and coupling to COPII for ER export (Zhang et al., 1998; Wang et al., 2004). The F508 residue resides in NBD1 (Fig. 1). The ΔF508-induced misfolding of CFTR starts during translation immediately after the NBD1 emerges from the ribosome (Hoelen et al., 2010). This conformational defect originates in NBD1 but spread throughout the whole molecule through domain-domain interactions, leading to a global conformation defect (Du et al., 2005; Du & Lukacs, 2009; Roy et al., 2010). Restoring wild-type-like global conformation is required for ΔF508 CFTR to pass the quality control and egress from the ER (Roy et al., 2010). Second site mutations in NBD1 have been identified that suppress the ΔF508 processing defect (Teem et al., 1993), and at least some of such suppressing mutations can act co-translationally on the NBD1 misfolding (Hoelen et al., 2010). Therefore, the de novo folding of ΔF508 CFTR at both co-translational and post-translational levels can be targeted for its rescue.

2.2 CFTR quality control in the ER

Newly synthesized CFTR undergo quality control before it can exit the ER. ER quality control starts even before CFTR is fully translated (Fig. 2). A membrane-associated ubiquitin ligase complex containing the E3 RMA1, the E2 Ubc6e and Derlin-1 mediates CFTR co-translational quality control (Sun et al., 2006; Younger et al., 2006). BAP31, an integral membrane protein that associates with Derlin-1 as well as the amino terminus of CFTR, promotes ΔF508 CFTR retrotranslocation from the ER and its subsequent degradation by the cytoplasmic 26S proteasome (B. Wang et al., 2008). P97/valosin-containing protein interacts with gp78/autocrine motility factor receptor in coupling CFTR ubiquitination to its retrotranslocation and proteasome degradation (Carlson et al., 2006; Vij et al., 2006). Interestingly, gp78 was found to cooperate with RMA1 in the ERAD of ΔF508 CFTR (Morito et al., 2008). Moreover, ubiquitin C-terminal hydrolase-L1 (UCH-L1) protects CFTR from co-translational ERAD (Henderson et al., 2010). This co-translational quality control of CFTR appears to be regulated by cytoplasmic Hsc70 as DNAJB12 was recently found to cooperate with Hsc70 and RMA1 in ΔF508 CFTR degradation (Grove et al., 2011). Consistent with this, we found that Hsp105, a nucleotide exchange factor (NEF) for Hsc70, promotes co-translational ERAD of CFTR (Saxena et al., 2011a).

A second ER quality control step occurs largely post-translationally, which is mediated through Hsc70 and cochaperone CHIP (Meacham et al., 2001) (Fig. 2). CHIP functions as a scaffold for the formation of multi-subunit E3 ubiquitin ligase for the post-translational ERAD of CFTR, and such degradation activity is also dependent upon Hsc70, Hdj-2 and the E2 UbcH5a (Younger et al., 2004). Interestingly, HspBP1 and BAG-2, two other NEFs for Hsc70, inhibits the CHIP-mediated post-translational ERAD of CFTR (Alberti et al., 2004; Arndt et al., 2005), suggesting a dual role for Hsc70 in regulating co-translational and post-translational ERAD of CFTR.

Nevertheless, inhibiting CFTR ERAD is not sufficient for ΔF508 CFTR to efficiently exit the ER (Jensen et al., 1995; Pagant et al., 2007). Obviously, another quality control system is responsible for the retention of the foldable pool of ΔF508 CFTR in the ER, the mechanism of which is less clear. We recently showed that the ER exit code and domain conformation both contribute significantly to the exportability of CFTR (Roy et al., 2010). Therefore, chaperone association and/or ER exit code presentation might be two important factors for this last checkpoint of the ER quality control of CFTR. A better understanding of its mechanism will lead to much greater improvement in ΔF508 CFTR maturation.

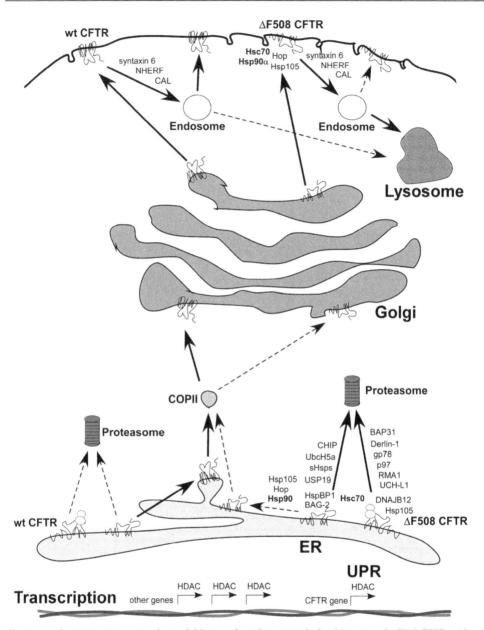

Shown are the transcription, synthesis, folding and quality control of wild-type and ΔF508 CFTR with a great number of regulators at both the ER and peripheral levels, which are potential molecular targets for ΔF508 CFTR rescue. Complete arrows indicate major pathways, and broken arrows denote minor pathways. Enhancement of some of the minor pathways for ΔF508 CFTR can effectively promote its rescue.

Fig. 2. Regulation of CFTR biogenesis and degradation.

2.3 ER-to-Golgi sorting signals within CFTR

Exit of proteins from the ER requires specific sorting signals on the cytoplasmic side of the ER membrane which is recognizable by the cargo selection complex (Sec23/24) of COPII (Aridor et al., 1998; Nishimura et al., 1999; Miller et al., 2002). A di-acidic ER exit motif (DAD) was identified in the NBD1 of CFTR (Fig. 1), and substitution of the second acidic residue (leading to DAA) abolishes CFTR association with Sec24 and dramatically reduces the export efficiency of CFTR (Wang et al., 2004). The ΔF508 mutation also reduces CFTR association with Sec24 (Wang et al., 2004) but the underlying mechanism might be different from the DAA mutant. Using in situ limited proteolysis to probe the domain conformation of CFTR (Zhang et al., 1998), we showed that the DAA mutant has similar domain conformation as wild-type CFTR despite its inability to efficiently exit the ER (Roy et al., 2010). This is in stark contrast to ΔF508 CFTR which displays global conformational defects including NBD1 (Du et al., 2005; Du & Lukacs, 2009; Roy et al., 2010). Furthermore, DAA CFTR displays lower chaperone association and higher post-ER stability when compared with ΔF508 CFTR (Roy et al., 2010). Therefore, the conformational defects in ΔF508 CFTR contribute significantly to its misprocessing.

ER retention/retrieval signals have been found in the cytoplasmic domains of multiple transmembrane cargo proteins (Nilsson et al., 1989; Zerangue et al., 1999). An RXR ER retention/retrieval signal serves as a quality control check point for the assembly of oligomeric cargo proteins in the ER (Zerangue et al., 1999; Margeta-Mitrovic et al., 2000). The RXR signals are exposed in individual subunits or in incompletely assembled oligomers but are concealed only when the proper assembly of the oligomer is achieved. This mechanism prevents the cell surface expression of improperly assembled cargo molecules. Multiple RXR motifs have been identified in the cytoplasmic domains of CFTR (Fig. 1), and the replacement of key arginine residues results in ΔF508 CFTR rescue, suggesting that the RXR motifs might contribute to the ER retention/retrieval of ΔF508 CFTR (Chang et al., 1999). It is proposed that such RXR motifs are shielded by domain-domain interactions in wild-type CFTR but become exposed when the F508 is deleted (Kim Chiaw et al., 2009). In fact, peptides designed to mimic such a sorting motif were found to functionally rescue ΔF508 CFTR (Kim Chiaw et al., 2009). As the key RXR motif in NBD1 contributes significantly to ΔF508 CFTR global conformation (Qu et al., 1997; Hegedus et al., 2006; Roy et al., 2010), it is unclear if the RXR-mimetics rescue ΔF508 CFTR by influencing ΔF508 CFTR conformation. Determining whether the RXR-mimetics are able to bind to the RXR sorting receptor or whether they block the retention/retrieval of other RXR-containing cargo molecules will provide a definitive answer.

3. Defining ΔF508 conformational defects

F508 resides in NBD1 (Fig. 1), and therefore the deletion of this residue should naturally affect the conformation of NBD1. Early in vitro studies using purified NBD1 revealed a kinetic folding defect in ΔF508 NBD1 (Qu & Thomas, 1996; Qu et al., 1997). However, the crystal structure of ΔF508 NBD1 revealed no major conformational change from the wild-type domain (Lewis et al., 2005). In the mean time, it was found that ΔF508 mutation causes major conformation changes in NBD2 (Du et al., 2005), highlighting the importance of domain-domain interactions in ΔF508 misfolding. This notion was strengthened by the finding that F508 side chain contributes significantly to NBD1 folding in the context of full-length CFTR (Thibodeau et al., 2005), and by the finding that F508 residue mediates the contact between NBD1 and cytoplasmic loop 4 (CL4) in MSD2 (Serohijos et al., 2008a). Therefore, deletion of F508 triggers a global conformational change in CFTR, leading to misprocessing (Du & Lukacs, 2009).

The apparent lack of a detectable NBD1 conformational change as a result of the ΔF508 mutation remains an enigma as how can the ΔF508 mutation trigger such a profound global conformational change without significantly impacting NBD1 conformation in the first place? The finding that some of the solubilization mutations included in ΔF508 NBD1 for crystallography studies actually rescue the ΔF508 processing defect in the context of full-length CFTR reopened this question (Pissarra et al., 2008). Another twist in our understanding of the impact of F508 deletion on NBD1 conformation came from the finding that the removal of the regulatory insert (RI), a 32-residue segment within NBD1 that is unique to CFTR but not shared by the NBD1's of other ABC transporters, renders ΔF508 NBD1 soluble, dimer-forming and displaying wild-type-like conformation (Atwell et al., 2010). Another study shows that, in the context of full-length CFTR protein, removal of the RI restores maturation, stability and function of ΔF508 CFTR, suggesting that the RI contributes significantly to ΔF508 misfolding in NBD1(Aleksandrov et al., 2010).

Using in situ limited proteolysis, we identified a definite conformational change within NBD1 as a result of ΔF508 mutation (Roy et al., 2010). The ΔF508 NBD1 conformation, like the conformation of other domains of ΔF508 CFTR, resembles the conformation of an earlier folding intermediate of wild-type CFTR (Zhang et al., 1998; Roy et al., 2010). Furthermore, rescue of ΔF508 CFTR using low temperature or R555K substitution leads to NBD1 as well as global conformational reversion, suggesting that conformational correction is prerequisite for the rescue of the folding and export defects of ΔF508 CFTR (Roy et al., 2010). Using crystallography and hydrogen/deuterium exchange mass spectrometry, Lewis, et al. showed that ΔF508 mutation increases the exposure of the 509-511 loop and increases the dynamics in its vicinity (Lewis et al., 2010). Consistent with the above, a conformational change in ΔF508 NBD1 was observed using a cysteine-labelling technique, and such conformational change is reversed by second site mutations in NBD1 (He et al., 2010). Interestingly, the second site mutations also restore the interactions between NBD1 and its contacting domains (He et al., 2010). Combination of G550E, R553M and R555K suppressor mutations in NBD1 produces a dramatic increase in ΔF508 CFTR processing, and this is accompanied by the enhanced folding of ΔF508 NBD1 both in isolation and in the context of full-length CFTR (Thibodeau et al., 2010). An interesting finding is that while NBD2 is not required for CFTR processing (Pollet et al., 2000), it contributes to ΔF508 CFTR rescue by second site mutations as well as by low temperature (Du & Lukacs, 2009; Cheng et al., 2010). Furthermore, the rescue of ΔF508 CFTR by suppressor mutations requires a continuous full-length CFTR peptide (Cheng et al., 2010), suggesting a role for peptide backbone tension in ΔF508 CFTR rescue (Thibodeau et al., 2005).

Taken together, ΔF508 mutation causes increased exposure of the 509-511 loop in NBD1 and increases its dynamics. These changes not only alter the conformation of NBD1, but through NBD1's interface with CL4 and NBD2, alter the conformation of other domains, leading to global conformational change. Second site mutations within NBD1 can partially correct the

ΔF508 NBD1 conformational defect, which spread to other domains through domain-domain interactions, leading to partial restoration of global conformation as well as processing. Conformation repair is at the heart of ΔF508 correction.

4. Elevating ΔF508 CFTR expression

The severe reduction in ΔF508 CFTR cell surface functional expression results from its defective export, reduced peripheral stability, and subnormal channel gating. Nevertheless, a small fraction of the mutant CFTR can leak from the ER and make its way to cell surface. One simple approach to enhance ΔF508 CFTR cell surface localization is to increase its expression. This can be achieved in cells heterologously expressing ΔF508 CFTR under the control of metallothionein promoter by treatment with sodium butyrate (Cheng et al., 1995). In CF airway epithelial cells, 4-phenylburyrate, a histone deacetylase (HDAC) inhibitor dramatically increases the expression of ΔF508 CFTR at the protein level (Rubenstein et al., 1997). Recently, a group of other HDAC inhibitors including Trichostatin A, suberoylanilide hydroxamic acid (SAHA) and Scriptaid were found to potently increase ΔF508 CFTR transcription in CFBE41o- cells (Hutt et al., 2010).

Interestingly, over-accumulation of ΔF508 CFTR in the ER induces the unfolded protein response (UPR) (Gomes-Alves et al., 2010), and induction of UPR inhibits CFTR endogenous transcription (Rab et al., 2007). The UPR-induced CFTR transcriptional repression is mediated through the transcription factor ATF6, and both DNA methylation and histone deacetylation contribute to this process (Bartoszewski et al., 2008). Therefore, there is a limit to which the transcription of endogenous ΔF508 CFTR can be increased but HDAC inhibitors may potentially alleviate the UPR-induced CFTR transcriptional repression (Fig. 2).

The expression of ΔF508 CFTR can also be regulated at the post-transcriptional level. A recent study revealed that the synonymous codon change of I507 in the ΔF508 allele can cause mRNA misfolding, leading to reduced rate of translation and/or impaired co-translational folding of ΔF508 CFTR (Bartoszewski et al., 2010). Therefore, codon-dependent mRNA folding represents a new mechanism by which ΔF508 CFTR expression can be regulated. Although it is not realistic to change the nucleotide sequence of ΔF508 CFTR in CF patients, identification of this novel mechanism opens up new opportunities for therapeutic intervention at the level of mRNA processing, folding, and stability.

5. Reducing ΔF508 CFTR ERAD

The vast majority of ΔF508 CFTR synthesized in the cells is degraded through the ERAD pathway (Jensen et al., 1995; Ward et al., 1995). Inhibition of ERAD will certainly increase the steady state level of ΔF508 CFTR in the ER and subsequently increase its cell surface localization (Fig. 2). Significant advance in understanding the mechanism of ERAD of ΔF508 CFTR has been achieved during the past 16 years. Hsc70 has been found to regulate both the co-translational and post-translational ERAD of ΔF508 CFTR with two distinct sets of cochaperones (Meacham et al., 2001; Zhang et al., 2001; Alberti et al., 2004; Arndt et al., 2005; Grove et al., 2011; Saxena et al., 2011a). While the functional relationship between the two remains unclear, multiple cochaperones, such as CHIP (Meacham et al., 2001), HspBP1

(Alberti et al., 2004), BAG-2 (Arndt et al., 2005), Hdj-2 (Younger et al., 2004), DNAJB12 (Grove et al., 2011) and Hsp105 (Saxena et al., 2011a) may be targeted for increasing the steady state levels of ΔF508 CFTR. Moreover, 4-phenylbutyrate, which rescues ΔF508 CFTR (Rubenstein et al., 1997), was found to reduce the expression level of Hsc70, subsequently decreases its association with ΔF508 CFTR, and therefore inhibits the ERAD of ΔF508 CFTR (Rubenstein & Zeitlin, 2000). More recently, a soluble sulfogalactosyl ceramide mimic that inhibits the Hsp40-activated Hsc70 ATPase activity, promotes the rescue of ΔF508 CFTR from ERAD (Park et al., 2009). In addition to Hsc70, small heat-shock proteins (sHsps) preferentially associate with ΔF508 CFTR and promote its ERAD (Ahner et al., 2007). It is believed that small heat-shock proteins bind to misfolded ΔF508 CFTR, prevent its aggregation and maintain its solubility during the ERAD (Ahner et al., 2007).

ERAD components such as RMA1 (Younger et al., 2006), gp78 (Morito et al., 2008), Derlin-1 (Sun et al., 2006; Younger et al., 2006), BAP31(B. Wang et al., 2008) and p97 (Carlson et al., 2006; Vij et al., 2006) can also be targeted. Although not essential for ERAD of CFTR (Carlson et al., 2006), interference of p97 expression in CF airway epithelial cells increases the steady state levels of ΔF508 CFTR in bands B and C, and enhances the CFTR-mediated chloride conductance across the plasma membrane (Vij et al., 2006). Interestingly, this effect is accompanied by reduction in interleukin-8 level which might alleviate the CF-associated airway inflammation (Vij et al., 2006). Other regulators of the p97-gp78 complex have been identified, which also influence the steady state level of ΔF508 CFTR (Nagahama et al., 2009; Ballar et al., 2010). Recently, ubiquitin-specific protease 19 (USP19), an ER-localized, membrane-anchored deubiquitinating enzyme, was shown to rescue ΔF508 CFTR from ERAD (Hassink et al., 2009), suggesting that deubiquitinating enzymes are another class of viable targets for rescuing ΔF508 CFTR (Fig. 2).

6. Enhancing ΔF508 CFTR maturation

Despite its obvious importance in rescuing ΔF508 CFTR, relatively little is known concerning how to improve the maturation of ΔF508 CFTR in the ER. The major reason is that ΔF508 CFTR hardly matures if at all at physiological temperature. However, at reduced temperature, ΔF508 CFTR does achieve conformational maturation much more efficiently, leading to greatly enhanced functional expression at the cell surface (Denning et al., 1992). Interestingly, such a temperature-sensitive phenotype is cell-dependent, suggesting that cellular machinery plays an essential role in the process (X. Wang et al., 2008). We found that the increased conformational stability provided by low temperature combines with chaperone actions in facilitating ΔF508 CFTR maturation at reduced temperature (Roy et al., 2010). Therefore, the temperature-dependent maturation of ΔF508 CFTR serves as an excellent model system in understanding the role of the cellular chaperone machinery in the forward folding of ΔF508 CFTR.

Mild heat shock greatly potentiates the temperature rescue of ΔF508 CFTR, and this is dependent upon transcription, suggesting that the upregulation of heat inducible chaperones promotes ΔF508 CFTR maturation (X. Wang et al., 2008). Using a series of chaperone- or cochaperone-deficient cell lines, we demonstrate that an Hsp70-Hsp90 chaperone network operates on the cytoplasmic face of the ER membrane facilitating the maturation of ΔF508 CFTR at reduced temperature. Cochaperone Hop, which physically and functionally links Hsp70 and Hsp90 through its multiple tetratricopeptide repeat (TPR) domains, is essential for the temperature-dependent maturation of ΔF508 CFTR, and Hsp105 is an integral player in the system (Saxena et al., 2011b). We also found that Hsc70, Hsp90β, Hop, Hsp105 and Hdj-2 are functionally linked during the temperature rescue of ΔF508 CFTR. Depletion of Hsp90β, Hop or Hsp105 also reciprocally reduces some or all of other chaperone components (Saxena et al., 2011b). It is highly likely that these folding components, and perhaps other yet unidentified chaperones or cochaperones, form a functionally organized chaperone network on the cytoplasmic side of the ER membrane, facilitating the conformational maturation of ΔF508 CFTR at reduced temperature. Given a clear role for Hsp90 in wild-type CFTR maturation at physiological temperature (Loo et al., 1998), we believe such a cytoplasmic chaperone network functions in the cell under physiological conditions. While its effect on ΔF508 CFTR maturation is more pronounced at reduced temperature, it should also impact ΔF508 CFTR maturation at the physiological temperature. Consistent with this prediction, overexpressing Hsp105 promotes ΔF508 CFTR processing at both the reduced and physiological temperatures (Saxena et al., 2011a). An in-depth analysis of this process will reveal novel molecular targets that promote the maturation of ΔF508 CFTR (Fig. 2).

Another approach to enhance ΔF508 CFTR maturation is through transcomplementation (Cormet-Boyaka et al., 2004). Such rescue requires co-expression of a sizeable segment of CFTR that contains wild-type sequence corresponding to the region where F508 is located. Such transcomplementation does not result in changes in Hsc70 association but is believed to improve ΔF508 CFTR forward folding through intra- and/or inter-molecular domain-domain interactions. A related but distinct approach to promote ΔF508 CFTR maturation is to co-express a fragment of ΔF508 CFTR containing NBD1 and R domains (Sun et al., 2008). This mutant fragment of CFTR can actually sequester key chaperone components from the endogenous ΔF508 CFTR and lead to its rescue. Moreover, co-expressing an N-terminal truncated CFTR mutant (Δ264) can not only transcomplement ΔF508 CFTR but also dramatically increases the protein expression levels of both wild-type and ΔF508 CFTR (Cebotaru et al., 2008). As the Δ264 mutant CFTR associates with VCP and HDAC6, two components involved in retrotranslocation of proteins from the ER, and is more efficiently degraded by the proteasome than ΔF508 CFTR, high level expression of this mutant may interfere with ΔF508 CFTR ERAD and hence increase its steady state level. Taken together, co-expression of CFTR fragments might rescue ΔF508 CFTR by improving its folding, helping it escape ER quality control and protecting it from ERAD. As these fragments have much lower molecular weight than full-length CFTR, they can be used as potential agents for CF gene therapy.

7. Increasing ΔF508 CFTR peripheral stability

The ΔF508 CFTR has reduced conformational stability in post-ER compartments and therefore turns over rapidly at the cell periphery (Lukacs et al., 1993; Sharma et al., 2001; Sharma et al., 2004). Increasing ΔF508 CFTR half-life at cell periphery is an important strategy for effective rescue of ΔF508 CFTR. CAL, a Golgi-associated, PDZ domain-containing protein that binds to the C-terminus of CFTR, reduces the half-life of CFTR at the cell surface (Cheng et al., 2002). RNA interference of endogenous CAL in CF airway epithelial cells increases plasma membrane expression of ΔF508 CFTR and enhances transepithelial chloride current (Wolde et al., 2007). The Na^+/H^+ exchanger regulatory factor (NHERF), a subplasma membrane PDZ domain protein, competes with CAL in associating with CFTR and promotes its plasma membrane localization (Cheng et al., 2002). Knockdown of NHERF1 promotes the degradation of temperature-rescued ΔF508 CFTR at the cell surface of human airway epithelial cells (Kwon et al., 2007). Expression of dominant-negative dynamin 2 mutant K44A increases CFTR cell surface expression, and counteracts the effect of CAL overexpression on CFTR cell surface stability (Cheng et al., 2004). SNARE protein syntaxin 6 binds to CAL and reduces CFTR cell surface stability in a CAL-dependent manner (Cheng et al., 2010). Therefore, CAL and its functional partners are viable molecular targets for increasing cell surface stability of ΔF508 CFTR (Fig. 2).

Cytoplasmic chaperone Hsc70 was shown to mediate the uncoating of clathrin-coated vesicles (Schmid & Rothman, 1985; Chappell et al., 1986) and hence regulates the peripheral trafficking of membrane bound cargo proteins such as CFTR. Recently, a more direct role for cytoplasmic Hsp70-Hsp90 chaperone network in regulating ΔF508 CFTR peripheral quality control was revealed, where Hsc70, Hsp90α, Hop and other chaperone components collaborate with the ubiquitin system in promoting the cell surface degradation of this mutant CFTR (Okiyoneda et al., 2010). This finding uncovers a great number of new potential chaperone targets for regulating cell surface stability of ΔF508 CFTR. However, as the cytoplasmic Hsp70-Hsp90 chaperone network also facilitates the maturation of CFTR in the ER (Loo et al., 1998; Meacham et al., 1999; Wang et al., 2006), a critical balance must be maintained between the two seemingly opposing effects of the Hsp70-Hsp90 chaperone network at the ER and the peripheral levels in order to effectively rescue ΔF508 CFTR (Fig. 2).

Of particular interest, we found that Hsp105 is involved in both processes. At the ER level, Hsp105 facilitates the Hsp70-Hsp90-mediated maturation of ΔF508 CFTR at reduced temperature (Saxena et al., 2011b). At the peripheral level, Hsp105 preferentially associates with the rescued ΔF508 CFTR, and stabilizes it in post-ER compartments (Saxena et al., 2011a). It is currently unclear whether Hsp105 functionally relates to Hsc70, Hop and Hsp90α at the cell periphery or it act on its own. While Hsp105 acts in the same direction as the cytoplasmic Hsp70-Hsp90 network at the ER level, it acts in opposite direction to Hsc70, Hop and Hsp90α at the cell periphery. Understanding these aspects is critical to the effective enhancement of ΔF508 CFTR cell surface functional expression by modulating cytoplasmic chaperone machinery.

8. Improving ΔF508 CFTR channel gating: Potentiator or corrector?

Although the primary defect in ΔF508 CFTR is impaired export (Cheng et al., 1990), it has aberrant channel gating as reflected in reduced channel open probability (Dalemans et al., 1991). Correcting such a defect will also improve the overall cell surface functional expression of ΔF508 CFTR. The G551D substitution in CFTR, a mutation causing severe CF, does not impact its export to plasma membrane but primarily impairs its channel opening (Tsui, 1995; Li et al., 1996). VX-770, a small molecule potentiator (improving channel gating) developed for G551D CFTR by the Vertex Pharmaceuticals Inc., also increases the channel open probability of ΔF508 CFTR (Van Goor et al., 2009). Interestingly, small molecule compound VRT-532 display both corrector (improving maturation) and potentiator activities for ΔF508 CFTR by binding directly to the mutant protein (Wellhauser et al., 2009). Recently, a fragment of a phenylglycine-type potentiator was successfully linked to a fragment of a bithiazole corrector to form a "hybrid" potentiator-corrector molecule, the cleavage of which by intestinal enzymes is able to release separate potentiator and corrector for ΔF508 rescue in vivo (Mills et al., 2010). Using high-throughput screen, multiple small molecules with independent potentiator and corrector activities for ΔF508 CFTR were also identified (Phuan et al., 2011). Using the above approaches, more efficient rescue of ΔF508 CFTR can be achieved.

9. Conformational repair: One stone and three birds

Given that the root cause of CF in the majority of patients lies in the conformational defects of ΔF508 CFTR, repairing its conformational defects will potentially lead to improved export, stability (both in the ER and at the cell periphery) and channel gating. Effective development of novel approaches in conformational repair relies on a thorough understanding of the conformational defects of ΔF508 CFTR and their correction. Given that F508 residue resides in NBD1, NBD1 is a central domain for the understanding of ΔF508 conformational repair. In addition, as domain-domain interactions within CFTR play an important role in altering or maintaining CFTR global conformation (Du et al., 2005; Du & Lukacs, 2009), key interfaces between different domains are also important in CFTR conformational repair (Serohijos et al., 2008a).

An excellent attempt was made early on in screening for suppressor mutations in NBD1 which restores the export of ΔF508 CFTR (Teem et al., 1993). This was made possible by swapping a portion of CFTR NBD1 into yeast *STE6* gene encoding an ABC transporter that delivers α-factor out of the cell which is necessary for mating. When ΔF508 mutation is included into the *STE6*-CFTR chimera, the yeast fails to transport α-factor. Using this system, second site mutations within the CFTR NBD1 portion were identified that rescue ΔF508 CFTR (Teem et al., 1993; Teem et al., 1996). Interestingly, R555K, one of such ΔF508 suppressor mutations, causes a global conformational reversion in ΔF508 CFTR, leading to increased export and enhanced post-ER stability (Roy et al., 2010). R555K, when combined with other rescue subsitutions, improves ΔF508 CFTR conformation and processing (Chang et al., 1999; Hegedus et al., 2006), and significantly increases the open probability of ΔF508 CFTR (Roxo-Rosa et al., 2006). These data support the notion that conformational repair is a highly effective approach for enhancing ΔF508 CFTR cell surface functional expression, ameliorating all three facets of ΔF508 defect.

Another approach for designing NBD1 conformational repair employs molecular dynamics simulation. Molecular dynamics has the advantage over structural biology in that it reveals information on folding kinetics and dynamics. Using this approach, key differences in the distribution of meta-stable intermediates have been identified between wild-type and ΔF508 NBD1, and additional rescue mutations can be designed (Serohijos et al., 2008b). These rescue mutations, if validated experimentally, will significantly advance our understanding of NBD1 folding both alone and in the context of full-length CFTR.

High resolution crystal structure of full-length CFTR is currently unavailable. However, the crystal structures of multiple ABC transporters including the p-glycoprotein have been solved (Locher et al., 2002; Dawson & Locher, 2006; Aller et al., 2009). Attempts to use these structures as bases for modeling full-length CFTR have provided new insights into the role of F508 residue in domain-domain interactions (Jordan et al., 2008; Loo et al., 2008; Serohijos et al., 2008a; Mornon et al., 2009). These studies, when backed up by biochemical analyses, are an excellent start point to probe ΔF508 global conformational defects and their repair.

10. Large-scale target identification for the rescue of ΔF508 CFTR

Aside from the above mechanism-based identification of therapeutic targets for ΔF508 rescue, several large-scale target identification regimes have been quite successful. The functional follow-up of these studies has yielded and will yield many novel molecular targets.

The first such attempt was to use proteomics to identify CFTR-interacting proteins between wild-type and ΔF508 CFTR (Wang et al., 2006), which revealed, among others, an ER-associated chaperone network facilitating CFTR biogenesis and quality control. In an attempt to gain information on the potential mechanism of ΔF508 chemical rescue by 4-phenylbutyrate, a pharmacoproteomic approach was used to identify changes in protein expression in CF airway epithelial cells in response to 4-phenylbutyrate treatment (Singh et al., 2006). This approach was then followed by a comparison of ΔF508 CFTR-interacting proteins between the chemically rescued (by 4-phenylbutyrate) and genetically repaired (by introducing wild-type CFTR) CF airway epithelial cells (Singh et al., 2008). Protein targets involved in the ERAD, protein folding and inflammatory response have been identified, and proteins that were modulated in the ER as well as on the plasma membrane have been isolated (Singh et al., 2008).

Recently, a high-throughput functional screen was designed to identify proteins that promote the rescue of ΔF508 CFTR (Trzcinska-Daneluti et al., 2009). In this study, 450 different proteins were fused to a chloride-senstive yellow fluorescent protein and were expressed in a ΔF508 CFTR-expressing stable cell line. The cells were screened for their ability to rescue the ΔF508 functional defect at the plasma membrane. Several proteins that are known to rescue ΔF508 CFTR as well as novel target proteins have been identified. Further functional characterization will reveal their usefulness as potential therapeutic targets.

Another excellent approach worth noting is the use of functional small interfering RNA screen to identify proteins that are involved in peripheral quality control of ΔF508 CFTR (Okiyoneda et al., 2010). This approach took advantage of a well developed cell surface ELISA assay measuring CFTR plasma membrane localization, where three HA-tags have been engineered in an extracellular domain of CFTR. The siRNAs targeting a great number of ubiquitin E3 ligases, ESCRT proteins, E2 enzymes and chaperone/cochaperones were introduced into the above cells, and the plasma membrane stability of the rescued ΔF508 CFTR-3HA was quantified. This study led to the identification of an Hsp70-Hsp90 chaperone network facilitating the peripheral quality control of ΔF508 CFTR. Functional followup of these chaperone proteins will not only reveal critical mechanistic information but also uncover yet unidentified molecular targets.

11. Small molecule modulators for ΔF508 CFTR

One of the major strategies for developing effective therapeutics for CF is to identify small molecule compounds that can improve ΔF508 CFTR cell surface functional expression. Using cell-based functional assay for CFTR-mediated chloride conductance combined with high-throughput screening of small molecule compound libraries, multiple CFTR modulators have been identified, affecting ΔF508 CFTR trafficking and/or channel function (Van Goor et al., 2006; Verkman et al., 2006). Once promising scafolds have been identified, structural optimization can be performed to enhance their biological activities, pharmacokinetics, and safety. In fact several of the above compounds are currently in clinical trial for treating CF.

While the functional screening as mentioned above has the benefit of identifying small molecule compounds that improve the aggregate endpoint readout on ΔF508 CFTR cell surface functional expression, the mechanisms by which these compounds do so are unknown. The compounds can either bind directly to CFTR to affect its folding and/or channel gating, or they can bind to other cellular proteins that regulate CFTR biogenesis, cell surface protein-protein interactions, or its degradation. Understanding these mechanistic aspects of a specific CFTR modulator will lead to the design and identification of additional molecular targets and CFTR modulators. This is especially important as only a limited number of efficacious CFTR modulators have been identified through the functional screen. In order to obtain an FDA-approved drug for CF, more of such compounds are desparately needed to feed into the CF drug discovery pipeline.

Recently, new screening strategies have been designed to improve the variety of workable lead compounds. These compounds might not have been identified during the functional screen because they do not provide the above-the-threshold functional readouts. However, if they have special properties that can enhance certain key aspects of ΔF508 CFTR rescue, such compounds can be further engineered or optimized to produce a much greater efficacy in terms of functional rescue of ΔF508 CFTR. A new strategry has been developed where small molecule compound libraries were screened by their ability to improve the plasma membrane localization of ΔF508 CFTR (Carlile et al., 2007).

A conformation-based virtual screen for ΔF508 CFTR modulators represents one step further as it aims at the core defect of ΔF508 CFTR (i.e. abberrant conformation). Recently, one attempt was made by the EPIX Pharmaceuticals Ltd to identify small molecule correctors for ΔF508 CFTR (Kalid et al., 2010). In this study, a total of three potential small molecule binding cavities were identified at a number of domain-domain interfaces of CFTR, and small molecule compounds were screened in silico for their ability to bind to these cavities. The initial hits derived from the virtual screen were then subjected to functional screen, which yielded a ten-fold increase in hit rate as compared to conventional screen regimes.

An alternative to the above high-throughput screening approach is to explore the possibility of using FDA-approved drugs for other conditions or other small molecule compounds that are safe for human use for rescuing ΔF508 CFTR. Sodium 4-phenylbutyrate is approved for clinical use in patients with urea cycle disorders. 4-Phenylbutyrate, like sodium butyrate, is also a transcriptional regulator that inhibits HDAC (Jung, 2001). 4-Phenylbutyrate was shown to rescue ΔF508 CFTR through a number of mechanisms including biosynthesis, folding and transport (Rubenstein et al., 1997; Rubenstein & Zeitlin, 2000; Choo-Kang & Zeitlin, 2001; Wright et al., 2004; Singh et al., 2006). More recently, SAHA (Vorinostat), an HDAC inhibitor approved by FDA for the treatment of cutaneous T cell lymphoma through epigenetic pathways (Monneret, 2007), was shown to restore cell surface functional expression of ΔF508 CFTR to 28% of wild-type level (Hutt et al., 2010). Doxorubicin (Adriamycin), a cancer chemotherapy agent, increases cell surface functional expression of ΔF508 CFTR through increasing its folding, promoting its chaperone dissociation and inhibiting its ubiquitination (Maitra et al., 2001; Maitra & Hamilton, 2007). Sildenafil (Viagra) was also shown to promote ΔF508 CFTR apical trafficking by unknown mechanism (Dormer et al., 2005). S-Nitrosoglutathione (GSNO), an endogenous bronchodilator (Gaston et al., 1993), was found to increase the expression and maturation of ΔF508 CFTR in airway epithelial cells (Zaman et al., 2006). Interestingly, GSNO was recently found to function at least in part through inhibiting Hop expression (Marozkina et al., 2010), suggesting that small molecules compound can promote ΔF508 CFTR rescue through modulating chaperone machinery.

12. Chaperone environment: A critical but complex part of the equation

Cellular chaperone machinery plays an important role in the synthesis, maturation, quality control of CFTR (Fig. 2). Due to misfolding, ΔF508 CFTR has more extensive association with molecular chaperones (Yang et al., 1993; Jiang et al., 1998; Meacham et al., 1999; Wang et al., 2006; Sun et al., 2008; Roy et al., 2010). Therefore, the impact of chaperone machinery on ΔF508 CFTR is greater than on wild-type CFTR. This notion is further underscored by the recent finding that cytoplasmic Hsp70-Hsp90 chaperone network promotes the peripheral quality control of ΔF508 CFTR (Okiyoneda et al., 2010). Modulating chaperone environment can not only impact the quality control of ΔF508 CFTR at either the ER or the peripheral level but also can dramatically influence its maturation (Loo et al., 1998; Zhang et al., 2002; Saxena et al., 2007; Saxena et al., 2011b).

Heat shock response is a transcriptional program by which cells upregulate the expression of an array of genes including those encoding molecular chaperones to cope with the massive need for protein folding and degradation as a result of elevated temperature or toxic agents (Morimoto et al., 1990). Therefore, conditions or agents that induce heat shock response will up-regulate the cellular chaperone machinery to enhance folding and ERAD of ΔF508 CFTR. Consistent with this finding, mild heat shock dramatically potentiates the temperature-rescue of ΔF508 CFTR (X. Wang et al., 2008). Another cellular response that up-regulate the cellular chaperone machinery is the unfolded protein response (UPR) (Sidrauski et al., 1998). This is particularly relevant to ΔF508 CFTR as over accumulation of this mutant protein in the ER induces such a response, leading to downregulation of CFTR endogenous transcription (Rab et al., 2007; Bartoszewski et al., 2008). Aside from the above two, the inherent variation in the cellular chaperone machinery among different tissues or cell types will also significantly affect the cell surface functional expression of ΔF508 CFTR (Varga et al., 2004; X. Wang et al., 2008; Rowe et al., 2010). Therefore, understanding the functional organization of the chaperone machinery in airway epithelial cells is highly relevant to the development of effective rescue strategies for ΔF508 CFTR.

Certain chemicals such as celastrol can globally influence the cellular chaperone machinery through inducing the heat shock response (Westerheide et al., 2004). Other epigentic modulators can also influence the expression of mutliple molecular chaperones (Wright et al., 2004; Hutt et al., 2010). Interfering with ER lumenal chaperone activities by depleting the ER calcium stores promotes the escape of ΔF508 CFTR from the ER quality control and enhances its cell surface expression (Egan et al., 2002). Certain small molecule compounds directly modulate the expression or activity of molecular chaperones (Jiang et al., 1998; Loo et al., 1998; Marozkina et al., 2010). Furthermore, small molecule compound can act as chemical chaperones to stabilize the conformation of ΔF508 CFTR, enhancing its cell surface functional expression (Brown et al., 1996; Fischer et al., 2001).

13. Conclusion

The ΔF508 mutation is present in over 90% of CF patients. This mutation impairs the conformational maturation of CFTR leading to defective export, reduced stability and abberant channel gating. Improving the cell surface functional expression of this mutant CFTR will benefit the vast majority of CF patients. While many approaches can be taken toward this goal, conformational rescue is the most effective, postitively impacting all three molecular defects of ΔF508 CFTR. The ΔF508 CFTR molecule is the most important target for the development of therapeutics. A clear understanding of its biogenesis, quality control and conformation is fundamental. In the cell, the synthesis, folding, quality control, trafficking and degradation of CFTR is dependent upon its interactions with multiple cellular machineries (Fig. 2). Such interactions provide additional opportunites for therapeutic interventions. The cellular protein homeostasis as regulated by the chapeorone machinery provides an important chemical environment for ΔF508 CFTR. Such an enironment is regulated by multiple cellular responses or epigenetic modulators. Understanding the relationship between such cellular environment and ΔF508 CFTR cell surface functional expression will provide additional molecular targets for intervention.

14. Acknowledgment

We thank the Cystic Fibrosis Foundation, the American Heart Association and the University of Toledo Health Science Campus for support.

15. References

Ahner, A., Nakatsukasa, K., Zhang, H., Frizzell, R. A. & Brodsky, J. L. (2007). Small heat-shock proteins select deltaF508-CFTR for endoplasmic reticulum-associated degradation. *Mol Biol Cell* Vol.18, No.3, (Mar 2007), pp.806-14

Alberti, S., Bohse, K., Arndt, V., Schmitz, A. & Hohfeld, J. (2004). The cochaperone HspBP1 inhibits the CHIP ubiquitin ligase and stimulates the maturation of the cystic fibrosis transmembrane conductance regulator. *Mol Biol Cell* Vol.15, No.9, (Sep 2004), pp.4003-10

Aleksandrov, A. A., Kota, P., Aleksandrov, L. A., He, L., Jensen, T., Cui, L., Gentzsch, M., Dokholyan, N. V. & Riordan, J. R. (2010). Regulatory insertion removal restores maturation, stability and function of DeltaF508 CFTR. *J Mol Biol* Vol.401, No.2, (Aug 13 2010), pp.194-210

Aller, S. G., Yu, J., Ward, A., Weng, Y., Chittaboina, S., Zhuo, R., Harrell, P. M., Trinh, Y. T., Zhang, Q., Urbatsch, I. L. & Chang, G. (2009). Structure of P-glycoprotein reveals a molecular basis for poly-specific drug binding. *Science* Vol.323, No.5922, (Mar 27 2009), pp.1718-22

Aridor, M., Weissman, J., Bannykh, S., Nuoffer, C. & Balch, W. E. (1998). Cargo selection by the COPII budding machinery during export from the ER. *J Cell Biol* Vol.141, No.1, (Apr 6 1998), pp.61-70

Arndt, V., Daniel, C., Nastainczyk, W., Alberti, S. & Hohfeld, J. (2005). BAG-2 Acts as an Inhibitor of the Chaperone-associated Ubiquitin Ligase CHIP. *Mol Biol Cell* Vol.16, No.12, (Dec 2005), pp.5891-900

Atwell, S., Brouillette, C. G., Conners, K., Emtage, S., Gheyi, T., Guggino, W. B., Hendle, J., Hunt, J. F., Lewis, H. A., Lu, F., Protasevich, II, Rodgers, L. A., Romero, R., Wasserman, S. R., Weber, P. C., Wetmore, D., Zhang, F. F. & Zhao, X. (2010). Structures of a minimal human CFTR first nucleotide-binding domain as a monomer, head-to-tail homodimer, and pathogenic mutant. *Protein Eng Des Sel* Vol.23, No.5, (May 2010), pp.375-84

Ballar, P., Ors, A. U., Yang, H. & Fang, S. (2010). Differential regulation of CFTRDeltaF508 degradation by ubiquitin ligases gp78 and Hrd1. *Int J Biochem Cell Biol* Vol.42, No.1, (Jan 2010), pp.167-73

Bartoszewski, R., Rab, A., Twitty, G., Stevenson, L., Fortenberry, J., Piotrowski, A., Dumanski, J. P. & Bebok, Z. (2008). The mechanism of cystic fibrosis transmembrane conductance regulator transcriptional repression during the unfolded protein response. *J Biol Chem* Vol.283, No.18, (May 2 2008), pp.12154-65

Bartoszewski, R. A., Jablonsky, M., Bartoszewska, S., Stevenson, L., Dai, Q., Kappes, J., Collawn, J. F. & Bebok, Z. (2010). A synonymous single nucleotide polymorphism in DeltaF508 CFTR alters the secondary structure of the mRNA and the expression of the mutant protein. *J Biol Chem* Vol.285, No.37, (Sep 10 2010), pp.28741-8

Brown, C. R., Hong-Brown, L. Q., Biwersi, J., Verkman, A. S. & Welch, W. J. (1996). Chemical chaperones correct the mutant phenotype of the delta F508 cystic fibrosis transmembrane conductance regulator protein. *Cell Stress Chaperones* Vol.1, No.2, (Jun 1996), pp.117-25

Carlile, G. W., Robert, R., Zhang, D., Teske, K. A., Luo, Y., Hanrahan, J. W. & Thomas, D. Y. (2007). Correctors of protein trafficking defects identified by a novel high-throughput screening assay. *Chembiochem* Vol.8, No.9, (Jun 18 2007), pp.1012-20

Carlson, E. J., Pitonzo, D. & Skach, W. R. (2006). p97 functions as an auxiliary factor to facilitate TM domain extraction during CFTR ER-associated degradation. *Embo J* Vol.25, No.19, (Oct 4 2006), pp.4557-66

Cebotaru, L., Vij, N., Ciobanu, I., Wright, J., Flotte, T. & Guggino, W. B. (2008). Cystic fibrosis transmembrane regulator missing the first four transmembrane segments increases wild type and DeltaF508 processing. *J Biol Chem* Vol.283, No.32, (Aug 8 2008), pp.21926-33

Chang, X. B., Cui, L., Hou, Y. X., Jensen, T. J., Aleksandrov, A. A., Mengos, A. & Riordan, J. R. (1999). Removal of multiple arginine-framed trafficking signals overcomes misprocessing of delta F508 CFTR present in most patients with cystic fibrosis. *Mol Cell* Vol.4, No.1, (Jul 1999), pp.137-42

Chappell, T. G., Welch, W. J., Schlossman, D. M., Palter, K. B., Schlesinger, M. J. & Rothman, J. E. (1986). Uncoating ATPase is a member of the 70 kilodalton family of stress proteins. *Cell* Vol.45, No.1, (Apr 11 1986), pp.3-13

Cheng, J., Cebotaru, V., Cebotaru, L. & Guggino, W. B. (2010). Syntaxin 6 and CAL mediate the degradation of the cystic fibrosis transmembrane conductance regulator. *Mol Biol Cell* Vol.21, No.7, (Apr 1 2010), pp.1178-87

Cheng, J., Moyer, B. D., Milewski, M., Loffing, J., Ikeda, M., Mickle, J. E., Cutting, G. R., Li, M., Stanton, B. A. & Guggino, W. B. (2002). A Golgi-associated PDZ domain protein modulates cystic fibrosis transmembrane regulator plasma membrane expression. *J Biol Chem* Vol.277, No.5, (Feb 1 2002), pp.3520-9

Cheng, J., Wang, H. & Guggino, W. B. (2004). Modulation of mature cystic fibrosis transmembrane regulator protein by the PDZ domain protein CAL. *J Biol Chem* Vol.279, No.3, (Jan 16 2004), pp.1892-8

Cheng, S. H., Fang, S. L., Zabner, J., Marshall, J., Piraino, S., Schiavi, S. C., Jefferson, D. M., Welsh, M. J. & Smith, A. E. (1995). Functional activation of the cystic fibrosis trafficking mutant delta F508-CFTR by overexpression. *Am J Physiol* Vol.268, No.4 Pt 1, (Apr 1995), pp.L615-24

Cheng, S. H., Gregory, R. J., Marshall, J., Paul, S., Souza, D. W., White, G. A., O'Riordan, C. R. & Smith, A. E. (1990). Defective intracellular transport and processing of CFTR is the molecular basis of most cystic fibrosis. *Cell* Vol.63, No.4, (Nov 16 1990), pp.827-34

Choo-Kang, L. R. & Zeitlin, P. L. (2001). Induction of HSP70 promotes DeltaF508 CFTR trafficking. *Am J Physiol Lung Cell Mol Physiol* Vol.281, No.1, (Jul 2001), pp.L58-68

Cormet-Boyaka, E., Jablonsky, M., Naren, A. P., Jackson, P. L., Muccio, D. D. & Kirk, K. L. (2004). Rescuing cystic fibrosis transmembrane conductance regulator (CFTR)-processing mutants by transcomplementation. *Proc Natl Acad Sci U S A* Vol.101, No.21, (May 25 2004), pp.8221-6

Dalemans, W., Barbry, P., Champigny, G., Jallat, S., Dott, K., Dreyer, D., Crystal, R. G., Pavirani, A., Lecocq, J. P. & Lazdunski, M. (1991). Altered chloride ion channel kinetics associated with the delta F508 cystic fibrosis mutation. *Nature* Vol.354, No.6354, (Dec 19-26 1991), pp.526-8

Dawson, R. J. & Locher, K. P. (2006). Structure of a bacterial multidrug ABC transporter. *Nature* Vol.443, No.7108, (Sep 14 2006), pp.180-5

Denning, G. M., Anderson, M. P., Amara, J. F., Marshall, J., Smith, A. E. & Welsh, M. J. (1992). Processing of mutant cystic fibrosis transmembrane conductance regulator is temperature-sensitive. *Nature* Vol.358, No.6389, (Aug 27 1992), pp.761-4

Dormer, R. L., Harris, C. M., Clark, Z., Pereira, M. M., Doull, I. J., Norez, C., Becq, F. & McPherson, M. A. (2005). Sildenafil (Viagra) corrects DeltaF508-CFTR location in nasal epithelial cells from patients with cystic fibrosis. *Thorax* Vol.60, No.1, (Jan 2005), pp.55-9

Du, K. & Lukacs, G. L. (2009). Cooperative assembly and misfolding of CFTR domains in vivo. *Mol Biol Cell* Vol.20, No.7, (Apr 2009), pp.1903-15

Du, K., Sharma, M. & Lukacs, G. L. (2005). The DeltaF508 cystic fibrosis mutation impairs domain-domain interactions and arrests post-translational folding of CFTR. *Nat Struct Mol Biol* Vol.12, No.1, (Jan 2005), pp.17-25

Egan, M. E., Glockner-Pagel, J., Ambrose, C., Cahill, P. A., Pappoe, L., Balamuth, N., Cho, E., Canny, S., Wagner, C. A., Geibel, J. & Caplan, M. J. (2002). Calcium-pump inhibitors induce functional surface expression of Delta F508-CFTR protein in cystic fibrosis epithelial cells. *Nat Med* Vol.8, No.5, (May 2002), pp.485-92

Fischer, H., Fukuda, N., Barbry, P., Illek, B., Sartori, C. & Matthay, M. A. (2001). Partial restoration of defective chloride conductance in DeltaF508 CF mice by trimethylamine oxide. *Am J Physiol Lung Cell Mol Physiol* Vol.281, No.1, (Jul 2001), pp.L52-7

Gaston, B., Reilly, J., Drazen, J. M., Fackler, J., Ramdev, P., Arnelle, D., Mullins, M. E., Sugarbaker, D. J., Chee, C., Singel, D. J. & et al. (1993). Endogenous nitrogen oxides and bronchodilator S-nitrosothiols in human airways. *Proc Natl Acad Sci U S A* Vol.90, No.23, (Dec 1 1993), pp.10957-61

Gelman, M. S. & Kopito, R. R. (2002). Rescuing protein conformation: prospects for pharmacological therapy in cystic fibrosis. *J Clin Invest* Vol.110, No.11, (Dec 2002), pp.1591-7

Gomes-Alves, P., Couto, F., Pesquita, C., Coelho, A. V. & Penque, D. (2010). Rescue of F508del-CFTR by RXR motif inactivation triggers proteome modulation associated with the unfolded protein response. *Biochim Biophys Acta* Vol.1804, No.4, (Apr 2010), pp.856-65

Grove, D. E., Fan, C. Y., Ren, H. Y. & Cyr, D. M. (2011). The endoplasmic reticulum-associated Hsp40 DNAJB12 and Hsc70 cooperate to facilitate RMA1 E3-dependent degradation of nascent CFTRDeltaF508. *Mol Biol Cell* Vol.22, No.3, (Feb 2011), pp.301-14

Hassink, G. C., Zhao, B., Sompallae, R., Altun, M., Gastaldello, S., Zinin, N. V., Masucci, M. G. & Lindsten, K. (2009). The ER-resident ubiquitin-specific protease 19 participates in the UPR and rescues ERAD substrates. *EMBO Rep* Vol.10, No.7, (Jul 2009), pp.755-61

He, L., Aleksandrov, L. A., Cui, L., Jensen, T. J., Nesbitt, K. L. & Riordan, J. R. (2010). Restoration of domain folding and interdomain assembly by second-site suppressors of the DeltaF508 mutation in CFTR. *Faseb J* Vol.24, No.8, (Aug 2010), pp.3103-12

Hegedus, T., Aleksandrov, A., Cui, L., Gentzsch, M., Chang, X. B. & Riordan, J. R. (2006). F508del CFTR with two altered RXR motifs escapes from ER quality control but its channel activity is thermally sensitive. *Biochim Biophys Acta* Vol.1758, No.5, (May 2006), pp.565-72

Henderson, M. J., Vij, N. & Zeitlin, P. L. (2010). Ubiquitin C-terminal hydrolase-L1 protects cystic fibrosis transmembrane conductance regulator from early stages of proteasomal degradation. *J Biol Chem* Vol.285, No.15, (Apr 9 2010), pp.11314-25

Hoelen, H., Kleizen, B., Schmidt, A., Richardson, J., Charitou, P., Thomas, P. J. & Braakman, I. (2010). The primary folding defect and rescue of DeltaF508 CFTR emerge during translation of the mutant domain. *PLoS One* Vol.5, No.11, (Nov 2010), pp.e15458

Hutt, D. M., Herman, D., Rodrigues, A. P., Noel, S., Pilewski, J. M., Matteson, J., Hoch, B., Kellner, W., Kelly, J. W., Schmidt, A., Thomas, P. J., Matsumura, Y., Skach, W. R., Gentzsch, M., Riordan, J. R., Sorscher, E. J., Okiyoneda, T., Yates, J. R., 3rd, Lukacs, G. L., Frizzell, R. A., Manning, G., Gottesfeld, J. M. & Balch, W. E. (2010). Reduced histone deacetylase 7 activity restores function to misfolded CFTR in cystic fibrosis. *Nat Chem Biol* Vol.6, No.1, (Jan 2010), pp.25-33

Jensen, T. J., Loo, M. A., Pind, S., Williams, D. B., Goldberg, A. L. & Riordan, J. R. (1995). Multiple proteolytic systems, including the proteasome, contribute to CFTR processing. *Cell* Vol.83, No.1, (Oct 6 1995), pp.129-35

Jiang, C., Fang, S. L., Xiao, Y. F., O'Connor, S. P., Nadler, S. G., Lee, D. W., Jefferson, D. M., Kaplan, J. M., Smith, A. E. & Cheng, S. H. (1998). Partial restoration of cAMP-stimulated CFTR chloride channel activity in DeltaF508 cells by deoxyspergualin. *Am J Physiol* Vol.275, No.1 Pt 1, (Jul 1998), pp.C171-8

Jordan, I. K., Kota, K. C., Cui, G., Thompson, C. H. & McCarty, N. A. (2008). Evolutionary and functional divergence between the cystic fibrosis transmembrane conductance regulator and related ATP-binding cassette transporters. *Proc Natl Acad Sci U S A* Vol.105, No.48, (Dec 2 2008), pp.18865-70

Jung, M. (2001). Inhibitors of histone deacetylase as new anticancer agents. *Curr Med Chem* Vol.8, No.12, (Oct 2001), pp.1505-11

Kalid, O., Mense, M., Fischman, S., Shitrit, A., Bihler, H., Ben-Zeev, E., Schutz, N., Pedemonte, N., Thomas, P. J., Bridges, R. J., Wetmore, D. R., Marantz, Y. & Senderowitz, H. (2010). Small molecule correctors of F508del-CFTR discovered by structure-based virtual screening. *J Comput Aided Mol Des* Vol.24, No.12, (Dec 2010), pp.971-91

Kerem, B., Rommens, J. M., Buchanan, J. A., Markiewicz, D., Cox, T. K., Chakravarti, A., Buchwald, M. & Tsui, L. C. (1989). Identification of the cystic fibrosis gene: genetic analysis. *Science* Vol.245, No.4922, (Sep 8 1989), pp.1073-80

Kim Chiaw, P., Huan, L. J., Gagnon, S., Ly, D., Sweezey, N., Rotin, D., Deber, C. M. & Bear, C. E. (2009). Functional rescue of DeltaF508-CFTR by peptides designed to mimic sorting motifs. *Chem Biol* Vol.16, No.5, (May 29 2009), pp.520-30

Kleizen, B., van Vlijmen, T., de Jonge, H. R. & Braakman, I. (2005). Folding of CFTR Is Predominantly Cotranslational. *Mol Cell* Vol.20, No.2, (Oct 28 2005), pp.277-87

Kwon, S. H., Pollard, H. & Guggino, W. B. (2007). Knockdown of NHERF1 enhances degradation of temperature rescued DeltaF508 CFTR from the cell surface of human airway cells. *Cell Physiol Biochem* Vol.20, No.62007), pp.763-72

Lewis, H. A., Wang, C., Zhao, X., Hamuro, Y., Conners, K., Kearins, M. C., Lu, F., Sauder, J. M., Molnar, K. S., Coales, S. J., Maloney, P. C., Guggino, W. B., Wetmore, D. R., Weber, P. C. & Hunt, J. F. (2010). Structure and dynamics of NBD1 from CFTR characterized using crystallography and hydrogen/deuterium exchange mass spectrometry. *J Mol Biol* Vol.396, No.2, (Feb 19 2010), pp.406-30

Lewis, H. A., Zhao, X., Wang, C., Sauder, J. M., Rooney, I., Noland, B. W., Lorimer, D., Kearins, M. C., Conners, K., Condon, B., Maloney, P. C., Guggino, W. B., Hunt, J. F. & Emtage, S. (2005). Impact of the deltaF508 mutation in first nucleotide-binding domain of human cystic fibrosis transmembrane conductance regulator on domain folding and structure. *J Biol Chem* Vol.280, No.2, (Jan 14 2005), pp.1346-53

Li, C., Ramjeesingh, M., Wang, W., Garami, E., Hewryk, M., Lee, D., Rommens, J. M., Galley, K. & Bear, C. E. (1996). ATPase activity of the cystic fibrosis transmembrane conductance regulator. *J Biol Chem* Vol.271, No.45, (Nov 8 1996), pp.28463-8

Locher, K. P., Lee, A. T. & Rees, D. C. (2002). The E. coli BtuCD structure: a framework for ABC transporter architecture and mechanism. *Science* Vol.296, No.5570, (May 10 2002), pp.1091-8

Loo, M. A., Jensen, T. J., Cui, L., Hou, Y., Chang, X. B. & Riordan, J. R. (1998). Perturbation of Hsp90 interaction with nascent CFTR prevents its maturation and accelerates its degradation by the proteasome. *Embo J* Vol.17, No.23, (Dec 1 1998), pp.6879-87

Loo, T. W., Bartlett, M. C. & Clarke, D. M. (2008). Processing mutations disrupt interactions between the nucleotide binding and transmembrane domains of P-glycoprotein and the cystic fibrosis transmembrane conductance regulator (CFTR). *J Biol Chem* Vol.283, No.42, (Oct 17 2008), pp.28190-7

Lukacs, G. L., Chang, X. B., Bear, C., Kartner, N., Mohamed, A., Riordan, J. R. & Grinstein, S. (1993). The delta F508 mutation decreases the stability of cystic fibrosis transmembrane conductance regulator in the plasma membrane. Determination of functional half-lives on transfected cells. *J Biol Chem* Vol.268, No.29, (Oct 15 1993), pp.21592-8

Lukacs, G. L., Mohamed, A., Kartner, N., Chang, X. B., Riordan, J. R. & Grinstein, S. (1994). Conformational maturation of CFTR but not its mutant counterpart (delta F508) occurs in the endoplasmic reticulum and requires ATP. *Embo J* Vol.13, No.24, (Dec 15 1994), pp.6076-86

Maitra, R. & Hamilton, J. W. (2007). Altered biogenesis of deltaF508-CFTR following treatment with doxorubicin. *Cell Physiol Biochem* Vol.20, No.52007), pp.465-72

Maitra, R., Shaw, C. M., Stanton, B. A. & Hamilton, J. W. (2001). Increased functional cell surface expression of CFTR and DeltaF508-CFTR by the anthracycline doxorubicin. *Am J Physiol Cell Physiol* Vol.280, No.5, (May 2001), pp.C1031-7

Margeta-Mitrovic, M., Jan, Y. N. & Jan, L. Y. (2000). A trafficking checkpoint controls GABA(B) receptor heterodimerization. *Neuron* Vol.27, No.1, (Jul 2000), pp.97-106

Marozkina, N. V., Yemen, S., Borowitz, M., Liu, L., Plapp, M., Sun, F., Islam, R., Erdmann-Gilmore, P., Townsend, R. R., Lichti, C. F., Mantri, S., Clapp, P. W., Randell, S. H., Gaston, B. & Zaman, K. (2010). Hsp 70/Hsp 90 organizing protein as a nitrosylation target in cystic fibrosis therapy. *Proc Natl Acad Sci U S A* Vol.107, No.25, (Jun 22 2010), pp.11393-8

Meacham, G. C., Lu, Z., King, S., Sorscher, E., Tousson, A. & Cyr, D. M. (1999). The Hdj-2/Hsc70 chaperone pair facilitates early steps in CFTR biogenesis. *Embo J* Vol.18, No.6, (Mar 15 1999), pp.1492-505

Meacham, G. C., Patterson, C., Zhang, W., Younger, J. M. & Cyr, D. M. (2001). The Hsc70 co-chaperone CHIP targets immature CFTR for proteasomal degradation. *Nat Cell Biol* Vol.3, No.1, (Jan 2001), pp.100-5

Miller, E., Antonny, B., Hamamoto, S. & Schekman, R. (2002). Cargo selection into COPII vesicles is driven by the Sec24p subunit. *Embo J* Vol.21, No.22, (Nov 15 2002), pp.6105-13

Mills, A. D., Yoo, C., Butler, J. D., Yang, B., Verkman, A. S. & Kurth, M. J. (2010). Design and synthesis of a hybrid potentiator-corrector agonist of the cystic fibrosis mutant protein DeltaF508-CFTR. *Bioorg Med Chem Lett* Vol.20, No.1, (Jan 1 2010), pp.87-91

Monneret, C. (2007). Histone deacetylase inhibitors for epigenetic therapy of cancer. *Anticancer Drugs* Vol.18, No.4, (Apr 2007), pp.363-70

Morimoto, R. I., Tissières, A., Georgopoulos, C. & Cold Spring Harbor Laboratory. (1990). *Stress proteins in biology and medicine*, Cold Spring Harbor Laboratory Press, 0879693371, Cold Spring Harbor, N.Y.

Morito, D., Hirao, K., Oda, Y., Hosokawa, N., Tokunaga, F., Cyr, D. M., Tanaka, K., Iwai, K. & Nagata, K. (2008). Gp78 cooperates with RMA1 in endoplasmic reticulum-associated degradation of CFTRDeltaF508. *Mol Biol Cell* Vol.19, No.4, (Apr 2008), pp.1328-36

Mornon, J. P., Lehn, P. & Callebaut, I. (2009). Molecular models of the open and closed states of the whole human CFTR protein. *Cell Mol Life Sci* Vol.66, No.21, (Nov 2009), pp.3469-86

Nagahama, M., Ohnishi, M., Kawate, Y., Matsui, T., Miyake, H., Yuasa, K., Tani, K., Tagaya, M. & Tsuji, A. (2009). UBXD1 is a VCP-interacting protein that is involved in ER-associated degradation. *Biochem Biophys Res Commun* Vol.382, No.2, (May 1 2009), pp.303-8

Nilsson, T., Jackson, M. & Peterson, P. A. (1989). Short cytoplasmic sequences serve as retention signals for transmembrane proteins in the endoplasmic reticulum. *Cell* Vol.58, No.4, (Aug 25 1989), pp.707-18

Nishimura, N., Bannykh, S., Slabough, S., Matteson, J., Altschuler, Y., Hahn, K. & Balch, W. E. (1999). A di-acidic (DXE) code directs concentration of cargo during export from the endoplasmic reticulum. *J Biol Chem* Vol.274, No.22, (May 28 1999), pp.15937-46

Okiyoneda, T., Barriere, H., Bagdany, M., Rabeh, W. M., Du, K., Hohfeld, J., Young, J. C. & Lukacs, G. L. (2010). Peripheral protein quality control removes unfolded CFTR from the plasma membrane. *Science* Vol.329, No.5993, (Aug 13 2010), pp.805-10

Pagant, S., Kung, L., Dorrington, M., Lee, M. C. & Miller, E. A. (2007). Inhibiting endoplasmic reticulum (ER)-associated degradation of misfolded Yor1p does not permit ER export despite the presence of a diacidic sorting signal. *Mol Biol Cell* Vol.18, No.9, (Sep 2007), pp.3398-413

Park, H. J., Mylvaganum, M., McPherson, A., Fewell, S. W., Brodsky, J. L. & Lingwood, C. A. (2009). A soluble sulfogalactosyl ceramide mimic promotes Delta F508 CFTR escape from endoplasmic reticulum associated degradation. *Chem Biol* Vol.16, No.4, (Apr 24 2009), pp.461-70

Phuan, P. W., Yang, B., Knapp, J., Wood, A., Lukacs, G. L., Kurth, M. J. & Verkman, A. S. (2011). Cyanoquinolines with Independent Corrector and Potentiator Activities Restore Δphe508-Cystic Fibrosis Transmembrane Conductance Regulator Chloride Channel Function in Cystic Fibrosis. *Mol Pharmacol* Vol.80, No.4, (Oct 2011), pp683-93

Pissarra, L. S., Farinha, C. M., Xu, Z., Schmidt, A., Thibodeau, P. H., Cai, Z., Thomas, P. J., Sheppard, D. N. & Amaral, M. D. (2008). Solubilizing Mutations Used to Crystallize One CFTR Domain Attenuate the Trafficking and Channel Defects Caused by the Major Cystic Fibrosis Mutation. *Chem Biol* Vol.15, No.1, (Jan 2008), pp.62-9

Pollet, J. F., Van Geffel, J., Van Stevens, E., Van Geffel, R., Beauwens, R., Bollen, A. & Jacobs, P. (2000). Expression and intracellular processing of chimeric and mutant CFTR molecules. *Biochim Biophys Acta* Vol.1500, No.1, (Jan 3 2000), pp.59-69

Qu, B. H., Strickland, E. H. & Thomas, P. J. (1997). Localization and suppression of a kinetic defect in cystic fibrosis transmembrane conductance regulator folding. *J Biol Chem* Vol.272, No.25, (Jun 20 1997), pp.15739-44

Qu, B. H. & Thomas, P. J. (1996). Alteration of the cystic fibrosis transmembrane conductance regulator folding pathway. *J Biol Chem* Vol.271, No.13, (Mar 29 1996), pp.7261-4

Rab, A., Bartoszewski, R., Jurkuvenaite, A., Wakefield, J., Collawn, J. F. & Bebok, Z. (2007). Endoplasmic reticulum stress and the unfolded protein response regulate genomic cystic fibrosis transmembrane conductance regulator expression. *Am J Physiol Cell Physiol* Vol.292, No.2, (Feb 2007), pp.C756-66

Riordan, J. R., Rommens, J. M., Kerem, B., Alon, N., Rozmahel, R., Grzelczak, Z., Zielenski, J., Lok, S., Plavsic, N., Chou, J. L., Drumm, M. L., Iannuzzi, M. C., Collins, F. S. & Tsui, L. C. (1989). Identification of the cystic fibrosis gene: cloning and characterization of complementary DNA. *Science* Vol.245, No.4922, (Sep 8 1989), pp.1066-73

Rowe, S. M., Pyle, L. C., Jurkevante, A., Varga, K., Collawn, J., Sloane, P. A., Woodworth, B., Mazur, M., Fulton, J., Fan, L., Li, Y., Fortenberry, J., Sorscher, E. J. & Clancy, J. P. (2010). DeltaF508 CFTR processing correction and activity in polarized airway and non-airway cell monolayers. *Pulm Pharmacol Ther* Vol.23, No.4, (Aug 2010), pp.268-78

Roxo-Rosa, M., Xu, Z., Schmidt, A., Neto, M., Cai, Z., Soares, C. M., Sheppard, D. N. & Amaral, M. D. (2006). Revertant mutants G550E and 4RK rescue cystic fibrosis mutants in the first nucleotide-binding domain of CFTR by different mechanisms. *Proc Natl Acad Sci U S A* Vol.103, No.47, (Nov 21 2006), pp.17891-6

Roy, G., Chalfin, E. M., Saxena, A. & Wang, X. (2010). Interplay between ER exit code and domain conformation in CFTR misprocessing and rescue. *Mol Biol Cell* Vol.21, No.4, (Feb 2010), pp.597-609

Rubenstein, R. C., Egan, M. E. & Zeitlin, P. L. (1997). In vitro pharmacologic restoration of CFTR-mediated chloride transport with sodium 4-phenylbutyrate in cystic fibrosis epithelial cells containing delta F508-CFTR. *J Clin Invest* Vol.100, No.10, (Nov 15 1997), pp.2457-65

Rubenstein, R. C. & Zeitlin, P. L. (2000). Sodium 4-phenylbutyrate downregulates Hsc70: implications for intracellular trafficking of DeltaF508-CFTR. *Am J Physiol Cell Physiol* Vol.278, No.2, (Feb 2000), pp.C259-67

Saxena, A., Banasavadi-Siddegowda, Y. K., Fan, Y., Bhattacharya, S., Liao, Y., Giovannucci, D. R., Frizzell, R. A. & Wang, X. (2011a). Hsp105 regulates CFTR biogenesis and quality control at multiple levels. *Pediatric Pulmonology* Vol.46, No.S34, (Oct 2011), pp.215-215

Saxena, A., Bhattacharya, S., Fan, Y., Banasavadi-Siddegowda, Y. K., Chalfin, E. M., Roy, G., Mai, J., Sanchez, E. R. & Wang, X. (2011b). Cochaperones Hop and Hsp105 functionally link Hsp70 and Hsp90 during DeltaF508 CFTR maturation at low temperature. *Pediatric Pulmonology* Vol.46, No.S34, (Oct 2011), pp.215-215

Saxena, A., Chalfin, E. M., Roy, G. & Wang, X. (2007). HSP105 reveals distinct conformational maturation pathways for wild-type and Delta F508 CFTR at reduced temperature. *Pediatric Pulmonology*, Vol.42, No.S30, (Aug 2007), pp.212-212

Schmid, S. L. & Rothman, J. E. (1985). Two classes of binding sites for uncoating protein in clathrin triskelions. *J Biol Chem* Vol.260, No.18, (Aug 25 1985), pp.10050-6

Serohijos, A. W., Hegedus, T., Aleksandrov, A. A., He, L., Cui, L., Dokholyan, N. V. & Riordan, J. R. (2008a). Phenylalanine-508 mediates a cytoplasmic-membrane domain contact in the CFTR 3D structure crucial to assembly and channel function. *Proc Natl Acad Sci U S A* Vol.105, No.9, (Mar 4 2008a), pp.3256-61

Serohijos, A. W., Hegedus, T., Riordan, J. R. & Dokholyan, N. V. (2008b). Diminished self-chaperoning activity of the DeltaF508 mutant of CFTR results in protein misfolding. *PLoS Comput Biol* Vol.4, No.2, (Feb 2008b), pp.e1000008

Sharma, M., Benharouga, M., Hu, W. & Lukacs, G. L. (2001). Conformational and temperature-sensitive stability defects of the delta F508 cystic fibrosis transmembrane conductance regulator in post-endoplasmic reticulum compartments. *J Biol Chem* Vol.276, No.12, (Mar 23 2001), pp.8942-50

Sharma, M., Pampinella, F., Nemes, C., Benharouga, M., So, J., Du, K., Bache, K. G., Papsin, B., Zerangue, N., Stenmark, H. & Lukacs, G. L. (2004). Misfolding diverts CFTR from recycling to degradation: quality control at early endosomes. *J Cell Biol* Vol.164, No.6, (Mar 15 2004), pp.923-33

Sidrauski, C., Chapman, R. & Walter, P. (1998). The unfolded protein response: an intracellular signalling pathway with many surprising features. *Trends Cell Biol* Vol.8, No.6, (Jun 1998), pp.245-9

Singh, O. V., Pollard, H. B. & Zeitlin, P. L. (2008). Chemical rescue of deltaF508-CFTR mimics genetic repair in cystic fibrosis bronchial epithelial cells. *Mol Cell Proteomics* Vol.7, No.6, (Jun 2008), pp.1099-110

Singh, O. V., Vij, N., Mogayzel, P. J., Jr., Jozwik, C., Pollard, H. B. & Zeitlin, P. L. (2006). Pharmacoproteomics of 4-phenylbutyrate-treated IB3-1 cystic fibrosis bronchial epithelial cells. *J Proteome Res* Vol.5, No.3, (Mar 2006), pp.562-71

Sun, F., Mi, Z., Condliffe, S. B., Bertrand, C. A., Gong, X., Lu, X., Zhang, R., Latoche, J. D., Pilewski, J. M., Robbins, P. D. & Frizzell, R. A. (2008). Chaperone displacement from mutant cystic fibrosis transmembrane conductance regulator restores its function in human airway epithelia. *Faseb J* Vol.22, No.9, (Sep 2008), pp.3255-63

Sun, F., Zhang, R., Gong, X., Geng, X., Drain, P. F. & Frizzell, R. A. (2006). Derlin-1 promotes the efficient degradation of the cystic fibrosis transmembrane conductance regulator (CFTR) and CFTR folding mutants. *J Biol Chem* Vol.281, No.48, (Dec 1 2006), pp.36856-63

Teem, J. L., Berger, H. A., Ostedgaard, L. S., Rich, D. P., Tsui, L. C. & Welsh, M. J. (1993). Identification of revertants for the cystic fibrosis delta F508 mutation using STE6-CFTR chimeras in yeast. *Cell* Vol.73, No.2, (Apr 23 1993), pp.335-46

Teem, J. L., Carson, M. R. & Welsh, M. J. (1996). Mutation of R555 in CFTR-delta F508 enhances function and partially corrects defective processing. *Receptors Channels* Vol.4, No.11996), pp.63-72

Thibodeau, P. H., Brautigam, C. A., Machius, M. & Thomas, P. J. (2005). Side chain and backbone contributions of Phe508 to CFTR folding. *Nat Struct Mol Biol* Vol.12, No.1, (Jan 2005), pp.10-6

Thibodeau, P. H., Richardson, J. M., 3rd, Wang, W., Millen, L., Watson, J., Mendoza, J. L., Du, K., Fischman, S., Senderowitz, H., Lukacs, G. L., Kirk, K. & Thomas, P. J. (2010). The cystic fibrosis-causing mutation deltaF508 affects multiple steps in cystic fibrosis transmembrane conductance regulator biogenesis. *J Biol Chem* Vol.285, No.46, (Nov 12 2010), pp.35825-35

Trzcinska-Daneluti, A. M., Ly, D., Huynh, L., Jiang, C., Fladd, C. & Rotin, D. (2009). High-content functional screen to identify proteins that correct F508del-CFTR function. *Mol Cell Proteomics* Vol.8, No.4, (Apr 2009), pp.780-90

Tsui, L. C. (1995). The cystic fibrosis transmembrane conductance regulator gene. *Am J Respir Crit Care Med* Vol.151, No.3 Pt 2, (Mar 1995), pp.S47-53

Van Goor, F., Hadida, S., Grootenhuis, P. D., Burton, B., Cao, D., Neuberger, T., Turnbull, A., Singh, A., Joubran, J., Hazlewood, A., Zhou, J., McCartney, J., Arumugam, V., Decker, C., Yang, J., Young, C., Olson, E. R., Wine, J. J., Frizzell, R. A., Ashlock, M. & Negulescu, P. (2009). Rescue of CF airway epithelial cell function in vitro by a CFTR potentiator, VX-770. *Proc Natl Acad Sci U S A* Vol.106, No.44, (Nov 3 2009), pp.18825-30

Van Goor, F., Straley, K. S., Cao, D., Gonzalez, J., Hadida, S., Hazlewood, A., Joubran, J., Knapp, T., Makings, L. R., Miller, M., Neuberger, T., Olson, E., Panchenko, V., Rader, J., Singh, A., Stack, J. H., Tung, R., Grootenhuis, P. D. & Negulescu, P. (2006). Rescue of ΔF508-CFTR trafficking and gating in human cystic fibrosis airway primary cultures by small molecules. *Am J Physiol Lung Cell Mol Physiol* Vol.290, No.6, (Jun 2006), pp.L1117-30

Varga, K., Jurkuvenaite, A., Wakefield, J., Hong, J. S., Guimbellot, J. S., Venglarik, C. J., Niraj, A., Mazur, M., Sorscher, E. J., Collawn, J. F. & Bebok, Z. (2004). Efficient intracellular processing of the endogenous cystic fibrosis transmembrane conductance regulator in epithelial cell lines. *J Biol Chem* Vol.279, No.21, (May 21 2004), pp.22578-84

Verkman, A. S., Lukacs, G. L. & Galietta, L. J. (2006). CFTR chloride channel drug discovery--inhibitors as antidiarrheals and activators for therapy of cystic fibrosis. *Curr Pharm Des* Vol.12, No.182006), pp.2235-47

Vij, N., Fang, S. & Zeitlin, P. L. (2006). Selective inhibition of endoplasmic reticulum-associated degradation rescues DeltaF508-cystic fibrosis transmembrane regulator and suppresses interleukin-8 levels: therapeutic implications. *J Biol Chem* Vol.281, No.25, (Jun 23 2006), pp.17369-78

Wang, B., Heath-Engel, H., Zhang, D., Nguyen, N., Thomas, D. Y., Hanrahan, J. W. & Shore, G. C. (2008). BAP31 interacts with Sec61 translocons and promotes retrotranslocation of CFTRDeltaF508 via the derlin-1 complex. *Cell* Vol.133, No.6, (Jun 13 2008), pp.1080-92

Wang, X., Koulov, A. V., Kellner, W. A., Riordan, J. R. & Balch, W. E. (2008). Chemical and biological folding contribute to temperature-sensitive DeltaF508 CFTR trafficking. *Traffic* Vol.9, No.11, (Nov 2008), pp.1878-93

Wang, X., Matteson, J., An, Y., Moyer, B., Yoo, J. S., Bannykh, S., Wilson, I. A., Riordan, J. R. & Balch, W. E. (2004). COPII-dependent export of cystic fibrosis transmembrane conductance regulator from the ER uses a di-acidic exit code. *J Cell Biol* Vol.167, No.1, (Oct 11 2004), pp.65-74

Wang, X., Venable, J., LaPointe, P., Hutt, D. M., Koulov, A. V., Coppinger, J., Gurkan, C., Kellner, W., Matteson, J., Plutner, H., Riordan, J. R., Kelly, J. W., Yates, J. R., 3rd & Balch, W. E. (2006). Hsp90 cochaperone Aha1 downregulation rescues misfolding of CFTR in cystic fibrosis. *Cell* Vol.127, No.4, (Nov 17 2006), pp.803-15

Ward, C. L., Omura, S. & Kopito, R. R. (1995). Degradation of CFTR by the ubiquitin-proteasome pathway. *Cell* Vol.83, No.1, (Oct 6 1995), pp.121-7

Wellhauser, L., Kim Chiaw, P., Pasyk, S., Li, C., Ramjeesingh, M. & Bear, C. E. (2009). A small-molecule modulator interacts directly with deltaPhe508-CFTR to modify its ATPase activity and conformational stability. *Mol Pharmacol* Vol.75, No.6, (Jun 2009), pp.1430-8

Westerheide, S. D., Bosman, J. D., Mbadugha, B. N., Kawahara, T. L., Matsumoto, G., Kim, S., Gu, W., Devlin, J. P., Silverman, R. B. & Morimoto, R. I. (2004). Celastrols as inducers of the heat shock response and cytoprotection. *J Biol Chem* Vol.279, No.53, (Dec 31 2004), pp.56053-60

Wolde, M., Fellows, A., Cheng, J., Kivenson, A., Coutermarsh, B., Talebian, L., Karlson, K., Piserchio, A., Mierke, D. F., Stanton, B. A., Guggino, W. B. & Madden, D. R. (2007). Targeting CAL as a negative regulator of DeltaF508-CFTR cell-surface expression: an RNA interference and structure-based mutagenetic approach. *J Biol Chem* Vol.282, No.11, (Mar 16 2007), pp.8099-109

Wright, J. M., Zeitlin, P. L., Cebotaru, L., Guggino, S. E. & Guggino, W. B. (2004). Gene expression profile analysis of 4-phenylbutyrate treatment of IB3-1 bronchial epithelial cell line demonstrates a major influence on heat-shock proteins. *Physiol Genomics* Vol.16, No.2, (Jan 15 2004), pp.204-11

Yang, Y., Janich, S., Cohn, J. A. & Wilson, J. M. (1993). The common variant of cystic fibrosis transmembrane conductance regulator is recognized by hsp70 and degraded in a pre-Golgi nonlysosomal compartment. *Proc Natl Acad Sci U S A* Vol.90, No.20, (Oct 15 1993), pp.9480-4

Younger, J. M., Chen, L., Ren, H. Y., Rosser, M. F., Turnbull, E. L., Fan, C. Y., Patterson, C. & Cyr, D. M. (2006). Sequential quality-control checkpoints triage misfolded cystic fibrosis transmembrane conductance regulator. *Cell* Vol.126, No.3, (Aug 11 2006), pp.571-82

Younger, J. M., Ren, H. Y., Chen, L., Fan, C. Y., Fields, A., Patterson, C. & Cyr, D. M. (2004). A foldable CFTRΔF508 biogenic intermediate accumulates upon inhibition of the Hsc70-CHIP E3 ubiquitin ligase. *J Cell Biol* Vol.167, No.6, (Dec 20 2004), pp.1075-85

Zaman, K., Carraro, S., Doherty, J., Henderson, E. M., Lendermon, E., Liu, L., Verghese, G., Zigler, M., Ross, M., Park, E., Palmer, L. A., Doctor, A., Stamler, J. S. & Gaston, B. (2006). S-nitrosylating agents: a novel class of compounds that increase cystic fibrosis transmembrane conductance regulator expression and maturation in epithelial cells. *Mol Pharmacol* Vol.70, No.4, (Oct 2006), pp.1435-42

Zerangue, N., Schwappach, B., Jan, Y. N. & Jan, L. Y. (1999). A new ER trafficking signal regulates the subunit stoichiometry of plasma membrane K(ATP) channels. *Neuron* Vol.22, No.3, (Mar 1999), pp.537-48

Zhang, F., Kartner, N. & Lukacs, G. L. (1998). Limited proteolysis as a probe for arrested conformational maturation of delta F508 CFTR. *Nat Struct Biol* Vol.5, No.3, (Mar 1998), pp.180-3

Zhang, H., Peters, K. W., Sun, F., Marino, C. R., Lang, J., Burgoyne, R. D. & Frizzell, R. A. (2002). Cysteine string protein interacts with and modulates the maturation of the cystic fibrosis transmembrane conductance regulator. *J Biol Chem* Vol.277, No.32, (Aug 9 2002), pp.28948-58

Zhang, Y., Nijbroek, G., Sullivan, M. L., McCracken, A. A., Watkins, S. C., Michaelis, S. & Brodsky, J. L. (2001). Hsp70 molecular chaperone facilitates endoplasmic reticulum-associated protein degradation of cystic fibrosis transmembrane conductance regulator in yeast. *Mol Biol Cell* Vol.12, No.5, (May 2001), pp.1303-14

6

CFTR Gene Transfer and Tracking the CFTR Protein in the Airway Epithelium

Gaëlle Gonzalez, Pierre Boulanger and Saw-See Hong
University of Lyon 1
France

1. Introduction

Cystic fibrosis (CF) is an autosomal recessive genetic disease caused by mutations in a single gene, the *cystic fibrosis transmembrane conductance regulator (CFTR)* gene. This disease primarily involves epithelial cells of the respiratory system, intestine, pancreas, gall bladder, and sweat glands. Although several organs are affected, the main cause of CF mortality and morbidity is due to pulmonary complications associated with impaired clearance and obstruction by viscous mucus secretions, which makes the lung epithelial cells the principle target for CF treatment. A monogenic disease such as CF was *a priori* an ideal candidate for gene therapy, as treatment of the disease was thought to be feasible with the introduction of the normal alleles of the *CFTR* gene into the airway epithelial cells to code for the functional protein.

2. CFTR gene transfer to the airway epithelium

The lung can be divided anatomically and physiologically into two regions, (i) the airways, consisting of the trachea, bronchi and bronchioles which brings air to the peripheral lung and (ii) the alveoli where the exchange of gas takes place. The airway epithelium is normally covered by a thin layer of mucus and acts as a natural barrier against foreign particles, including pathogens. In CF individuals, the airways are filled with sputum consisting of inflammatory cells, cell debris, highly viscous mucus and DNA, causing obstruction of the airways, constituting the major barrier for gene transfer as it prevents the cellular uptake of the vectors by the airway epithelial cells (Griesenbach, Alton et al., 2009; Hida et al., 2011).

The main target tissue for CF gene therapy is believed to be the airway epithelium, which exhibits all ion transport functions of CFTR and is easily accessible. However, the nature of the cells which are the best target for CF gene therapy is still debatable. The transfer of genes to the airway results in gene expression primarily in lung epithelial cells, and the transgene is localised to the lung without much systemic distribution. The highest level of CFTR gene expression is found in the bronchial submucosal gland cells (Merten et al., 1996; Kammouni et al., 1999; Chow et al., 2000) and it was suggested that these glandular cells may be better reached by vasculature and systemic application of the vector rather than by the airways (Boucher, 1999 ; Kolb et al., 2006).

There are several ways of introducing therapeutic genes into human cells but the most efficient method of gene transfer into human cells is by the use of viral vectors. Viruses have evolved and developed natural strategies to enter, transfer their genetic material and reproduce in specific tissues of their hosts, making them highly adapted as vectors to transfer genes into their natural target cells. Since 1989, twenty-nine clinical trials for CF have been carried out using adenovirus or adeno-associated virus vectors and non-viral vectors. In these gene therapy protocols, the major site of vector administration was the respiratory airways such as the nasal and lung epithelium. Unfortunately, the somewhat disappointing results of these clinical trials showed that CF gene therapy was more difficult than originally anticipated. The viral and non-viral vectors used in these trials revealed their limitations and inefficacy in gene transfer to the human airway epithelium.

2.1 Adenovirus (Ad) vector

The adenovirus as a gene transfer vector has several advantages over other vectors : (i) its capacity to incorporate large transgenes; (ii) its ease for genetic manipulation (Hong et al., 2003; Magnusson et al., 2007; Magnusson et al., 2001); and (iii) its facility to be produced to high titres. The efficiency of Ad vectors in gene transfer has been demonstrated in numerous systems (Henning et al., 2002; Gaden et al., 2004; Toh et al., 2005) and the functional analysis of transgenes expressed by Ad can be tested *in vitro* in cell lines, *ex vivo* in tissues and *in vivo* in animal models. *In vitro* studies demonstrated that recombinant Ad vectors can express CFTR in cultured CF airway epithelial cells and correct the Cl- transport defect (Zabner et al., 1993). Following this, a number of *in vivo* studies in animals and in tracheal explants showed that Ad vectors can express CFTR as well as reporter genes in the airway epithelia (Rosenfeld et al., 1992; Harvey et al., 1999; Scaria et al., 1998).

Ten CF clinical trials involving Ad vectors were conducted during the period 1993-2001 (available in Clinical Trials website : http://www.wiley.com//legacy/wileychi/ genmed/clinical/). The first Ad vector used in CF gene therapy trials involving CF patients was a serotype 2 (Ad2) vector, genetically modified in the E1 region to carry the CFTR cDNA, under the E1a promoter and had the same polyadenylation addition site as the E1b and pIX transcripts (Zabner et al., 1993). The results obtained from the early clinical trials with Ad vector administration in the nasal and pulmonary tissues showed that the Ad vectors were well-tolerated at low to intermediate doses in humans, and partially corrected the chloride transport (Zabner et al., 1993, Crystal, 1995; Welsh et al., 1995;).

One major difficulty which was revealed from the clinical trials was the inefficient *CFTR* gene transfer to the airway epithelium of CF patients (Perricone et al., 2001). It is known today that several factors were responsible for the low efficiency of *CFTR* gene transfer (Crystal, 1995): (*i*) the nonspecific inflammatory reactions (Otake et al., 1998) and immune response to the Ad-CFTR vector (Gahery-Segard et al., 1998 ; Piedra et al., 1998); (*ii*) the airway epithelial cells lack high affinity receptors for Ad (Zabner et al., 1997), as these receptors have a basolateral localization, which makes them inaccessible to Ad-CFTR vectors (Walters et al., 1999); (*iii*) mechanical factors, like bronchial mucus (Arcasoy et al., 1997 ; Perricone et al., 2000; Hida et al., 2011), or local bacterial infections, can negatively influence the effective binding of Ad vectors to the surface of epithelial cells, and the subsequent delivery of the therapeutic gene; (*iv*) a combination of the above different mechanisms, or/and intrinsic properties of differentiated airway epithelial cells (Gaden et al., 2002). Another hurdle encountered with Ad vectors was that gene transfer to the airway epithelia was transient and the use of recombinant adenovirus vectors would require repeated administration. The requirement for repeated vector administration is a major concern as this will generate neutralizing antibodies against the vector in gene therapy recipients which would subsequently reduce gene transfer efficacy.

2.2 Adeno-associated virus (AAV) vector

AAV gene transfer vectors have attracted much interest due to their good safety profile (no known pathology has been found to be associated with AAV in humans), broad tissue tropism and more importantly prolonged gene expression due to the integration of their DNA into the cellular genome. These vectors are thought to exhibit less inflammatory and immune reactions than the adenovirus. However, there are still technical problems concerning the small cloning capacity which could barely accommodate the CFTR gene (4.7 kb), and the difficulty in achieving high titers during AAV vector production.

Six CF gene therapy clinical trials using AAV vectors were carried out from 1999 – 2007 (Clinical Trials website : http://www.wiley.com//legacy/wileychi/genmed/clinical/). The first AAV-CFTR vector used showed physiological correction of chloride transport in nasal epithelial cells in gene therapy recipients, even in those with low CFTR mRNA expression (Wagner JA et al, 1999). The more recent clinical trials used the AAV vector, TgAAV-CFTR, developed by Targeted Genetics Corp, which carried the weak AAV long terminal repeat (LTR) promoter to drive CFTR gene expression (Griesenbach et al., 2009). The clinical data showed that repeated doses of aerosolised AAV-CFTR vector treatment did not result in significant therapeutic improvement (Moss et al., 2007). The reasons for these disappointing results could likely be that (i) AAV was inefficient in transducing airway epithelial cells via the apical membrane, (ii) the LTR promoter used to drive CFTR expression was too weak, or (iii) repeated administration of AAV to the lung resulted in the development of an anti-viral immune response (Griesenbach et al., 2009). In brief, the vector was well tolerated but there are still concerns about the toxicity and immunological responses related to the repeated administration of this vector. In addition, it was reported recently that insertional mutagenesis was observed in neonatal mice models treated with recombinant AAV vectors : the mice developed hepatocellular carcinoma which was associated with AAV vector integration (Dosante et al., 2007).

2.3 Non-viral vectors

Nine CF gene therapy clinical trials have been carried out using non-viral or synthetic vectors from 1995-2004 (Clinical Trials website : http://www.wiley.com//legacy /wileychi/genmed/clinical/). There are three main non-viral vector systems : cationic liposomes, DNA-polymer conjugates and naked DNA. Non-viral vectors have their limitations such as (i) low efficiency in gene transfer as compared to viral vectors, and (ii) loss of efficacy with repeated administrations. However, the major advantage of these vectors is that they are less immunogenic compared to Ad and AAV vectors. Their inefficacy is mainly due to intracellular barriers such as endosomal sequestration and cytoplasmic degradation, where Ca^{2+}-sensitive cytosolic nucleases restrict the half-life of DNA to 50-90 mins (Pollard et al., 2001). The nuclear membrane of non-dividing, airway epithelial cells constitutes another intracellular barrier as the nuclear entry of exogenous DNA occurs only in cells that are actively dividing (Ferrari et al., 2002).

To date, only cationic liposome-based systems have been tested in CF clinical trials. The first cationic liposome vector used was DC-Chol (3β{N-[N',N'-dimethylaminoethane]carbamoyl} cholesterol) mixed with DOPE (dioleoylphosphatidyl ethanolamine), complexed to CFTR plasmid DNA, and administered to patients via the nose. Cationic liposomes facilitate gene transfer by their interaction with DNA via their positively charged side chains and enhancing fusion with the host cell membrane via the hydrophobic lipid portion. The results obtained were encouraging as partial restoration of CFTR function was observed. However, the transfection efficiency and the duration of expression would need to be increased for therapeutic benefit (Caplen et al., 1995). Improvements to non-viral vector gene transfer efficiency to the lung have been proposed by using DNA condensed to molecular conjugates carrying a 17 amino acid peptide ligand which targets the serpin-enzyme complex receptor expressed on the apical surface of airway epithelial cells (Ziady et al., 2002).

Recently, three non-viral gene transfer agents : (i) cationic liposome (GL67A), (ii) compacted DNA nanoparticle with polyethyleneglycol-substituted lysine 30-mer (NP) and, (iii) 25kDa-branched polyethyeneimine (PEI) were evaluated *in vivo* in a sheep lung model. The efficacy profile of these agents to deliver a plasmid carrying the CFTR cDNA to the ovine airway epithelium by aerosol administration was compared. The results showed that GL67A was overall the best gene transfer agent for aerosol delivery to the sheep lung, and was selected for clinical trials in CF patients (McLachlan et al., 2011). In an ongoing clinical trial by the UK CF Gene Therapy Consortium and funded by the CF Trust, CF patients were given a single dose of a plasmid carrying the CFTR cDNA, complexed to the cationic lipid GL67A. This initial single-dose clinical trial will assess the safety and duration of CFTR expression in patients. Another clinical trial is planned for to determine whether repeated non-viral CFTR gene transfer (12 doses over 12 months) will improve CF lung disease (Sinn et al., 2011).

3. Tracking the CFTR in cells using GFP-CFTR fusion protein

The green fluorescent protein (GFP) is a 27-kDa protein from the jellyfish *Aequorea victoria*, discovered by Shimomura and co-workers in the 1960's and was shown to emit bright green fluorescence under UV light (Shimomura et al., 1962). It took another 30 years before this protein was cloned and its functionality demonstrated in different organisms (Prasher et al., 1994 ; Chalfie et al. 1994; Inouye and Tsuji 1994 ; Tsien, 1998). The GFP is widely used today as a biological marker in cell biology and gene transfer technology. The GFP can be detected in living cells without selection or staining, and be genetically fused to other proteins to produce fluorescent chimeras and generally does not alter the function or cellular localization of the fusion protein (Gerdes and Kaether, 1996 ; Lippincott-Schwartz and Smith, 1997). It is used as a reporter protein for studying complex biological processes such as organelle dynamics and protein trafficking. In gene transfer experiments, the GFP serves an *in vivo* marker, allowing for the determination of gene transfer efficiency and for selection of cells positive for the transgene. Other applications of GFP in gene therapy involve the use of GFP-tagged therapeutic proteins to determine the site, level and duration of expression, or for the correlation between gene transfer efficiency and therapeutic outcome (Wahlfors et al., 2001).

3.1 Construction and *in vitro* applications of GFP-CFTR

The CFTR protein is a 1,480 residue glycosylated molecule with 12 transmembrane domains and 3 intracytoplasmic domains (Figure 1). The protein is highly glycosylated at two asparagine residues on the extracellular loop 4, in both the immature and mature-glycosylated forms (Sheppard and Welsh, 1999). The immature CFTR has a high content of oligosaccharides of the mannoside type, and exists in the endoplasmic reticulum as a precursor before its transit to the trans-Golgi network. During the transit, the CFTR is processed into its mature form with the addition of complex carbohydrate chains containing polylactosaminoglycan sequences (O'Riordan et al., 2000). A functional CFTR requires the protein to be fully glycosylated, and its function as a chloride channel in epithelial cells is dependent on its cellular trafficking and transport to the apical membrane.

The first direct visualization of the CFTR protein within cells was made possible by the genetic fusion of the green fluorescent protein (GFP) to the N-terminus of the CFTR protein. The choice of adding the GFP-tag at the N-terminus (Figure 1) was such that it would have minimal interference with the membrane-targeting signal thought to be encoded in the C-terminus of the protein (Milewski et al., 2001; Moyer et al., 1998). Functional and cell trafficking studies of the CFTR protein and its mutants were made possible with the expression of the GFP-fused protein in different cell lines, using expression plasmids (Moyer et al., 1999; Loffing-Cueni et al., 2001; Haggie, Stanton, and Verkman, 2002). The GFP-CFTR fusion construct displayed functionality in terms of apical membrane localisation in Madin-Darby Canine Kidney (MDCK) cells. Short circuit current measurements showed that the protein mediated cAMP-activated transepithelial chloride transport across monolayers of stably transfected MDCK cells (Moyer et al., 1998). Studies of the dynamics of CFTR protein responses to bacterial infections, the manner by which the CFTR protein responds to, interacts with, and mediates translocation of *P. aeruginosa* and serovar *S. typhi* from the cell surface into the cell were also done using a GFP-CFTR fused protein (Gerçeker et al., 2000).

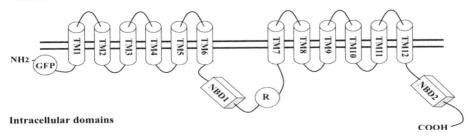

Fig. 1. Schematic representation of the GFP-CFTR fusion protein and the topology of the different domains. The GFP is located on the N-terminus of the CFTR protein. GFP, green fluorescent protein ; TM, transmembrane domain ; NBD1, nucleotide binding domain 1 ; NBD2, nucleotide binding domain 2 ; R, regulatory domain ; NH2, protein aminoterminus ; COOH, protein carboxyterminus.

3.2 *Ex vivo* applications of GFP-CFTR

The GFP-CFTR fusion constructs have also been inserted into viral vectors such as Adenovirus (Vais, 2004; Granio et al., 2007; Granio et al., 2010) and Sendai virus (Ban et al., 2007) to facilitate the detection and direct tracking of the protein after gene transfer. When the Ad vectors, Ad5-GFP-CFTR and Ad5-GFP-CFTRΔF508, were used to transduce reconstituted airway epithelium from ΔF508 CF patients, the biologically active GFP-CFTR and the mutant GFP-CFTRΔF508 proteins could be directly tracked in the epithelial cells by confocal fluorescence microscopy due to their GFP-tag (Granio et al., 2007 ; see Figure 2, A and B). The GFP-CFTR protein (green) was observed to be located on the apical membrane of the reconstituted airway epithelium, at the same plane as the ZO-1 protein (red) which is the marker for tight junctions at the apical membrane. The nuclei of the cells were stained blue with DAPI (Figure 2, A and B). In epithelial cells infected with the Ad5 expressing the GFP-CFTRΔF508, the fluorescence was observed in the central and basal areas of the cytoplasm and none expressed at the apical surface (Figures 2, B and D). This was the first report showing the direct localization of an exogenous GFP-tagged CFTR protein on reconstituted human epithelial cells after Ad-mediated gene transfer (Granio et al., 2007).

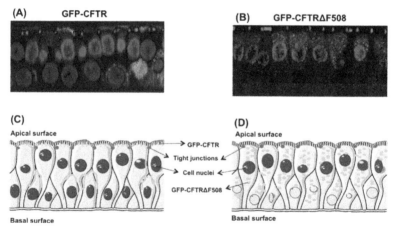

Fig. 2. Cellular localisation of the GFP-CFTR and GFP-CFTRΔF508 protein in *ex vivo* reconstituted human airway epithelium after gene transfer with Ad5-GFP-CFTR (A) and Ad5-GFP-CFTRΔF508 (B). (A), (B) : reconstructed images of sagittal sections of transduced epithelia generated from the z-stack images obtained in confocal fluorescence microscopy. (C), (D) : schematic representation of the images shown in (A) and (B), respectively.

The availability of appropriate cell receptors at the apical surface of airway epithelial cells is a crucial factor for the efficient uptake of viral vectors. A majority of viral vectors such as Adenovirus, AAV, Measles virus and pseudotyped retroviruses can only infect airway epithelial cells via the basal membrane (Kremer et al., 2007; Sinn et al., 2002; Teramoto et al., 1998; Zabner et al., 1997). Airway epithelial cells are not easily transduced by Ad5-based vectors as the Coxsackie-Adenovirus Receptor (CAR), a high affinity receptor for Ad5 and many other Ad serotypes vectors are mainly localised in the tight junctions and not at the apical surface (Walters et al., 1999), and thus not accessible to Ad vectors. One strategy of overcoming this physical barrier was to design an Ad vector which will recognise a receptor expressed on the apical surface of airway epithelium. The Ad serotype 35 (Ad35) or a chimeric Ad5F35 vector (a serotype 5 capsid carrying serotype 35 fibers), which both recognise CD46 as receptor, a molecule found on the apical surface of human airway epithelium (Gaggar, Shayakhmetov, and Lieber, 2003; Sinn et al., 2002; Corjon et al., 2011) would be capable of directly infecting the airway epithelia from the apical membrane .

The demonstration was recently made with a chimeric Ad5F35 vector expressing GFP-CFTR. This chimeric vector transduced efficiently well-differentiated human airway epithelium via the apical membrane and showed stable expression of the GFP-CFTR protein. Measurements of transepithelial ion transport showed the correction of the chloride channel function at relatively low vector doses in ΔF508 CF airway epithelial cells (Granio et al., 2010). This is a successful example of a viral vector which was genetically modified to target a receptor on the apical surface of the airway epithelial cells for efficient gene transduction. In a separate study using an *in vivo* mice model, the Ad5F35 vector was found to preferentially target the lungs of CD46-transgenic mice after systemic administration of the vector (Greig et al., 2009). The chimeric Ad5F35 vector therefore shows promise as an efficient lung targeted gene transfer vector for CF.

3.3 *In vivo* applications of GFP-CFTR

A study was conducted to determine whether a GFP-CFTR fusion protein was functional as a transgene when expressed *in vivo*, in colonic and airway epithelial cells of CF mice, and had the capacity to correct the CF defect. To assess the *in vivo* function of the GFP-CFTR, bitransgenic mice *cftr ~Ss1D/~551D KI8-GFP-CFTR +/-* were obtained by breeding K 18-GFP-CFTR mice to *cftr c551D/c551D* CF mice. The analysis of transcripts, protein and electrolyte transport in the colon and airways indicated that the K18-GFP-CFTR was expressed and partially restored the ion transport in the G551D CF mice model. Thus, it appeared that *in vivo*, the GFP-CFTR fusion protein was capable of supporting the complex interactions required to regulate epithelial chloride transport (Oceandy et al., 2003).

4. Development of new vectors for CFTR transfer

4.1 Human parainfluenza virus

The human parainfluenza virus type 3 (PIV3) can infect the human airway epithelium and specifically targets ciliated epithelial cells (Zhang et al., 2005). *In vitro* studies using PIV3-based vectors for *CFTR* gene transfer to CF epithelial cells resulted in the complete reversal of the CF phenotype, with the transepithelial ion transport, airway surface liquid volume regulation and mucus transport, restored to levels observed in non-CF epithelial cells (Zhang et al., 2009). *In vivo* administration of a PIV3 vector carrying a transgene coding for the rhesus α-fetoprotein (rhAFP) to the nasal epithelium of the rhesus macaque (*Macaca mulatta*) showed expression and secretion of the rhAFP in the mucosal and serosal compartments. The transgene expression was transient and paralleled vector persistance, suggesting that as PIV3 was cleared, rhAFP expression was lost (Zhang et al., 2010). The specificity of the PIV3 vectors for the airways make them particularly interesting as gene transfer vectors for CF therapy.

4.2 Respiratory syncytial virus

The respiratory syncytial virus (RSV) can infect the lungs of CF patients, despite the physical barriers of the respiratory tract, such as the sticky and mucus-rich environment of the CF lung. In addition, this virus has a natural tropism for the luminal ciliated cells of the airways (Zhang et al., 2002). It was suggested that since RSV has the capacity for reinfections, repeated administrations of an RSV-based vector would be possible. Recently, it was demonstrated that a RSV vector carrying the *CFTR* gene can infect both non-CF and CF airway epithelium, and in particular the ciliated cells. In CF cells, the CFTR was expressed at the apical surface and showed correction of chloride channel activity which was equivalent in level observed in normal human airway epithelial cultures. Further studies in animal models are needed to determine the immune response to this vector, as well as its persistence in single and repeated administration (Kwilas et al., 2010).

4.3. Integrative vectors

The major goal of gene therapy is to have the delivered transgene safely and stably maintained in replicating cells. One approach to achieve genetic stability is via integration of the transgene into the host cell genome, using integrating vectors such as retrovirus and AAV vectors. The main dangers of integrative vectors are their uncontrolled or random integration which can cause (i) transgene silencing if the insertion occurs in condensed heterochromatin, or (ii) insertional mutagenesis if the integration event occurs near growth-promoting genes leading to oncogenesis. The latter was encountered with lentivirus and AAV vectors, in animal models as well as in human clinical trials (Donsante et al., 2007; Hacein-Bey-Abina S, 2003).

Just as for Ad vectors, lentiviral gene transfer to the human airway epithelium is inefficient due to the lack of receptors. The strategy of "pseudotyping" or substitution of the lentivirus envelope with the envelope protein of another virus, such as Ebola virus (Kobinger et al., 2003), baculovirus (Sinn et al., 2008) or Sendai virus (Mitomo et al., 2010) have demonstrated increase in gene transfer efficiency to the airway epithelium. Before the application of lentiviral vectors for pulmonary gene transfer, preclinical studies in large animal models will need to be carried out to carefully assess their efficacy and safety.

4.4 Episomal vectors

Extrachromosomal or episomal vectors are gene transfer agents which has the capacity of persisting in the nucleus of transduced cells without integrating into the host genome. Due to their nonintegrative nature, there is theoretically no risk of the physical disruption of the cell genome. In addition, episomal vectors can persist in multiple copies per cell, resulting in high expression of the therapeutic gene (Lufino, Edser, and Wade-Martins, 2009). Many of the episomal systems which has been developed are based on sequences derived from viruses such as the Epstein-Barr and Polyoma viruses, which have certain phases of their viral life cycle maintained episomally. The two major requirements of episomal vectors are the presence of a viral origin of replication and the expression of a virally encoded protein which is necessary for vector replication and its repartition into the daughter cells upon cell division.

4.4.1 Polyoma-derived episomal vectors

The first stable episomal plasmid vector described in the literature contained sequences derived from the BK virus which belongs to the polyomavirus family. This episomal vector which carried most of the BK viral genome could persist at a stable copy number of 20–120 copies/cell, depending on the cell line used, and showed low percentage of integration events (Milanesi et al., 1984). Its replication depended on the presence of the BK-derived origin of replication and a *trans*activating factor, a viral protein called large T antigen, which is responsible for binding to the viral origin of replication and mediating the vector replication. Replicating vectors based on Simian Vacuolating virus 40 (SV40) were among the first viral-based episomal systems to be developed. SV40 is a nonenveloped DNA virus with a double-stranded genome belonging to the family of polyomaviruses (Vera and Fortes, 2004). The SV40-derived vectors are composed of a *cis*-acting elements, essentially the SV40 origin of replication, and the sequence encoding for the SV40 T antigen.

4.4.2 Epstein-Barr-derived episomal vector

The major progress toward the development of an efficient episomal gene transfer vector came from plasmids based on the Epstein-Barr virus (EBV), a member of the family of herpesviruses. The EBV is capable of life-long persistence as an extrachromosomal, circular multicopy plasmid carried by B-lymphocytes in a latent state (Lindahl et al., 1976). The origin of replication (*oriP*, origin of plasmid replication) of EBV requires the *trans*-acting factor EBV Nuclear Antigen-1 (EBNA-1) for replication (Rawlins et al., 1985; Yates, Warren, and Sugden, 1985). The EBNA-1 binds to metaphase chromosomes and interphase chromatin, and this interaction facilitates the partition of *oriP* plasmids into daughter cells during mitosis (Ito et al., 2002). Plasmid constructs containing EBV episomal elements have been tested in pre-clinical animal models for treatment of diseases such as hemophilia and diabetes. The delivery of the EBV-based episomes were made by injections to the target tissues. Although the efficacy of transduction was less efficient *in vivo* compared to viral vectors, long term expression of the therapeutic gene was obtained (Mei et al., 2006 ; Yoo et al., 2006).

4.4.3 Adeno-EBV hybrid episomal vector

A hybrid Adenovirus-EBV (Ad-EBV) episomal vector has a major interest as it exploits the advantages of both vectors, combining the efficiency of gene transfer of the Ad vector with the episomal replicative nature of the EBV vector. Helper-dependent adenovirus (HD-Ad) vectors which are deleted of all viral coding regions, also known as gutless Ad, (Kochanek et al., 1996 ; Parks et al., 1996), are also interesting vectors as they are less immunogenic. The use of HD-Ad vectors for the development of episomal Ad-EBV vector brings further advantage to these vectors for their use in gene therapy.

Circular replicating Ad-EBV vectors can be obtained by co-infecting an adenovirus carrying EBNA-1 and *oriP* elements with a *loxP* site at both ends, with a second adenovirus encoding Cre recombinase, whose expression will result in the circularisation of the first virus (Dorigo et al., 2004; Gallaher et al., 2009). Another strategy described for obtaining circular Ad episomes which does not rely on the expression of a viral protein such as EBNA-1, was based on the human origin of replication derived from the *lamin B2* locus with the site-specific FLPe recombinase and *Frt* recognition sites. This vector system produces circular episomes free of viral coding or bacterial DNA sequences (Kreppel and Kochanek, 2004). A more recent study described the development of an HD-Ad-EBV vector in which Cre recombinase is transiently expressed from a hepatocyte-specific promoter such that the vector generation and transgene expression are tissue specific. The results obtained using this strategy were highly promising as long-term persistence of the circularized vector DNA and stable transgene expression in hepatocytes was observed in immunocompetent mice (Gil et al., 2010).

5. Conclusions

Profitable lessons have been drawn from the past two decades of CF gene therapy trials using different transfer vectors. The numerous difficulties and problems encoutered have helped in the improvement and design of future gene transfer vectors. New viral vectors such as RSV and PIV which specifically targets cilliated lung epithelial cells have been developed for pulmonary gene transfer. Significant improvement have been made for high-density Ad episomal vectors to achieve efficiency and specificity of transduction, coupled to long-term vector persistance and stable transgene expression. In parallel, the GFP has served as a very useful *in vivo* marker for the evaluation of gene transfer vectors. The visualization of CFTR protein *in situ* by means of the GFP fluorescent tag has contributed towards a better comprehension of CFTR multiple functions such as its cellular trafficking and the dynamics of its interactions with intracellular as well as extracellular partners.

6. Acknowledgments

The authors are grateful to the French Cystic Fibrosis Foundation (Vaincre la Mucoviscidose, VLM) and the University of Lyon 1 for their support. GG is financially supported by a doctoral fellowship from VLM. SSH is an INSERM Research Associate. PB is Emeritus Professor of the University of Lyon 1.

7. References

Arcasoy, S.M., Latoche, J., Gondor, M., Watkins, S. C., Henderson, A., Hughey, R., Finn, O.J., & Pilewski, J.M. (1997). MUC1 and other sialoglycoconjugates inhibit adenovirus-mediated gene transfer to epithelial cells. *Am. J. Respir. Cell Mol. Biol.* 17, 422-435.

Ban, H., Inoue, M., Griesenbach, U., Munkonge, F., Chan, M., Iida, A., Alton, E.W.F. W., & Hasegawa, M. (2007). Expression and maturation of Sendai virus vector-derived CFTR protein: functional and biochemical evidence using a GFP-CFTR fusion protein. *Gene Ther.* 14, 1688-1694.

Boucher, R. C. (1999). Status of gene therapy for cystic fibrosis lung disease. *J. Clin. Invest.* 103, 441-445.

Caplen, N.J., Alton, E.W., Middleton, P.G., Dorin, J.R., Stevenson, B.J., Gao, X., Durham, S.R., Jeffery, P.K., Hodson, M.E., Coutelle, C., Huang, L., Porteous, D.J., Williamson

R., & Geddes. D.M. (1995). Liposome-mediated CFTR gene transfer to the nasal epithelium of patients with cystic fibrosis. *Nat. Med.* 1, 39–46

Chalfie, M., Tu, Y., Euskirchen, G., Ward, W.W. & Prasher, D.C. (1994). Green fluorescent protein as a marker for gene expression. *Science* 263, 802-805.

Chow, Y.H., Plumb, J., Wen, Y., Steer, B.M., Lu, Z., Buchwald, M., & Hu, J. (2000). Targeting transgene expression to airway epithelia and submucosal glands, prominent sites of human CFTR expression. *Mol. Ther.* 2, 359-367.

Corjon, S., Gonzalez, G., Henning, P., Grichine, A., Lindholm, L., Boulanger, P., Fender, P. & Hong, S.S. (2011). Cell entry and trafficking of human adenovirus bound to blood factor X is determined by the fiber serotype and not hexon:heparan sulfate interaction. *PLoS One*, 6, e18205.

Crystal, R. G. (1995). Transfer of genes to humans: early lessons and obstacles to success. *Science* 270, 404-410.

Donsante, A., Miller, D.G., Li, Y., Vogler, C., Brunt, E. M., Russell, D.W., & Sands, M.S. (2007). AAV vector integration sites in mouse hepatocellular carcinoma. *Science* 317, 477.

Dorigo, O., Gil, J. S., Gallaher, S.D., Tan, B.T., Castro, M.G., Lowenstein, P.R., Calos, M. P., & Berk, A.J. (2004). Development of a novel helper-dependent adenovirus-Epstein-Barr virus hybrid system for the stable transformation of mammalian cells. *J. Virol.* 78, 6556-6566.

Ferrari, S., Geddes, D.M., & Alton, E.W.F.W. (2002). Barriers to and new approaches for gene therapy and gene delivery in cystic fibrosis. *Adv. Drug Deliv. Rev.* 54, 1373-1393.

Gaden, F., Franqueville, L., Hong, S.S., Legrand, V., Figarella, C., & Boulanger, P. (2002). Mechanism of restriction of normal and cystic fibrosis transmembrane conductance regulator-deficient human tracheal gland cells to adenovirus infection and ad-mediated gene transfer. *Am. J. Respir. Cell Mol. Biol.* 27, 628-640.

Gaden, F., Franqueville, L., Magnusson, M.K., Hong, S.S., Merten, M.D., Lindholm, L., & Boulanger, P. (2004). Gene transduction and cell entry pathway of fiber-modified adenovirus type 5 vectors carrying novel endocytic peptide ligands selected on human tracheal glandular cells. *J. Virol.* 78, 7227-7247.

Gaggar, A., Shayakhmetiv, D.M., & Lieber, A. (2003). CD46 is a cellular receptor for group B adenoviruses. *Nat. Med.* 9, 1408-1412.

Gahery-Segard, H., Farace, F., Godfrin, D., Gaston, J., Lengagne, R., Tursz, T., Boulanger, P., & Guillet, J. G. (1998). Immune response to recombinant capsid proteins of adenovirus in humans: antifiber and anti-penton base antibodies have a synergistic effect on neutralizing activity. *J. Virol.* 72, 2388-2397.

Gallaher, S.D., Gil, J.S., Dorigo, O., & Berk, A.J. (2009). Robust in vivo transduction of a genetically stable Epstein-Barr virus episome to hepatocytes in mice by a hybrid viral vector. *J. Virol.* 83, 3249-3257.

Gerçeker, A.A., Zaidi, T., Marks, P., Golan, D.E., & Pier, G.B. (2000). Impact of heterogeneity within cultured cells on bacterial invasion: analysis of *Pseudomonas aeruginosa* and *Salmonella enterica* Serovar Typhi entry into MDCK cells by using green fluorescent protein-labelled cystic fibrosis transmembrane conductance regulator receptor. *Infect. Immun.* 68, 861-870.

Gerdes, H.H., & Kaether, C. (1996). Green fluorescent protein: applications in cell biology. *FEBS Lett.* 389, 44-47.

Gil, J.S., Gallaher, S.D., & Berk, A.J. (2010). Delivery of an EBV episome by a self-circularizing helper-dependent adenovirus: long-term transgene expression in immunocompetent mice. *Gene Ther.* 17, 1288-1293.

Granio, O., Ashbourne Excoffon, K.J.D., Henning, P., Melin, P., Norez, C., Gonzalez, G., Karp, P.H., Magnusson, M.K., Habib, N., Lindholm, L., Becq, F., Boulanger, P., Zabner, J., & Hong, S.S. (2010). Adenovirus 5-fiber 35 chimeric vector mediates efficient apical correction of the cystic fibrosis transmembrane conductance regulator defect in cystic fibrosis primary airway epithelia. *Hum. Gene Ther.* 21, 251-269.

Granio, O., Norez, C., Ashbourne Excoffon, K.J.D., Karp, P.H., Lusky, M., Becq, F., Boulanger, P., Zabner, J., & Hong, S.S. (2007). Cellular localization and activity of Ad-delivered GFP-CFTR in airway epithelial and tracheal cells. *Am. J. Respir. Cell Mol. Biol.* 37, 631-639.

Greig, J.A., Buckley, S.M., Waddington, S.N., Parker, A.L., Bhella, D., Pink, R., Rahim, A.A., Morita, T., Nicklin, S.A., McVey, J.H., & Baker, A.H. (2009). Influence of coagulation factor X on in vitro and in vivo gene delivery by adenovirus (Ad) 5, Ad35, and chimeric Ad5/Ad35 vectors. *Mol. Ther.* 17, 1683-1691.

Griesenbach, U., Alton, E.W.F.W., & Consortium., o. b. o. t. U. C. F. G. T. (2009). Gene transfer to the lung: Lessons learned from more than 2 decades of CF gene therapy. *Adv. Drug Del. Rev.* 61, 128-139.

Griesenbach, U., Geddes, D.M., & Alton, E.W.F.W. (2004). Gene therapy for cystic fibrosis: an example for lung gene therapy. *Gene Therapy* 11, S43-S50.

Hacein-Bey-Abina, S., Von Kalle C., Schmidt, M., McCormack, M.P., Wulffraat, N., Leboulch, P., Lim, A., Osborne, C.S., Pawliuk, R., Morillon, E., Sorensen, R., Forster, A., Fraser, P., Cohen, J.I., de Saint Basile, G., Alexander, I., Wintergerst, U., Frebourg, T., Aurias, A., Stoppa-Lyonnet, D., Romana, S., Radford-Weiss, I., Gross, F., Valensi, F., Delabesse, E., Macintyre, E., Sigaux, F., Soulier, J., Leiva, L.E., Wissler, M., Prinz, C., Rabbitts, T.H., Le Deist, F., Fischer, A., & Cavazzana-Calvo, M. (2003). LMO2-associated clonal T cell proliferation in two patients after gene therapy for SCID-X1. *Science* 302, 415-419.

Haggie, P.M., Stanton, B.A., & Verkman, A.S. (2002). Diffusional mobility of the cystic fibrosis transmembrane conductance regulator mutant, dF508-CFTR, in the endoplasmic reticulum measured by photobleaching of GFP-CFTR chimeras. *J. Biol. Chem.* 277, 16419-16425.

Harvey, B.G., Leopold, P.L., Hackett, N.R., Grasso, T.M., Williams, P.M., Tucker, A.L., Kaner, R.J., Ferris, B., Gonda, I., Sweeney, T.D., Ramalingam, R., Kovesdi, I., Shak, S., & Crystal, R.G. (1999). Airway epithelual CFTR mRNA expression in cystic fibrosis patients after repetitive administration of a recombinant adenovirus. *J. Clin. Invest.* 104, 1245-1255.

Henning, P., Magnusson, M.K., Gunneriusson, E., Hong, S.S., Boulanger, P., Nygren, P. A., & Lindholm, L. (2002). Genetic modification of Ad5 tropism by a novel class of ligands based on a three-helix bundle scaffold derived from staphylococcal protein A. *Hum. Gene Ther.* 13, 1427-1439.

Hida, K., Lai, S. K., Suk, J.S., Won, S.Y., Boyle, M.P., & Hanes, J. (2011). Common gene therapy viral vectors do not efficiently penetrate sputum from cystic fibrosis patients. *PLoS One* 6(5), e19919.

Hong, S.S., Magnusson, M.K., Henning, P., Lindholm, L., & Boulanger, P. (2003). Adenovirus (Ad) stripping: a novel method to generate liganded Ad vectors with new cell target specificity. *Mol. Ther.* 7, 692-699.

Inouye, S. & Tsuji, F.I. (1994). *Aequorea* green fluorescent protein. Expression of the gene and fluorescence characteristics of the recombinant protein. *FEBS Lett.* 341, 277-280.

Ito, S., Gotoh, E., Ozawa, S., & Yanagi, K. (2002). Epstein-Barr virus nuclear antigen-1 is highly colocalized with interphase chromatin and its newly replicated regions in particular. *J. Gen. Virol.* 83, 2377-2383.

Kammouni, W., Moreau, B., Becq, F., Saleh, A., Pavirani, A., Figarella, C., & Merten, M.D. (1999). A cystic fibrosis tracheal gland cell line, CF-KM4. Correction by adenovirus-mediated CFTR gene transfer. *Am. J. Respir. Cell Mol. Biol.* 20, 684-691.

Kobinger, G.P., Schumer, G.P., Medina, M.F., Weiner, D.J. & Wilson, J.M. (2003). Stable and efficient gene transfer in airway of non-human primates with HIV vector pseudotyped with deletion mutant of the Ebola envelope glycoproteins. *Pediatr. Pulmonol. Suppl.* 25, 256.

Kochanek, S., Clemens, P.R., Mitani, K., Chen, H.H., Chan, S., & Caskey, C.T. (1996). A new adenoviral vector: replacement of all viral coding sequences with 28 kb of DNA independently expressing both full-length dystrophin and beta-galactosidase. *Proc. Natl. Acad. Sci. USA* 93, 5731-5736.

Kolb, M., Martin, G., Medina, M., Ask, K., & Gauldie, J. (2006). Gene therapy for pulmonary diseases. *Chest* 130, 879-884.

Kremer, K.L., Dunning, K.R., Parsons, D.W., & Anson, D.S. (2007). Gene delivery to airway epithelial cells in vivo: a direct comparison of apical and basolateral transduction strategies using pseudotyped lentivirus vectors. *J. Gene Med.* 9, 362-368.

Kreppel, F., & Kochanek, S. (2004). Long-term transgene expression in proliferating cells mediated by episomally maintained high-capacity adenovirus vectors. *J. Virol.* 78, 9-22.

Kwilas, A.R., Yednak, M.A., Zhang, L., Liesman, R., Collins, P.L., Pickles, R.J. & Peeples, M.E. (2010). Respiratory syncytial virus engineered to express the cystic fibrosis transmembrane conductance regulator corrects the bioelectric phenotype of human cystic fibrosis airway epithelium *in vitro. J. Virol.* 84, 7770-7781.

Lindahl, T., Adams, A., Bjursell, G., Bornkamm, G.W., Kasch-Dierich, C., & Jehn, U. (1976). Covalently closed circular duplex DNA of Epstein-Barr virus in a human lymphoid cell line. *J. Mol. Biol.* 102, 511-530.

Lippincott-Schwartz, J., & Smith, C.L. (1997). Insights into secretory and endocytic membrane traffic using fluorescent protein chimeras. *Curr. Opin. Neurobiol.* 7, 631-639.

Loffing-Cueni, D., Loffing, J., Shaw, C., Taplin, A.M., Govindan, M., Stanton, C.A., & Stanton, B.A. (2001). Trafficking of GFP-tagged dF508-CFTR to the plasma membrane in a polarized epithelial cell line. *Am. J. Physiol. Cell Physiol.* 281, C1889-C1897.

Lufino, M.M.P., Edser, P.A.H., & Wade-Martins, R. (2009). Advances in high-capacity extrachromosomal vector technology: episomal maintenance, vector delivery and transgene expression. *Mol. Ther.* 16, 1525-1538.

Magnusson, M.K., Henning, P., Myhre, S., Wikman, M., Uil, T. G., Friedman, M., Andersson, K.M.E., Hong, S.S., Hoeben, R.C., Habib, N.A., Stahl, S., Boulanger, P., & Lindholm, L. (2007). An Ad5 vector genetically re-targeted by an AffibodyTM molecule with specificity for tumor antigen HER2/neu. *Cancer Gene Ther.* 14, 468-479.

Magnusson, M.K., Hong, S.S., Boulanger, P., & Lindholm, L. (2001). Genetic re-targeting of adenovirus: a novel strategy employing 'de-knobbing' of the fiber. *J. Virol.* 75, 7280-7289.

McLachlan, G., Davidson, H., Holder, E., Davies, L.A., Pringle, I.A., Sumner-Jones, S.G., Baker, A., Tennant, P., Gordon, C., Vrettou, C., Blundell, R., Hyndman, L., Stevenson, B., Wilson, A., Doherty, A., Shaw, D.J., Coles, R.L., Painter, H., Cheng, S.H., Scheule, R.K., Davies, J.C., Innes, J.A., Hyde, S.C., Griesenbach, U., Alton, E.W., Boyd, A.C., Porteous, D.J., Gill, D.R., & Collie, D.D. Pre-clinical evaluation of three non-viral gene transfer agents for cystic fibrosis after aerosol delivery to the ovine lung. (2011). *Gene Ther.* Epub ahead of print, doi:10.1038/gt.2011.55

Mei, W. H., Qian, G. X., Zhang, X. Q., Zhang, P., and Lu, J. (2006). Sustainied expression of Epstein-Barr virus episomal vector mediated factor VIII in vivo following muscle electroporation. *Haemophilia* 12, 271-279.

Merten, M.D., Kammouni, W., Renaud, W., Birg, F., Mattei, M.G., & Figarella, C. (1996). A transformed human tracheal gland cell line, MM-39, that retains serous secretory functions. *Am. J. Respir. Cell Mol. Biol.* 15, 520-528.

Milanesi, G., Barbanti-Brodano, G., Negrini, M., Lee, D., Corallini, A., Caputo, A., Grossi, M.P., & Ricciardi, R.P. (1984). BK virus-plasmid expression vector that persists episomally in human cells and shuttles into Escherichia coli. *Mol. Cell Biol.* 4, 1551-1560.

Milewski, M.I., Mickle, J.E., Forrest, J.K., Stafford, D.M., Moyer, B.D., Cheng, J., Guggino, W.B., Stanton, B.A., & Cutting, G.R. (2001). A PDZ-binding motif is essential but not sufficient to localize the C terminus of CFTR to the apical membrane. *J. Cell Sci.* 114, 719-726.

Mitomo, K., Griesenbach, U., Inoue, M., Somerton, L., Meng, C., Akiba, E., Tabata, T., Ueda, Y., Frankel, G.M., Farley, R., Singh, C., Chan, M., Munkonge, F., Brum, A., Xenariou, S., Escudero-Garcia, S., Hasegawa, M., & Alton, E.W. (2010). Toward gene therapy for cystic fibrosis using a lentivirus pseudotyped with Sendai virus envelopes. *Mol. Ther.*, 18, 1173–1182.

Moss, R.B., Milla, C., Colomba, J., Accurso, F., Zeitlin, P.L., Clancy, J.P., Spencer, L.T., Pilewski, J., Waltz, D.A., Dorkin, H.L., Ferkol, T., Pian, M., Ramsey, B., Carter, B.J., Martin, D.B., & Heald, A.E. (2007). Repeated aerosolized AAV-CFTR for treatment of cystic fibrosis: a randomised placebo-controlled phase 2B trial. *Hum. Gene Ther.* 18, 726-732.

Moyer, B.D., Loffing, J., Schwiebert, E.M., Loffing-Cueni, D., Halpin, P.A., Karlson, K.H., Ismailov, I.I., Guggino, W.B., Langford, G.M., & Stanton, B.A. (1998). Membrane trafficking of the cystic fibrosis gene product, cystic fibrosis transmembrance conductance regulator, tagged with green fluorescent protein in Madin-Darby canine kidney cells. *J. Biol. Chem.* 273, 21759-21768.

Moyer, B.D., Loffing-Cueni, D., Loffing, J., Reynolds, D., & Stanton, B.A. (1999). Butyrate increases apical membrane CFTR but reduces chloride secretion in MDCK cells. *Am. J. Physiol. Renal Physiol.* 277, F271-276.

O'Riordan, C.R., Lachapelle, A.L., Marshall, J., Higgins, E.A., & Cheng, S.H. (2000). Characterization of the oligosaccharide conductance regulator. *Glycobiology* 10, 1225-1233.

Oceandy, D., McMorran, B., Schreiber, R., Wainwright, B.J., & Kunzelmann, K. (2003). GFP-tagged CFTR transgene is functional in the G551D cystic fibrosis mouse colon. *J. Membrane Biol.* 192, 159-167.

Otake, K., Ennist, D.L., Harrod, K., & Trapnell, B.C. (1998). Nonspecific inflammation inhibits adenovirus-mediated pulmonary gene transfer and expression independent of specific acquired immune responses. *Hum. Gene Ther.* 9, 2207-2222.

Parks, R.J., Chen, L., Anton, M., Sankar, U., Rudnicki, M.A., & Graham, F.L. (1996). A helper-dependent adenovirus vector system: removal of helper virus by Cre-mediated excision of the viral packaging signal. *Proc. Natl. Acad. Sci. USA* 93, 13565-13570.

Perricone, M.A., Morris, J.E., Pavelka, K., Plog, M.S., O'Sullivan, B.P., Joseph, P.M., Dorkin, H., Lapey, A., Balfour, R., Meeker, D.P., Smith, A.E., Wadsworth, S.C., & St George, J.A. (2001). Aerosol and lobar administration of a recombinant adenovirus to individuals with cystic fibrosis. ii. transfection efficiency in airway epithelium. *Hum. Gene Ther.* 12, 1383-1394.

Perricone, M.A., Rees, D.D., Sacks, C.R., Smith, K.A., Kaplan, J.M., & St George, J.A. (2000). Inhibitory effect of cystic fibrosis sputum on adenovirus-mediated gene transfer in cultured epithelial cells. *Hum. Gene Ther.* 11, 1997-2008.

Piedra, P.A., Poveda, G.A., Ramsey, B., McCoy, K., & Hiatt, P.W. (1998). Incidence and prevalence of neutralizing antibodies to the common adenoviruses in children with cystic fibrosis: implication for gene therapy with adenovirus vectors. *Pediatrics* 101, 1013-1019.

Pollard, H., Toumaniantz, G., Amos, J.L., Avet-Loiseau, H., Guihard, G., Behr, J.P. & Escande, D. (2001). Ca^{2+}-sensitive cytosolic nucleases prevent efficient delivery to the nucleus of injected plasmids. *J. Gene Med.* 3, 153-164.

Prasher, D.C., Eckenrode, V.K., Ward, W.W., Prendergast, F.G. & Cormier, M.J. (1992). Primary structure of the *Aequorea victoria* green-fluorescent protein. *Gene* 111, 229-233.

Rawlins, D.R., Milman, G., Hayward, S.D., & Hayward, G.S. (1985). Sequence-specific DNA binding of the Epstein-Barr virus nuclear antigen (EBNA-1) to clustered sites in the plasmid maintenance region. *Cell* 42, 859-868.

Rosenfeld, M.A., Yoshimura, K., Trapnell, B.C., Yoneyama, K., Rosenthal, E.R., Dalemans, W., Fukayama, M., Bargon, J., Stier, L.E., Stratford-Perricaudet, L., Perricaudet, M., Guggino, W.B., Pavirani, A., Lecocq, J.-P., & Crystal, R.G. (1992). In vivo transfer of the human cystic fibrosis transmembrane conductance regulator gene to the airway epithelium. *Cell* 68, 143-155.

Scaria, A., St George, J.A., Jiang, C., Kaplan, J.M., Wadsworth, S.C., & Gregory, R.J. (1998). Adenovirus-mediated persistent cystic fibrosis transmembrane conductance regulator expression in mouse airway epithelium. *J. Virol.* 72, 7302-7309.

Sheppard, D., & Welsh, M.J. (1999). Structure and function of the CFTR chloride channel. *Physiol. Rev.* 79, S23-S45.

Shimomura, O., Johnson, F.H., & Saiga, Y. (1962). Extraction, purification and properties of aequorin, a bioluminescent protein from the luminous hydromedusan, *Aequorea. J. Cell Comp. Physiol.* 59, 223-239.

Sinn, P.L., Williams, G., Vongpunsawad, S., Cattaneo, R., & McCray Jr, P.B. (2002). Measles virus preferentially transduces the basolateral surface of well-differentiated human airway epithelia. *J. Virol.* 76, 2403-2409.

Sinn, P.L., Arias, A.C., Brogden, K.A. & McCray, P.B. Jr (2008). Lentivirus vector can be readministered to nasal epithelia without blocking immune responses. *J. Virol.,* 82, 10684-10692.

Sinn, P.L., Reshma, M.A., & McCray Jr, P.B. (2011). Genetic therapies for cystic fibrosis lung disease. *Human Mol. Genetics,* 20, R79-R86.

Teramoto, S., Bartlett, J.S., McCarty, D., Xiao, X., Samulski, R.J., & Boucher, R.C. (1998). Factors influencing adeno-associated virus-mediated gene transfer to human cystic fibrosis airway epithelial cells: comparison with adenovirus vectors. *J. Virol.* 72, 8904-8912.

Toh, M.L., Hong, S.S., van de Loo, F., Franqueville, L., Lindholm, L., van den Berg, W., Boulanger, P., & Miossec, P. (2005). Enhancement of Ad-mediated gene delivery to rheumatoid arthritis synoviocytes and synovium by fiber modifications: role of RGD and non-RGD-binding integrins. *J. Immunol.* 175, 7687-7698.

Tsien, R.Y. (1998). The green fluorescent protein. *Ann. Rev. Biochem.* 67, 509-544.

Vais, H., Gao, G.P., Yang, M., Tran, P., Louboutin, J.P., Somanathan, S., Wilson, J.M., & Reenstra, W.W. (2004). Novel adenoviral vectors coding for GFP-tagged wtCFTR and deltaCFTR: characterization of expression and electrophysiological properties in A549 cells. *Pflugers Arch.,* 449, 278-287.

Vera, M., & Fortes, P. (2004). Simian virus-40 as a gene therapy vector. *DNA Cell Biol.* 23, 271-282.

Wagner, J.A., Messner, A.H., Moran, M.L., Daifuku, R., Kouyama, K., Desch, J.K., Manley, S., Norbash, A.M., Conrad, C.K., Friborg, S., Reynolds, T., Guggino, W.B., Moss, R.B., Carter, B.J., Wine, J.J., Flotte, T.R., & Gardner, P. (1999). Safety and biological efficacy of an adeno-associated virus vector-cystic fibrosis transmembrane regulator (AAV-CFTR) in the cystic fibrosis maxillary sinus. *Laryngoscope* 109, 266-274.

Wahlfors, J., Loimas, S., Pasanen, T., & Hakkarainen, T. (2001). Green fluorescent protein (GFP) fusion constructs in gene therapy research. *Histochem. Cell Biol.* 115, 59-65.

Walters, R.W., Grunst, T., Bergelson, J.M., Finberg, W., Welsh, M.J., & Zabner, J. (1999). Basolateral localization of fiber receptors limits adenovirus infection from the apical surface of airway epithelia. *J. Biol. Chem.* 274, 10219-10226.

Welsh, M.J., Zabner, J., Graham, S.M., Smith, A.E., Moscicki, R.A., & Wadsworth, S.C. (1995). Adenovirus-mediated gene transfer for cystic fibrosis. Part A. Safety of dose and repeat administration in the nasal epithelium. Part B. Clinical efficacy in the maxillary sinus. *Hum. Gene Ther.* 6, 205-218.

Yates, J.L., Warren, N., & Sugden, B. (1985). Stable replication of plasmids derived from Epstein-Barr virus in various mammalian cells. *Nature* 313, 812-815.

Yoo, H. S., Mazda, O., Lee, H. Y., Kim, J. C., Kwon, S. M., Lee, J. E., Kwon, I. C., Jeong, H., Jeong, Y. S., and Jeong, S. Y. (2006). In vivo gene therapy of type I diabetic mellitus using a cationic emulsion containing an Epstein-Barr virus-based plasmid vector. *J. Control Release* 112, 139-144.

Zabner, J., Couture, L.A., Gregory, R.J., Graham, S.M., Smith, A.E., & Welsh, M.J. (1993). Adenovirus-mediated gene transfer transiently corrects the chloride transport defect in nasal epithelia of patients with cystic fibrosis. *Cell* 75, 207-216.

Zabner, J., Freimuth, P., Puga, A., Fabrega, A., & Welsh, M.J. (1997). Lack of high affinity fiber receptor activity explains the resistance of ciliated airway epithelia to adenovirus infection. *J. Clin. Invest.* 100, 1144-1149.

Ziady, A.G., Kelley, T.J., Milliken, E., Ferkol, T., & Davis, P.B. (2002). Functional evidence of CFTR gene transfer in nasal epithelium of cystic fibrosis mice *in vivo* following luminal application of DNA complexes targeted to the serpin-enzyme complex receptor. *Mol. Ther.* 5, 413-419.

Zhang, L., Peeples, M.E., Boucher, R.C., Collins, P.L., & R. J. Pickles. (2002). Respiratory syncytial virus infection of human airway epithelial cells is polarized, specific to ciliated cells, and without obvious cytopathology. *J. Virol.* 76, 5654–5666.

Zhang, L., Bukreyev, A., Thompson, C.I., Watson, B., Peeples, M.E., Collins, P.L., & Pickles, R.J. (2005). Infection of ciliated cells by human parainfluenza virus type 3 in an in vitro model of human airway epithelium. *J. Virol.* 79, 1113–1124.

Zhang, L., Button, B., Gabriel, S.E., Burkett, S., Yan, Y., Skiadopoulos, M.H., Dang, Y.L., Vogel, L.N., McKay, T., Mengos, A., Boucher, R.C., Collins, P.L., & Pickles, R.J. (2009). CFTR delivery to 25% of surface epithelial cells restores normal rates of mucus transport to human cystic fibrosis airway epithelium. *PLoS Biol.* 7, e1000155.

Zhang, L., Limberis, M.P., Thompson, C., Antunes, M.B., Luongo, C., Wilson J.M., Collins, P.L. & Pickles, R.J. (2010). α-fetoprotein gene delivery to the nasal epithelium of nonhuman primates by human parainfluenza viral vectors. *Hum. Gene Ther.* 21, 1657-1664.

7

Pharmacological Modulators of Sphingolipid Metabolism for the Treatment of Cystic Fibrosis Lung Inflammation

M.C. Dechecchi et al.*
Laboratory of Molecular Pathology, Laboratory of Clinical Chemistry and Haematology,
University Hospital of Verona, Verona,
Italy

1. Introduction

Cystic Fibrosis (CF) lung disease is characterised by progressive chronic infection and inflammation of the airways. This prolonged airway inflammatory response leads to irreversible lung damage and fibrosis which is believed to be driven by two distinct, coordinated events: *a)* a defective cystic fibrosis transmembrane regulator (CFTR) causes airway surface dehydration and increased mucus viscosity leading to chronic colonization with *Pseudomonas aeruginosa* (*P.aeruginosa*) (Boucher, 2007); *b)* mutated CFTR triggers the generation of pro-inflammatory and chemotactic cytokines orchestrated by bronchial epithelial cells, independently of infection (Rubin, 2007; Elizur et al., 2008). The chemokine IL-8, abundantly expressed at sites of chronic inflammation, seems to play a major role in driving the formation of neutrophil (PMN)-rich exudates into the lung of CF patients (Khan et al., 1995; Noah et al., 1997; DiMango et al., 1998; Puchelle et al., 2001; Joseph et al., 2005; Perez et al., 2007). Therefore, reduction of the exaggerated production of IL-8 is key therapeutic target in CF. Anti-inflammatory drugs are an attractive therapeutic tool in CF aimed to decrease the rate of decline in lung function. However, the inherent complexity of the inflammatory response combined with the obvious dependency on this response to contain infection and the side effect profiles of common anti-inflammatories, have made identifying the most suitable therapy a major priority.

*E. Nicolis[1], P. Mazzi[2], M. Paroni[3], F. Cioffi[4], A. Tamanini[1],V. Bezzerri[1], M. Tebon[1], I. Lampronti[5], S. Huang[6], L. Wiszniewski[6], M.T. Scupoli[4], A. Bragonzi[3], R. Gambari[5], G. Berton[2] and G. Cabrini[1]
[1]Laboratory of Molecular Pathology, Laboratory of Clinical Chemistry and Haematology, University Hospital of Verona, Verona, Italy
[2]Department of Pathology, University of Verona, Italy
[3]Infections and Cystic Fibrosis Unit, San Raffaele Scientific Institute, Milano, Italy
[4]Interdepartmental Laboratory for Medical Research (LURM) and Department of Clinical and Experimental Medicine - Section of Haematology, University of Verona, Italy
[5]Department of Biochemistry and Molecular Biology, University of Ferrara, Ferrara, Italy
[6]Epithelix Sàrl, Genève, Switzerland*

Consensus is growing on sphingolipids (SLs) as novel targets to cure pulmonary disorders including CF, since modulation of cellular ceramide reduces lung inflammation (Lahiri and Futerman, 2007; Uhlig and Gulbins, 2008). The results in the area of ceramide and CF pathophysiology are very interesting, although contradicting due to the animal models used and methods of ceramide detection (Wojewodka , 2011). The accumulation of ceramide has been identified as one of the key regulators of inflammation in CF airways in different CFTR-/- mouse models (Teichgraber, 2008). On the contrary, decreased ceramide levels have been shown in CFTR ko mice (Guibault, 2008). The possible explanation for this discrepancy seems to be the special diet required for CFTR ko mice, that severely affects the concentration of SLs. Other possible causes, such as genetic determinants, could influence individual levels of SLs (Hicks, 2009). In a different study, no significant difference has been found in basal ceramide levels in immortalised CF bronchial epithelial cells and lung homogenate from CFTR ko mice compared to wild type cells and mice (Yu, 2009). Very importantly, ceramide has been demonstrated to accumulate in the lower airways of CF patients and to be positively associated with neutrophilic inflammation (Brodlie, 2010), supporting the hypothesis that reduction of ceramide may be a therapeutic target for CF lung inflammation.

Extending our previous study (Dechecchi, 2008), we have recently demonstrated that the iminosugar N-butyldeoxynojirimycin (miglustat), an inhibitor of the first step in glycosphingolipid (GSL) biosynthesis, reducing the *P.aeruginosa* induced immunoreactive ceramide expression, produces an anti-inflammatory effect in human bronchial epithelial cells *in vitro* and down-regulates the neutrophil chemotaxis in murine lungs *in vivo* (Dechecchi, 2011). These findings strengthen the notion that the metabolism of SLs can be manipulated as a therapeutic option for CF lung disease. With regard to new treatments for CF lung pathology, miglustat deserves great attention since it restores CFTR function in respiratory and pancreatic cells *in vitro* (Norez, 2006; Dechecchi, 2008) and in CF mice (Lubamba, 2009) and produces an anti-inflammatory effect *in vitro* and *in vivo* (Dechecchi, 2011). Notably, miglustat is a FDA-approved and EMA-designated orally bioavailable orphan drug, used in Europe and USA for the treatment of Gaucher disease and other GSL storage diseases.

In this chapter we review the pre-clinical evidence on the anti-inflammatory effect of miglustat in comparative effectiveness studies with the SL inhibitor amitriptyline and the glucocorticoid (GC) dexamethasone. Importance will be placed on the efficacy of each anti-inflammatory molecule to balance between the anti-inflammatory activity and possible impairment of the host defence.

2. CF bronchial cells seem to be resistant to the treatment with glucocorticoids

Chronic inflammation is commonly treated by a number of approaches including fast-acting symptomatic drugs, such as non-steroidal anti-inflammatory drugs (NSAIDs), glucocorticoids and slow-acting disease-modifying anti-rheumatic drugs, such as low-dose methotrexate. In the treatment of chronic lung inflammation of CF patients, corticosteroids and NSAIDs have garnered the most attention, to date. Although traditional treatments with corticosteroids and ibuprofen have demonstrated potential benefits in CF patients, their use is limited by severe adverse effects, as for high doses of prednisone, or by a narrow pharmacological window, as in the case of ibuprofen (Birke, 2001; Koehler, 2004; Konstan, 2005). The endobronchial location makes CF pulmonary inflammation potentially amenable to inhaled therapies, thus achieving much higher concentrations in the airway epithelium and limiting the adverse effects of long term systemic use. As the airway epithelium is targeted by inhaled agents, bronchial epithelial cells *in vitro* have been widely used to prove the efficacy of these drugs. The glucocorticoid dexamethasone, largely used in the treatments of inflammatory conditions is scarcely effective in reducing the expression of the chemokine IL-8 in CF bronchial epithelial cells (Figure 1). As a matter of fact, it produces inhibitory effect only at the higher dose (30 μM) (Figure1A) in CF bronchial epithelial IB3-1 cells whereas it fails to reduce the transcription of IL-8 in Cufi-1 cells (Figure 1B). Different from the results obtained in CF CuFi-1 cells, treatment with dexamethasone results in reducing the inflammatory response, in non CF NuLi-1 cells (Figure 1C). These findings suggest that CF bronchial cells seem to be resistant to GC treatment, consistent with scarce efficacy of GC treatment observed in CF patients.

3. *P.aeruginosa* stimulated IL-8 mRNA expression is reduced in CF bronchial epithelial cells treated with inhibitors of SL metabolism miglustat and NB-DGJ

The role of CFTR deficiency in promoting inflammation remains unclear. Inhibition of function of wild type CFTR by CFTR$_{inh172}$ (Perez, 2007) or correction of F508del mutated CFTR function by MPB-07 or miglustat (Dechecchi, 2007; 2008) regulates the inflammatory response to *P. aeruginosa*, suggesting that the pro-inflammatory circuitry in CF airways could be initiated from those epithelial cells lacking CFTR function. However the galactose analogue *N*-butyldeoxygalactonojirimycin (NB-DGJ), which is not a corrector of F508del-CFTR function (Norez, 2006), similarly reduces the PAO1 stimulated IL-8 mRNA expression in CF cells (Figure 2). Additionally this reduction has been obtained both in CF and non CF cells with both miglustat and NB-DGJ (Dechecchi, 2008). Therefore, miglustat affects the inflammatory response to *P. aeruginosa* through a mechanism which, at least partly, is independent of the correction of F508del-CFTR function. As far as the effect of miglustat and NB-DGJ on immune response is concerned, they could affect the host response to *P.aeruginosa* through the regulation of SL metabolism, in particular CerGlcT and/or non lysosomal glucosylceramidase, an activity shared by both compounds (Butters, 2005), thus strengthening the notion that metabolism of SLs can be manipulated as a therapeutic option for CF lung disease.

4. Amitriptyline reduces IL-8 gene expression in CF bronchial cells

Two main routes have been defined for the generation of ceramide: hydrolysis of sphingomyelin (SM) by acid sphingomyelinase (ASM) and *de novo* biosynthesis (Hannun, 2008). Ceramide generated by ASM plays an important role in the infection by *P. aeruginosa* since it reorganizes into rafts required to internalize bacteria, induce apoptosis and regulate the cytokine response (Grassme', 2003). Treatment of CF mice by ASM inhibitors, such as amitriptyline and others tricyclic antidepressants, has been shown to reduce the degree of inflammation (Teichgraber, 2008; Becker, 2010). Notably, amitriptyline results in dose dependent inhibition of IL-8 transcription by bronchial epithelial cell lines IB3-1 and CuFi-1, infected with *P.aeruginosa* (Figure 3), consistent with the overall anti-inflammatory

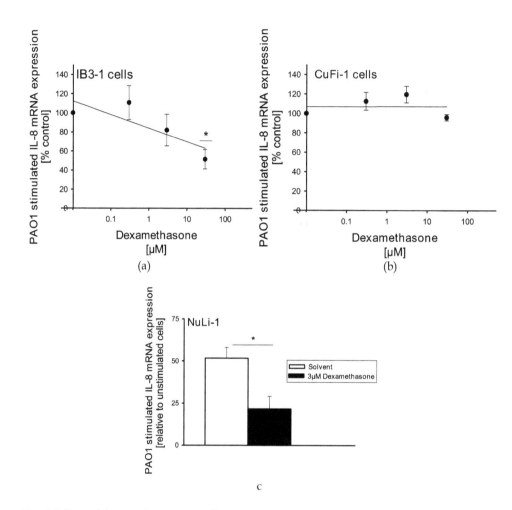

Fig. 1. Effect of dexamethasone on inflammatory response to *P.aeruginosa* in CF and non CF bronchial epithelial cells.

IB3-1 (human bronchial epithelial cell line) (Zeitlin, 1991) (*A*), CuFi-1 (F508del/F508del CFTR mutant genotype) (*B*) and NuLi-1 (*C*), (wild type CFTR) (Zabner, 2003) cell lines were treated with dexamethasone, at doses indicated in the figure, or solvent alone, for 24 hours and then infected with *P.aeruginosa* strain PAO1 (kindly provided by A. Prince, Columbia University, New York)(50CFU/cell) for 4 hours at 37° C. The inflammatory response was evaluated by studying the expression of mRNA of IL-8, measured by Real-time qPCR as described (Dechecchi, 2008) and obtained by comparing the ratio IL-8 and the housekeeping gene GAPDH between non infected and infected cells. Results are expressed as mean ± standard error of the mean (n=5). Comparisons between groups were made by using Student's *t* test. Statistical significance was defined with $p<0.05$. * , *p* value <0.05.

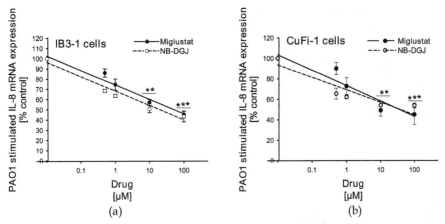

Fig. 2. Result of miglustat and NB-DGJ on *P.aeruginosa* stimulated IL-8 mRNA expression in CF bronchial cell lines IB3-1 and CuFi-1 cells.

IB3-1 (*A*) and CuFi-1 (*B*) cells were treated with miglustat, NB-DGJ, at doses indicated in the figure, or solvent alone for 24 hours and then infected with PAO1 as in Figure 1. Stimulated IL-8 mRNA expression was calculated as indicated in the legend of Figure 1 and expressed as % of untreated cells. Data reported are mean ± standard error of the mean of 3 independent experiments, performed in duplicate. **, p value < 0.01; ***, p value < 0.001.

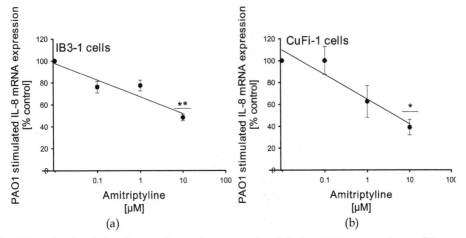

Fig. 3. Result of amitriptyline on *P.aeruginosa* stimulated IL-8 mRNA expression in CF bronchial cell lines IB3-1 and CuFi-1 cells

IB3-1 (*A*) and CuFi-1 (*B*) cells were treated with amitriptyline, at doses indicated in the figure, or solvent alone for 24 hours and then infected with PAO1 as in Figure 1. Stimulated IL-8 mRNA expression was calculated as indicated in the legend of Figure 1 and expressed as % of untreated cells. Data reported are mean ± standard error of the mean of 8 (IB3-1) or 6 (CuFi-1) independent experiments, performed in duplicate. *, *p* value <0.05; **, p value < 0.01.

effect reported in CF murine lungs (Teichgraber, 2008; Becker, 2010). Interestingly, we have recently demonstrated that, besides inhibiting IL-8 transcription, both miglustat and amitriptyline reduce the *P.aeruginosa* induced immunoreactive ceramide expression (Dechecchi, 2011), by targeting different pathways of SL metabolism: CerGlcT and/or non-lysosomal glucosylceramidase (miglustat) and ASM (amitriptyline). As far as the effect on immune response is concerned, the same overall decrease of ceramide could regulate the transmembrane signaling between the receptors for pathogens and the transcription of the inflammatory genes, thus reducing inflammation.

5. Miglustat and amitriptyline inhibit the pro-inflammatory signaling downstream the receptors for *P.aeruginosa* and for pro-inflammatory cytokines

The importance of ceramide as a pro-inflammatory mediator derives from its capability to activate protein kinases and phosphatases in different downstream pathways and from the generation of second messengers (Hannun, 2008). Ceramide is produced in response to various stimulants such as cytokines, heat, UV radiation, lipopolysaccharide (LPS) and other agents thus leading to specific and overlapping events that include the activation of a common set of kinases and transcription factors. Both miglustat and amitriptyline inhibit the expression of IL-8 mRNA stimulated by either *P.aeruginosa* or TNFα or IL-1β (Figure 4), indicating that they affect the pro-inflammatory signaling downstream and in common with the receptors for *P. aeruginosa* and for these pro-inflammatory cytokines. Importantly, ceramide-induced activation of the transcription factor NF-kB and p38 kinase amplifies the production of several inflammatory mediators and adhesion molecules (Won, 2004). Therefore, it can be hypothesized that miglustat and amitriptyline, decreasing plasma membrane ceramide, generated by *P.aeruginosa* infection or pro-inflammatory cytokines, attenuate the activation of NF-kB mediated signaling cascade which in turn down-regulates the immune response.

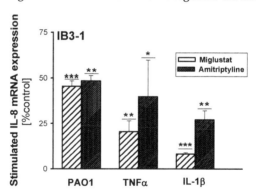

Fig. 4. Effect of miglustat and amitriptyline on IL-8 gene expression stimulated by *P.aeruginosa*, TNFα or IL-1β.

IB3-1 cells were treated with miglustat (100μM), amitriptyline (10μM) or solvent alone for 24 hours and then infected with PAO1 or stimulated by the pro-inflammatory cytokines TNF α (10ng/ml) or IL-1 β (50 ng/ml) for 4 hours at 37°C as in Figure 1. Stimulated IL-8 mRNA expression was calculated as indicated in the legend of Figure 1 and expressed as % of untreated cells. Data reported are mean ± standard error of the mean of 3 independent experiments performed in duplicate. *, p value <0.05; **, p value < 0.01; ***, p value < 0.001.

6. Miglustat down-regulates the expression of key genes involved in neutrophil chemotaxis in human bronchial CF epithelial cells

The infection of a host by a pathogenic microorganism initiates complex cascade of events directed toward the recruitment of defence mechanisms. Parallel analysis of gene expression provides a new tool for studying interplay of signals and transcriptional responses in biological systems. Infection of IB3-1 cells with the *P.aeruginosa* strain PAO1, for a short time (4 hours), up-regulates the expression of genes involved in the inflammatory response, mainly neutrophil chemotaxis, such as the chemokines IL-8, Gro-$\alpha/\beta/\gamma$, GCP-2, the adhesion molecule ICAM-1, the cytokines IL-1α/β, IL-6, TNF-α, the antimicrobial peptide HBD-4, Toll-like receptor 2 and NFKB1 (Figure 5A). These results obtained in CF cell line correlate with findings in cultured human bronchial epithelial primary cells derived from the bronchi of CF patients (Figure 5B), which exhibit many of the morphological and functional characteristics believed to be associated with CF airway disease (Neuberger, 2011) and recall many features of the colonization of the respiratory epithelium by pathogens. As far as host defence mechanisms are concerned, bronchial epithelium is not simply a physical barrier against invading pathogens but is also an important source of inflammatory mediators, actively involved in the immune response. Therefore cultured CF bronchial cells provide a useful tool for the pre-clinical testing of novel pharmacotherapies. Indeed, miglustat has an anti-inflammatory effect in CF bronchial cells, since it reduces the expression of key genes induced by *P.aeruginosa* and IL-8 protein release (Dechecchi, 2011). Also amitriptyline has an anti-inflammatory effect in CF bronchial cell lines (Figure 5A) and at lower extent in CF primary cells (Figure 5B). Regarding the therapeutic activity of amitriptyline, it should be noted that systemic inhibition of ASM might negatively affect the host defence, as demonstrated by studies on mice completely lacking ASM which were found to be unable to control infections (Grassme', 2003). Moreover, since amitriptyline inhibits serotonin and noradrenaline uptake in presynaptic nerve ending (Maubach, 1999), it might cause severe adverse effects in long term use in CF children. As with all treatments, utility will largely depend on the balance between potential risks and benefits.

7. Miglustat up-regulates the transcription of the antimicrobial peptide HBD-4

The treatment of CF patients with drug aimed to limit the excessive inflammatory response could mean that they become vulnerable to infections. As a matter of fact, dexamethasone down-regulates the expression of HBD-4 (Figure 6), an antimicrobial peptide induced by infectious or inflammatory stimuli, that plays an important role in the host innate immune response, with strong activity against *P.aeruginosa* (Yanagi, 2005). This result is consistent with suppression of *b*-defensins by GC treatment, already reported (Jang, 2007). On the other hand, well known huge side effects of long term use of steroids limit their clinical utility in CF patients (Nichols, 2008). On the contrary, miglustat up-regulates the expression of HBD-4, both in cell lines and primary cells (Figures 5 and 6), adding ground to the suggestion that miglustat could not compromise the ability to resist infection with pathogens in CF patients. Additionally, results on the safety of miglustat obtained during the first 5 years of the clinical studies, do not report any increased susceptibility to bacterial infections in patients affected by Gaucher disease (Hollak, 2009). All this considered the proximity to a treatment of CF lung inflammation with miglustat is real and promising.

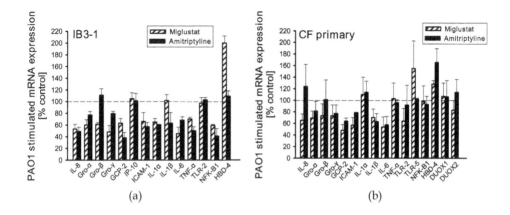

(a)   (b)

Fig. 5. Inflammatory response to *P.aeruginosa* in IB3-1 and CF primary cells treated with miglustat or amitriptyline.

IB3-1 cells (*A*) and human airway epithelium reconstituted in vitro with cells isolated from CF patients and cultivated on micro-porous filters at air-liquid interface (MucilAir™, Epithelix Sàrl, Genève, Switzerland) (*B*) were treated with miglustat (100μM), amitriptyline (10μM) or solvent alone for 24 hours and then infected with PAO1. The inflammatory response was evaluated by studying the expression of several genes known to be associated with host immune defences by RNA macroarrays (TaqMan Low Density Array, Applied Biosystems, Foster City, CA) as detailed (Dechecchi, 2011). Stimulated mRNA expression was calculated as indicated in the legend of Figure 1 and expressed as % of untreated cells. (*A*) IB3-1 cells. Miglustat significantly reduces the expression of IL-8, ICAM-1, TNF-α (**, p value<0.01), gro-α/β/γ, GCP-2, IL-1α, IL-6 and NFKB1(*, *p* value<0.05) and increases the expression of HBD-4 (**, p value<0.01). Amitriptyline significantly reduces the expression of IL-8, Gro-α, ICAM-1 (**, p value<0.01), gro-γ, GCP-2, IL-1α/1β, IL-6, TNF-α and NFKB1(*, *p* value<0.05) (n=6). (*B*) CF primary cells. Miglustat significantly reduces the expression of IL-8, GCP-2, ICAM-1, TNF-α, IL-6 (*, *p* value<0.05) and increases the expression of HBD-4 (*, p value<0.05). Amitriptyline significantly reduces the expression of GCP-2, ICAM-1, IL-1β, IL-6 (*, *p* value<0.05) and increases the expression of HBD-4 (*, p value<0.05) (n=4).

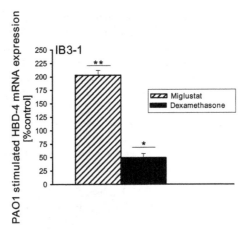

Fig. 6. *P.aeruginosa* stimulated transcription of the antimicrobial peptide HBD-4 in IB3-1 cells: result of miglustat and dexamethasone.

IB3-1 cells were treated with miglustat (100μM), dexamethasone (30μM) or solvent alone for 24 hours and then infected with PAO1 as in Figure 1. Stimulated HBD-4 mRNA expression was measured by Real-time qPCR as described (Dechecchi, 2011), calculated as indicated in the legend of Figure 1 and expressed as % of untreated cells. Data reported are mean ± standard error of the mean of 5 independent experiments performed in duplicate. **, p value<0.01 (miglustat); *, p value<0.05 (dexamethasone).

8. Miglustat down-regulates neutrophil chemotaxis in the early inflammatory response *in vivo*

The pressing challenge for the discovery of new drugs is to transform findings from bench studies into effective therapies. The success of results obtained with CFTR correctors and potentiators suggests that primary coltures of human airway epithelia will likely be the model system of choice for future proof of principle studies of experimental therapeutics (Neuberger, 2011). With regard to miglustat, the anti-inflammatory effect observed in CF primary cells (Dechecchi, 2011) provides a significant body of evidence concerning the utility of miglustat in modifying lung inflammation. However, an essential requirement for entering clinical trial is a thorough testing in pre-clinical animal models. As a matter of fact development of new animal models of CF such as CFTR knock-out pigs (Rogers, 2008), raises the possibility to employ these animals to evaluate new treatments. Murine models of acute and chronic infection with *P.aeruginosa*, along with mice genetically modified for the CFTR gene, are a key asset in CF research and mimic many of the characteristic features of CF lung pathology (Bragonzi, 2010). Additionally, mice with the airway specific over expression of the Na+ channel βENaC, develop a CF−like lung inflammation (Mall, 2004). These models have provided insights in the effectiveness of anti-inflammatory therapy in reducing lung damage. Interestingly, lung inflammation of βENaC over expressing mice seems to be resistant to GC treatment (Livraghi, 2009) and amitriptyline reduces the degree of inflammation in CFTR-/- mice (Teichgraber, 2008; Becker 2010). As far as the effectiveness of miglustat is concerned, it reduces the recruitment of PMN into the bronchoalveolar space induced by intranasal instillation of LPS (Figure 7A) (Dechecchi, 2011). The pharmacokinetic profile and tissue distribution of miglustat, after oral dosing in small rodents, demonstrate that it is well absorbed, exhibits a bioavailability of 40-60%, is widely distributed within the body and, notably, it is present at high concentrations in the lung 1 hour after administration (Treiber, 2007). Indeed, a treatment schedule of an oral administration with miglustat one hour before the intra tracheal inoculum with *P. aeruginosa* is effective in reducing the inflammatory response associated to acute pneumonia in terms of leukocyte recruitment and myeloperoxidase (MPO) activity in the airways (Figure 7B and Figure 7C). Taken together, these results indicate that miglustat may down-regulates neutrophil recruitment in the early phase of the inflammatory response.

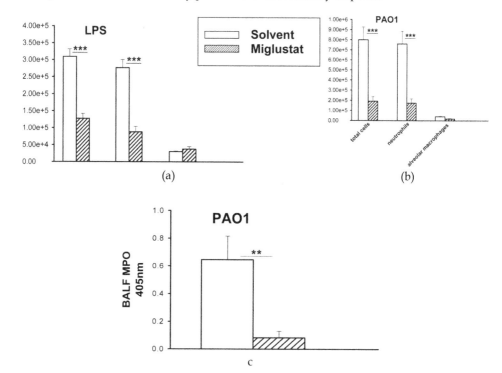

Fig. 7. Effect of miglustat on murine models of lung inflammation.

(A). Aqueous solution of miglustat (100 mg/Kg) or vehicle alone was administered once daily in wild type C57BL/6J mice by intraesophageal gavage, for a period of three consecutive days before pro-inflammatory challenge with LPS by intranasal instillation. Bronchoalveolar lavage fluid (BALF) was examined 4 hrs after challenge, as described (Dechecchi, 2011). Data reported are mean ± standard error of the mean. n=6(vehicle), n=12 (miglustat). ***, p value < 0.001. (B and C). C57BL/6 mice were infected by intra-tracheal injection with the reference *P. aeruginosa* strain PAO1 (1x10^5 CFU) one hour after oral injection with miglustat (400mg/kg), or vehicle. Mice were sacrificed 4 hours after PAO1 injection and the inflammatory response associated to PAO1-induced acute pneumonia in terms of leukocyte recruitment (B) and MPO activity (C) in the airways was analyzed as described (Bragonzi, 2009, Moalli, 2011). Data reported are mean

± standard error of the mean. n=5 (vehicle), n=6 (miglustat). ***, p value < 0.001(leukocyte recruitment); **, p value < 0.01(MPO activity).

9. Conclusions

Strategies aimed to limit the excessive inflammatory response by targeting neutrophil recruitment are a relevant approach for CF patients. In general, each anti-inflammatory molecule should balance between the anti-infective role of neutrophils and the detrimental effects that they produce in the course of chronic inflammation due to the release of proteases and reactive oxygen species. In this respect, while others anti-inflammatory based therapies have failed in humans with CF in the past, the regulation of SLs may represent a useful potential target for pharmacotherapy. This review summarizes evidence derived from the validation of the anti-inflammatory properties of miglustat in bronchial epithelial cells *in vitro* and in murine models of lung inflammation and infection *in vivo*, demonstrating a down-regulation of neutrophils chemotactic signaling. Recalling that miglustat is an orally bioavailable FDA-approved and EMA−designated orphan available drug, therapeutic trials for CF patients could be envisioned in the near future.

10. Acknowledgment

We are very grateful to A. Tamanini for helpful discussions, F. Quiri and V. Lovato for excellent technical assistance, A. Prince (Columbia University, New York) for the *P.aeruginosa* laboratory strain PAO1, In Vitro Model and Cell Culture Care of the University of Iowa for providing NuLi-1 and CuFi-1 cells.

This research was supported by Italian Cystic Fibrosis Research Foundation (grant FFC # 16/2010) with the contribution of "Assistgroup", "Latteria Montello SpA" and "Delegazione FFC di Imola" (to MCD).

11. References

Becker K.A.; Riethmüller J.; Lüth A.; Döring G.; Kleuser B.; Gulbins E. (2010). Acid Sphingomyelinase Inhibitors Normalize Pulmonary Ceramide and Inflammation in Cystic Fibrosis. Am J Respir Cell Mol Biol. 42(6):716-24

Birke F.W.; Meade C.J.; Anderskewitz R.; Speck G.A.; Jennewein H.M. (2001). In vitro and in vivo pharmacological Characterization of BIIL 284, a novel and potent leukotriene B(4) receptor antagonist. *J Pharmacol Exp Ther.* 297:458-66

Boucher R.C. (2007). Evidence for airway surface dehydration as the initiating event in CF airway disease. *J Intern Med* 261:5−16

Bragonzi A.; Worlitzsch D.; Pier G.B.; Timpert P.; Ulrich M.; Hentzer M.; Andersen J.B.; Givskov M.; Conese M.; Doring G. (2005). Nonmucoid *Pseudomonas aeruginosa* expresses alginate in the lungs of patients with cystic fibrosis and in a mouse model. *J Infect Dis* 192:410-9

Bragonzi A.; Paroni M.; Nonis A.; Cramer N.; Montanari S.; Rejman J.; Di Serio C.; Döring G.; Tümmler B. (2009). *Pseudomonas aeruginosa* microevolution during cystic fibrosis lung infection establishes clones with adapted Virulence. *Am J Respir Crit Care Med.* 180(2):138-45.

Bragonzi A. (2010). Murine models of acute and chronic lung infection with cystic fibrosis pathogens. Int J Med Microbiol. 300(8):584-93.

Brodlie M.; McKean M.C.; Johnson G.E.; Gray J.; Fisher A.J.; Corris P.A.; Lordan J.L.; Ward C. (2010). Ceramide is Increased in the Lower Airway Epithelium of People with Advanced Cystic Fibrosis Lung Disease. Am J Respir Crit Care Med 182 (3): 369-75

Butters T.D.; Dwek R.A. and Platt F.M. (2005). Imino sugar inhibitors for treating the lysosomal Glycosphingolipidoses. Glycobiology 15, 43R-52R.

Dechecchi M.C.; Nicolis E.; Bezzerri V.; Vella A.; Colombatti M.; Assael B.M.; Mettey Y.;Borgatti M.; Mancini I.; Gambari R.; Becq F. and Cabrini G. (2007). MPB-07 reduces the inflammatory response to Pseudomonas aeruginosa in cystic fibrosis bronchial cells. Am J Respir Cell Mol Biol 36, 615-624

Dechecchi M.C.; Nicolis E.; Norez C.; Bezzerri V.; Borgatti M.; Mancini I.; Rizzotti P.; Ribeiro C.M.; Gambari R.; Becq F.;Cabrini G. (2008). Anti-inflammatory effect of miglustat in bronchial epithelial cells. J Cyst Fibros. 7(6):555-65

Dechecchi M.C.; Nicolis E.; Mazzi P.; Cioffi F.; Bezzerri V.; Lampronti I.; Huang S.; Wiszniewski L.; Gambari R.; Scupoli M.T.; Berton G.; Cabrini G. (2011). Modulators of Sphingolipid Metabolism Reduce Lung Inflammation. Am J Respir Cell Mol Biol. Jun 9. [Epub ahead of print]

DiMango E.;Ratner A.J.; Bryan R.; Tabibi S.; Prince A. (1998) Activation of NF-kB by adherent Pseudomonas aeruginosa in normal and cystic fibrosis respiratory epithelial cells. J Clin Invest 101:2598-2605

Elizur A.; Cannon C.L. ; Ferkol T.W. (2008). Airway inflammation in cystic fibrosis. Chest 133:489–495

Grassme' H.; Jendrossek V.; Riehle A.; von Kürthy G.; Berger J.; Schwarz H.; Weller M.; Kolesnick R.; Gulbins E. (2003). Host defense against Pseudomonas aeruginosa requires ceramide-rich membrane rafts. Nature Medicine 9:322-330

Guilbault C.; De Sanctis J.B.; Wojewodka G.; Saeed Z.; Lachance C.; Skinner T.A.; Vilela R.M.; Kubow S.; Lands L.C.; Hajduch M.; Matouk E.; Radzioch D. (2008). Fenretinide corrects newly found ceramide deficiency in cystic fibrosis. Am J Respir Cell Mol Biol. 38(1):47-56

Hannun YA. and Obeid L.M. (2008). Principles of bioactive lipid signaling: lessons from sphingolipids. Nat Rew Mol Cell Biol 9:139-150

Hicks A.A.; Pramstaller P.P.; Johansson A.; Vitart V.; Rudan I.; Ugocsai P.; Aulchenko Y.; Franklin C.; Liebisch G.; Erdmann J.; Jonasson I.; Zorkoltseva I.V.; Pattaro C.; Hayward C.; Isaacs A.; Hengstenberg C.; Campbell S.; Gnewuch C.; Janssens A.C.; Kirichenko A.V.; König I.R.; Marroni F.; Polasek O.; Demirkan A.; Kolcic I.; Schwienbacher C.; Igl W.; Biloglav Z.; Witteman J.C.; Pichler I.; Zaboli G.; Axenovich T.I.; Peters A.; Schreiber S.; Wichmann H.E.; Schunkert H.; Hastie N.; Oostra B.A.; Wild S.H.; Meitinger T.; Gyllensten U.; van Duijn C.M.; Wilson J.F.; Wright A.; Schmitz G.; Campbell H.; (2009). Genetic determinants of circulating sphingolipid concentrations in European populations. PLoS Genet. 5:1-11

Hollak C.E.; Hughes D.; van Schaik I.N.; Schwierin B.; Bembi B. (2009). Miglustat (Zavesca) in type 1 Gaucher disease: 5- year results of a post-authorization safety surveillance programme. Pharmacoepidemiol Drug Saf. 18(9):770-7

Jang B-C.; Lim K-J.; Suh M-H.; Park J-G. and Suh S. (2007). Dexamethasone suppresses interleukin-1B-induced human β-defensin 2 mRNA expression: involvement of p38

MAPk, JNK, MKP-1 and NF-kB transcriptional factor in A549 cells. FEMS Immunol Med Microbiol 51: 171-184

Joseph T.; Look D.; Ferkol T. (2005). NF-kB activation and sustained IL-8 gene expression in primary cultures of cystic fibrosis airway epithelial cells stimulated with *Pseudomonas aeruginosa*. *Am J Physiol Lung Cell Mol Physiol* 288: L471-L479

Khan T.Z. ; Wagener J.S. ; Bost T. ; Martinez J. ; Accurso F.J. ; Riches D.W. ; (1995). Early pulmonary inflammation in infants with cystic fibrosis. *Am J Respir Crit Care Med* 151:1075-1082

Koehler D.R.; Downey G.P.; Sweezey N.B.; Tanswell A.K.; Hu J. (2004) Lung inflammation as a therapeutic target in cystic fibrosis. *Am J Respir Cell Mol Biol* 31:377-381

Konstan M.W.; Doring G. ;Lands L.C.; Hilliard K.A.; Koker P.; Bhattacharya .; Staab A.; Hamilton A.L. (2005). Results of a phase II clinical trial of BIIL284 BS for the treatment of CF lung disease. *Pediatric Pulmonol S* 28: 125-126

Lahiri S. and Futerman A.H. (2007).The metabolism and function of sphingolipids and glycosphingolipid. *Cell Mol Life Sci.* 64: 2270-2284.

Livraghi A.; Grubb B.R.; Hudson E.J.; Wilkinson K.J.; Sheehan J.K.; Mall M.A. O'Neal W.K. Boucher R.C.; Randell S.H. (2009). Airway and lung pathology due to mucosal surface dehydration in {beta}-epithelial Na+ channel- overexpressing mice: role of TNF-{alpha} and IL-4R{alpha} signaling, influence of neonatal development, and limited efficacy of glucocorticoid treatment.J Immunol. 182(7):4357-67

Lubamba B.; Lebacq J.; Lebecque P.; Vanbever R.; Leonard A.; Wallemacq P.; Leal T. (2009). Airway delivery of low-dose miglustat normalizes nasal potential difference in F508del cystic fibrosis mice. *Am J Respir Crit Care Med.* 179:1022-8.

Mall M.; Grubb B.R.; Harkema J.R.; O'Neal W.K.; Boucher R.C. (2004). Increased airway epithelial Na+ absorption produces cystic fibrosis–like lung disease in mice. Nat Med 10:487–493

Maubach K.A.; Rupniak N.M.; Kramer M.S.; Hill R.G. (1999). Novel strategies for pharmacotherapy of depression. Curr Opin Chem Biol. 481-8

Moalli F, Paroni M, Véliz Rodriguez T, Riva F, Polentarutti N, Bottazzi B, Valentino S, Mantero S, Nebuloni M, Mantovani A, Bragonzi A, Garlanda C. The therapeutic potential of the humoral pattern recognition molecule PTX3 in chronic lung infection caused by Pseudomonas aeruginosa. J Immunol. 2011 May 1;186(9):5425-34.

Neuberger T.; Burton B.; Clark H. and Van Goor F. (2011). Use of primary cultures of human bronchial epithelial cells Isolated from cystic fibrosis patients for the pre-clinical testing of CFTR modulators, In: Cystic Fibrosis, Methods in Molecular Biology, M.D. Amaral and K. Kunzelmann (eds), 39-54, Springer Science

Nichols D.P; Konstan M.W. and Chmiel J.F. (2008) Anti-inflammatory therapies for cystic fibrosis-related lung disease. Clinic Rev Aller Immunol 35: 135-153

Noah T.L.; Black H.R.; Cheng P.W,; Wood R.E.; Leigh M.W. (1997) Nasal and bronchoalveolar lavage fluid cytokines in early cystic fibrosis. *J Infect Dis* 175: 638-647

Norez C.; Noel S.; Wilke M.; Bijvelds M.; Jorna H.; Melin P.; DeJonge H. and Becq F. (2006). Rescue of functional delF508- CFTR channels in cystic fibrosis epithelial cells by the α-glucosidase inhibitor miglustat. FEBS Lett. 580:2081- 2086.

Perez A.; Issler A.C.; Cotton C.U.; Kelley T.J.; Verkman A.S.; Davis P.B. (2007). CFTR inhibition mimics the cystic fibrosis inflammatory profile. *Am J Physiol Lung Cell Mol Physiol* 292:L383–395

Puchelle E. ; De Bentzmann S. ; Hubeau C. ; Jacquot J. ; Gaillard D. (2001). Mechanisms involved in cystic fibrosis airway inflammation. *Pediatr Pulmonol* S23:143-5

Rogers C.S.; Stoltz D.a,; Meyerholz D.K. et al (2008). Disruption of the CFTR gene produces a model of cystic fibrosis in newborn pigs. Science 321: 1837-41

Rubin BK. (2007). CFTR is a modulator of airway inflammation. *Am J Physiol Lung Cell Mol Physiol* 292:L381–382.

Teichgraber V.; Ulrich M.; Endlich N.; Riethmüller J.;Wilker B.; De Oliveira-Munding C.C.; van Heeckeren A.M.; Barr M.L.; von Kürthy G.; Schmid K.W.; Weller M.; Tümmler B.; Lang F.; Grassme H.; Döring G.; Gulbins E (2008). Ceramide accumulation mediates inflammation, cell death and infection susceptibility in cystic fibrosis. *Nature Med* 14:382-391

Treiber A.; Morand O. and Clozel M. (2007) The pharmacokinetics and tissue distribution of the glucosylceramide synthase inhibitor miglustat in the rat. Xenobiotica 37:298-314.

Uhlig S.; Gulbins E. (2008). Sphingolipids in the lungs. *Am J Respir Crit Care Med.* 178(11):1100-14

Vicentini L.P.; Mazzi L.; Caveggion E.; Continolo S.; Fumagalli L.; Lapinet-Vera J.A.; Lowell C.A.; Berton G. (2002). Fgr deficiency results in defective eosinophil recruitment to the lung during allergic airway inflammation. *J Immunol* 168: 6446

Wojewodka G.; De Sanctis J.B. and Radzioch D. (2011). Ceramide in Cystic Fibrosis : A potential new target for therapeutic intervention. J of Lipids 2011: 1-13

Won J.S.; Im Y.B.; Khan M.; Singh A.K.; Singh I. (2004). The role of neutral sphingomyelinase produced ceramide in lipopolysaccharide-mediated expression of inducible nitric oxide synthase.J Neurochem. 88:583-93

Yanagi S.; Ashitani J.; Ishimoto H.; Date Y.; Mukae H.; Chino N.; Nakazato M. (2005). Isolation of human beta-defensin-4 in lung tissue and its increase in lower respiratory tract infection. Respir Res. 6:130

Yu H.; Zeidan Y.H.; Wu B.X.; Jenkins R.W.; Flotte T.R.; Hannun Y.A.; Virella-Lowell I. (2009). Defective acid sphingomyelinase pathway with *Pseudomonas aeruginosa* infection in cystic fibrosis. *American Journal of Respiratory Cell and Molecular Biology* 41:367-375

Zabner J.; Karp P.; Seiler M.; Phillips S.L. Mitchell C.J.; Saavedra M.; Welsh M.; Klingelhutz A.J. (2003). Development of cystic fibrosis and non cystic fibrosis airway cell lines. *Am. J. Physiol. Lung Cell Mol. Physiol.* 284:L844-L854.

Zeitlin P.L.; Lu L.; Rhim J.; Cutting G.; Stetten G.; Kieffer K.A.; Craig R.; Guggino W.B. (1991). A cystic fibrosis bronchial epithelial cell line: immortalization by adeno-12-SV40 infection. *Am. J.Respir. Cell Mol Biol* 4: 313-319.

Part 2

Disease Management

8

The Importance of Adherence and Compliance with Treatment in Cystic Fibrosis

Rosa Patricia Arias-Llorente,
Carlos Bousoño García and Juan J. Díaz Martín
Cystic Fibrosis Unit. University Central Hospital of Asturias
Spain

1. Introduction

Over the last few years, the survival of cystic fibrosis (CF) patients has increased markedly. This is attributed to earlier diagnoses of the disease, the improvement of patient care involving multidisciplinary teams and more effective therapeutic options.

The therapeutic requirements of patients with CF are highly complex. Many patients require continuous care at home with many prophylactic medications, such as nebulised or oral antibiotics, pancreatic enzymes, mucolytic agents, vitamin and nutritional supplements as well as daily physiotherapy and a healthy lifestyle with adequate nutrition and exercise. These treatments are intensified and become more complicated during the exacerbation of the disease. Throughout its evolution, other pathologies associated with CF may also occur which require extra treatment regimens.

The complexity of the therapeutic requirements of these patients has added to their longevity. The life-long duration of the treatment and their complexity, have been pointed to as the main determinants of therapeutic adherence. Preventative management and symptomatic treatment are introduced in early childhood for most people with CF, and so management and treatment routines have been a daily concern for most adults for many years. (Kettler et al., 2002; Modi et al., 2006).

All of these difficulties have been identified as determinants of adherence and they are shared with the patients of other chronic diseases. Accordingly, the compliance rate in CF cases is very similar as that of the other chronically ill. In 1979, Sackett and Snow reviewed 537 studies on adherence in chronic disease cases, indicating that the range of adherence for long term preventative regimens was 33-94% with a mean adherence rate of 57% and for long term treatment the range was 41-61% with a mean adherence rate of 54%. Later, poor compliance with medical advice and prescribed treatments in the chronically ill in general is well-documented in the literature, and adherence rarely exceeds 80% and more often it is between 30% and 70%. (Abbott et al., 1996; Conway et al., 1996; Daniels et al., 2011; Kettler et al., 2002; Michaud et al., 1991; Modi et al., 2006).

2. The definition of adherence and compliance

The term compliance is applied when patients follow closely and correctly all the therapeutic indications prescribed by physicians. So, the definition of compliance is "the extent to which patients are obedient and follow the instructions, proscriptions and prescriptions of health professionals". We talk about adherence meaning the extent to which the patient responds to these indications, taking them and 'endorsing' them as his own. This refers not only to medication, but it also includes non-pharmacological measures, such as hygiene, diet controls, etc. (Kettler et al., 2002, as cited in Meichenbaum & Turk, 1987). So, adherence is defined as an "active, voluntary, collaborative involvement of the patient in a mutually acceptable course of behaviour to produce a desired preventative or therapeutic result". However, both terms receive general use and so are treated indifferently in the literature. No doubt the results of adherence are influenced by the definition adopted. Lots of different classifications of adherence – and extent of this has been described – have been assessed from different points of view. Some authors have suggested that patients should be described as fully-adherent, partially-adherent or non-compliant (Lask, 1994). Koocher differentiates the term non-compliant into three groups: those who have an inadequate understanding of the disease, those who present a psychological resistance to disease, and those who – when properly educated – choose not to be compliant (Koocher et al., 1990).

On the other hand, it has been found to be very difficult to classify an individual as compliant. Studies have found that despite compliance, significantly less than 100% could achieve the desired health outcomes (Kettler et al., 2002). However, the cut off point at which they would stop objectifying favourable results and should promote greater compliance is very difficult to define.

Poor adherence can lead to more rapid disease progression. (Abbott et al., 2001; Patterson et al., 1993). Nonetheless, there are studies that reject the existence of a conclusive association between poor compliance and disease progression (Abbott et al., 1994). However, a lack of compliance may increase the number of consultations and hospital admissions with a consequent increase in health spending. In addition, it may hinder the knowledge of the effectiveness of treatments. On the other hand, it is believed that total adherence may not be necessary, as the complete fulfilment of all of the components of a treatment does not guarantee good health. (Abbott et al., 2001). It is known that a patient with poor compliance may stay well, perhaps because of individual responses to different treatments. It is reasonable, therefore, be able to find a balance between the two sides, but is not an easy task for the specialist in relation to these patients.

3. The measurement of adherence

The measure of treatment adherence is not an easy task. We must find a balance between the errors obtained using certain procedures – such as personal interview – and the difficulty in performing other more objective technical procedures.

The methods most commonly used to study adherence in patients with CF include:

3.1 Personal interview

The most frequently used method is to ask directly or take a survey of the patient as to whether the treatment takes place and to what extent it does so. However, patients often tend to overestimate their compliance (Abbott et al., 1996; Conway et al., 1996, Kettler et al., 2002) and frequently this does not reflect the opinion of the specialist. This data can be compared by asking the opinion of the medical team responsible for the patient or else their family. Although this is the easiest and most accessible system for assessing adherence to all kinds of treatments, it cannot be denied that the results are not entirely objective.

3.2 Therapeutic response

Using this method of measuring adherence in such a complex disease as CF and the many variants of treatment can lead to errors. In particular, knowledge of the desired effect achieved by taking a certain drug is almost impossible given the significant interaction between the different treatments.

3.3 Serum or urinary excretion of drugs or their metabolites

The first thing to note is that this is an invasive method and as such it is highly uncomfortable for the patient, who would have to undergo a large number of extractions in order to verify their genuine compliance. This problem is compounded by the pharmacokinetic variations of the substances studied, and it allows the analysis of only certain medications and reports only those drugs that have been recently consumed by the patient.

3.4 Monitoring with electronics, such as aerosol dispensers or nebulisers, that record the date and time of each dispensation

This data would be periodically downloaded for analysis so as to give an idea of adherence. Amongst its advantages it is worth noting that it allows us to guess the behaviour of patients, it is non-invasive, and it allows the collection of data over a long period of time without the patient having to attend hospital. On the other hand, this type of monitoring has its limitations. With its high cost we must also add the fact that data provide information about the use of a medication removed from dispenser. However, it is reasonable to assume that most patients who make the effort to remove medication from the dispenser in the prescribed way will also consume the medication. This technology is limited when used for evaluating physical therapy, and it gives no information on adherence to such treatment regimens as exercise or diet (Kettler et al., 2002; McNamara et al., 2009; Modi et al., 2006).

4. Predictors of compliance

Once the degree of compliance of a patient is measured, it is interesting to know the reasons for why compliance might not be adequate and identify the motivations for good adherence. Understanding the factors that may be related to adherence will enable us to act on them to some degree and so improve compliance and impact upon the course of the disease.

Described below are the factors that have often been studied as predictors of compliance in the literature.

4.1 The relationship between the patient and health professionals

In a chronic disease with a complex treatment such as CF, the relationship of patients with their health professionals is very important. This can have a positive or negative impact on compliance, and so it should foster an environment of trust that allows for good communications between them. Numerous studies have shown that those who believe that it is important to follow your doctor's instructions and those who have confidence in the benefits of their treatment are more compliant. (Abbott et al., 2001; Patterson et al., 1993) The level of adherence has been linked with the knowledge of the specifics associated with prescribed medical treatments. Therefore, the physician must strive to convey adequate information which is detailed yet easy to understand. After all, in many cases the patient has not properly understood the reason for each prescription, as made clear by the fact that 12%-32% of mothers do not fully understand the medical advice concerning their child (Ievers et al., 1999).

Such appropriate information must convince patients that their actions when performing the treatment will impact on the course of their disease. The fact of involving the patient will give us with the ability to schedule a treatment plan together with them and which allows us to improve adherence. To do this, we must recognise that there is no single treatment for all patients and it should be individualised and simplified wherever possible.

Moreover, the maintenance of adequate adherence to prescribed treatments is very important for care monitoring and the provision of adequate supervision, and we should always try not to judge and accept that a lack of enforcement is, to a certain extent, normal with this type of disease (Conway et al., 1996; Lask et al., 1994).

4.2 The severity of the disease

The perception of the severity of the disease differs between doctors and patients. From the doctor's point of view, the patients underestimate the severity of their disease and overestimate their care.

Some authors suggest that adherence is worse amongst those patients with more severe cases due to a lack of positive reinforcement in that they do not notice any beneficial effect resulting from adherence to their treatment (Kettler et al., 2002). However, the severity of the disease has often been evaluated as a possible predictor of adherence in CF cases with conflicting results (Abbott et al., 1994, 1996, 2001; Conway et al., 1996; Gudas et al., 1991; Kettler et al., 2002).

4.3 Social and family relationships

It is very important that patients with CF receive good socio-familial support. Strong family cohesion and adequate social support have been associated with better adherence to treatment. A special importance is attached to the family in the care of patients during childhood, where the burden of treatment compliance during this time of life is maintained by the parents (Battistini et al., 1998; Eddy et al., 1998; Foster et al., 2001; Moise et al., 1987).

However, there are other difficult times, such as adolescence, where receiving strong family support and positive reinforcement is central to maintaining good adhesion to the different treatments that have to meet the needs of these patients. The stresses between parents and children, and poor relationships between parents, are associated with low compliance and could have an adverse impact on the disease and health status of children with CF (Dziuban et al., 2010; Eddy et al., 1998; Foster et al., 2001; Smith et al., 2010).

4.4 Types of treatment

There is wide agreement in the literature over the differences in adherence to the different components of the treatment of patients with CF. While the adherence to antibiotic therapy (80-95%) and intake of enzymes (65-90%) is high, we cannot say the same for habitual physiotherapy, exercise and the taking of vitamins and nutritional supplements, for which compliance is found to be about 40-55%. The high compliance found in relation to certain aspects of the treatment of patients with CF probably reflects the short-term benefit associated with a given treatment or else any immediate unpleasant symptoms which may result from non-compliance. An example of this would be the appearance of steatorrhea as a consequence of ending the intake of pancreatic enzymes in patients with exocrine pancreatic insufficiency. (Abbott et al., 1994; Conway et al., 1996; Daniels et al., 2011; McNamara et al., 2009).

4.5 Age

Treatment adherence tends to decrease with age. Younger children show greater compliance, perhaps because during this time the responsibility for treatment lies with their parents. However, later on during adolescence, adherence decreases when the patient takes responsibility for their own treatment (Bucks et al., 2009; Dziuban et al., 2010; Gudas et al., 1991; Zindani et al., 2006).

The overall compliance of adolescents with CF is around 50%. Several factors, such as the family environment, staff perceptions about their illness, shame of displaying their problem in front of friends, and their relationship with their doctor are all classically associated with compliance, which is difficult to predict at this age due to the multiple factors involved (Michaud et al., 1991). All these factors occur at the time when the adolescent is transferred to the adult specialist (Kettler et al., 2002), and many patients experience suspicion and insecurity which also often tends to affect adherence.

In chronic diseases, the normal behaviour of denial and a reduction of anxiety tend to increase with age in facilitating emotional adjustment in adulthood. So, while these attitudes improve the mental health of these patients they also often negatively affect their adherence (Lask, 1994).

4.6 Epidemiological factors

Demographic factors such as sex, level of educational, knowledge of the disease, socioeconomic status and occupation, and clinical factors such as the age of diagnosis and the frequency of clinical visits, have all been evaluated as possible predictors of adherence in CF cases, and have met with conflicting results (Abbott et al., 1994, 1996, 2001; Dziuban et al., 2010; Gudas et al., 1991; Oerman et al., 2000).

4.7 Ways of coping with the disease

Psychological factors are beginning to emerge as strong predictors of adherence. Classically, it was said that the incidence of mental health disorders in people with CF is recognisably similar to that of the general population. However, high levels of stress are common and require recognition and attention (Abbott et al., 2001; Dziuban et al., 2010; Kettler et al., 2002).

A large percentage of patients with CF and their parents reported elevated symptoms of depression. In a recent study, rates of depressive symptoms were elevated in children with CF and their parents (29% for children, 35% for mothers and 23% for fathers). In addition, child depressive symptoms were significantly associated with lower rates of adherence to airway clearance (Smith et al., 2010).

Moise claims that there are lower levels of psychological distress and better adjustment in patients who use avoidance as a way of coping with illness, and those who use more direct methods and are positive (Moise et al., 1987).

It is well-documented that poor psychological well-being can influence a detrimental physiological function and a disease's progression, morbidity and mortality (Abbott et al., 2001). Perhaps it should be admitted that a degree of non-compliance is normal in these patients.

Concern about their illness and the perception that they have little personal control over its course has been shown to be a facilitator of adherence. The way of coping with CF has a potential influence on the direction and course of their disease. In particular, denial has been associated with rebellion and persistent non-compliance, while the adopting of an attitude of optimism and hope is associated with greater compliance (Abbott et al., 1996, 2001; Dziuban et al., 2010).

Currently, there is a major dilemma amongst health professionals with regard to promoting good mental health, whether they should allow denial and avoidance strategies for the patient to cope with the disease, or else whether they should promote compliance, which is dependent upon the recognition of the disease and the need for treatment.

5. Treatment compliance in children and adults with CF

The irregular adherence to treatment of patients with CF can alter the course of their illness. There are a number of important consequences of a failure to comply in treating CF, namely: deaths from cardiovascular diseases and infections, hospital admissions, increased visits, additional diagnostic testing requirements, additional alternative or unnecessary treatments, the home storage of medications and increased health spending. Knowledge of these aspects which motivate a patient in meeting certain treatments, and the discovery of the reasons given to justify the failure of others, can help the physician to promote adherence among their patients and influence the course of their disease.

In 2008, we published a study designed to determine treatment compliance and how it was perceived by patients, parents and by a team of specialists in CF. We also analysed the relative importance given to each of the prescribed treatments and the reasons that were given for non-adherence, and we investigated the possible predictors of therapeutic compliance. We also looked at the reasons for non-adherence, so as to determine possible predictors of therapeutic compliance (Arias-Llorente et al., 2008).

5.1 Patients and methods

5.1.1 Patients

Thirty-four CF patients controlled by the outpatient CF clinic of the University Central Hospital of Asturias and which attended periodic revisions (one each trimester) participated in the study. Up until the age of 14 they are controlled by paediatric gastroenterologists and pneumologists and by an adult specialist from that age on.

5.1.2 Study protocol

Data was collected by reviewing the clinical histories of the patients and it included epidemiologic data (age, gender, age at the diagnosis of CF, the timing of the evolution of the disease and CFTR mutation), a respiratory evaluation (the treatment received at the time of the interview, spirometric values, Bhalla score, lung transplantation) and a digestive evaluation (body mass index (BMI), nutritional index (NI), blood levels of alkaline phosphatase, transaminases, gamma-glutamyl transpeptidase, fat soluble vitamins, folic acid, albumin, β-carotene, faecal elastase, and immunoreactive trypsin, 72-hour faecal fat) and global evaluation (associated co-morbidities, Shwachman-Kulczycki score).

5.1.3 Questionnaire

A self-administered questionnaire was given to each patient when attending a routine visit to be answered in the clinic. Patients older than 12 years completed the questionnaire themselves, while it was filled out by the parents of younger patients. The questionnaire included four different subsets of questions, one for each of the different treatments usually given to CF patients, namely: physiotherapy, respiratory medication (including DNase, antibiotics and inhaled corticosteriods), digestive medication (including pancreatic enzymes, vitamins, deoxycholic acid and antacids) and nutritional supplements.

For each subset of therapeutic options, the CF patients were asked multiple questions on treatment compliance, the frequency of treatment, the importance attached to the treatment, their personal opinion about their own treatment compliance and the reasons given for non-compliance. At the end of the questionnaire, the CF patients score (from 0 to 100%) their global therapeutic compliance, considering all the treatments received.

According to the score obtained by the questionnaire, patients were then grouped according to their compliance or non-compliance for each of the therapeutic options and globally.

In addition, the paediatric and adult gastroenterologists, pneumologists and nurses of the CF clinic were also asked to subjectively classify the treatment compliance of the CF patients in terms of compliance and non-compliance.

5.2 Results

Thirty-four CF patients (21 of which were female) with an age range of 1.6 to 40.6 years (mean 14.5) were included in the study. Fourteen patients were under 10 years of age, 11 between 10 and 20, and 9 were older than 20. The average time of the evolution of the disease was 12.2 years (range from 1.3 to 40.6).

5.2.1 Adherence for each type of treatment

At the time of the study the average number of digestive and respiratory medications to be taken by the patients were 3.5 (range 0 to 7) and 4.5 (range 1 to 9) respectively.

Treatment compliance was greater for digestive (88.2%) and respiratory medication (61.8%), compared to physiotherapy (41.2%) and nutritional supplements (59%). This data is shown in Table 1, as well as that extracted from the views of the health professionals with regard to adherence of the patients to each type of treatment. The questionnaire results show a global compliance of 59%, whereby only 56% were compliant according to the opinion of the clinicians. Moreover, when the patient was directly asked, at the end of the questionnaire, to indicate their adherence to the therapy in their opinion, the treatment compliance was higher both for each type of treatment and globally.

	QUESTIONNAIRE	SPECIALISTS	PATIENTS
Physiotherapy	41.2%	35.3%	62.%
Respiratory	61.8%	59%	75.8%
Nutritional	59%	56%	77.7%
Digestive	88.2%	70.4%	91.2%
Global	59%	56%	84.8%

Table 1. The percentage of therapeutic adherence for each type of treatment based upon a questionnaire and specialist opinions and the perception of patients.

In conclusion, CF patients had a greater treatment adherence when prescribed digestive and respiratory medications as opposed to physiotherapy and nutritional supplements.

5.2.2 Degree and frequency of compliance

All of the CF patients take their digestive medications daily, although 64.7% admitted that they only consume pancreatic enzymes during principal meals and not during snacks. 50% of the CF patients indicated daily treatment compliance with respiratory medication and nutritional supplements. On the other hand, 14.7% only took their respiratory medications when they felt worse and 5.8% never took them, and nearly 30% of the patients said that they never consume their nutritional supplements.

The data from our questionnaire about physiotherapy is quite remarkable. Only 38.2% admitted to practising physiotherapy daily, while nearly 45% of patients reported as having physiotherapy only when they felt worse, occasionally or else never.

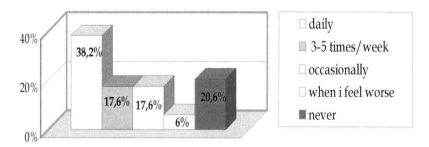

Fig. 1. Frequency of practice of physiotherapy (percentage of patients).

5.2.3 The importance given to different types of treatment and their impact on quality of life

The importance attached by patients to each type of treatment (average scores between 1 and 10): physiotherapy, 7.17; respiratory medication, 8; digestive, 9.4; nutritional support, 6.2) influenced compliance, and the treatments with the highest score saw the best level of adherence.

CF patients considered their digestive medication to be indispensable (94.1%) compared to respiratory medications, physiotherapy and nutritional supplements (70.6%, 59% and 44.1% respectively).

Type of treatment effect on quality of life was evaluated by the CF patients, and Table 2 shows the results of this evaluation. While 85.3% of the patients thought that digestive medications significantly improve their quality of life, half of the CF patients considered that physiotherapy plays little or no role on their perceived quality of life.

	Much	Enough	Little	Nothing
Physiotherapy	35.2%(25–45)	17.6%(5–31)	17.6%(5–31)	29.4% (14–44)
Respiratory	26.5% (11–41)	29.4% (14–44)	11.7% (3–28)	14.7% (3–27)
Digestive	38.2% (20–52)	44.1% (27–61)	2.9% (0.08–17)	8.8% (2–27)
Nutritional	11.7% (3–28)	38.2% (20–52)	11.7% (3–28%)	14.7% (3–27)

Table 2. The impact of treatments on quality of life of the patients (95% confidence interval limits in brackets).

5.2.4 Satisfaction

Patient satisfaction about their own treatment adherence was significantly higher for digestive medication, with 70.6 % of the CF patients considering that they were taking the correct dose of digestive medication, while only 8.8% considered that they should have been more compliant. By way of contrast, only 29.4% of the CF patients considered that they were practising as much physiotherapy as they needed, in comparison to 41.2% who thought that they should practise more frequently.

5.2.5 Reasons for poor compliance

The main reason given for not taking digestive medications was forgetfulness. However, the most repeated excuses for not complying with respiratory medication and nutritional supplements were the belief that they didn't need the medications (11.7% and 14.7% respectively), together with a lack of time for respiratory medication (8.8%) and the unpleasant taste or texture for nutritional supplements (14.7%).

The reasons given for not doing physiotherapy exercises included not having enough time (23.5%), not needing the treatment (20.6%) and substitution by other exercises (20.6%). Actually, the median time that our patients employ in practising physiotherapy is noticeably less than the ageing of sickness evolution (7.6 years vs. 12.2 years). A considerable number of patients believe that physiotherapy is not necessary after receiving lung transplantation.

	% patients
Physiotherapy	
Not enough time	29.4%
I don´t think need it, I feel well without treatment.	20.6%
Exercise instead	20.6%
I don´t believe that it does my any good	14.7%
It interferes with my social life	11.8%
Simply forget	8.8%
Transplantation	5.9%
Respiratory medication	
I don´t think need it	11.7%
Not enough time	8.8%
Only when I feel worse	8.8%
It interferes with my social life	5.9%
Simply forget	5.9%
Exercise instead	2.9%
Nutritional supplements	
I don´t think need it	14.7%
I don´t like the taste or texture	14.7%
Simply forget	8.8%
I don´t believe in it	5.9%

Table 3. The predominant reasons for poor compliance with different treatments (percentage of patients).

5.2.6 Differences between compliant and non-compliant CF patients

It was objectified that treatment adherence decreases with age. We have observed that 23.8% of patients younger than 15 years were non-compliant, while this percentage rose to 69.2% for those older than 15 years, up to 89% for those older than 20 years. Non-compliant patients were significantly older (the average age of compliant patients was 10.4 years; that of non-compliant patients was 20.5 years, p=0.008) and had a longer time of evolution for their disease (compliant 9.4 years; non-compliant 16.8 years, p = 0.025). In our study, we have observed that adherence to treatment decreases with the severity of the CF disease (Shwachman score compliant 83.2 vs. non-compliant 73.9 points, p = 0.048).

No gender differences were observed. Moreover, compliant CF patients attached more importance to all of the different therapeutic options than non-compliant CF patients (Table 4). Nutritional parameters were also analysed, and compliant CF patients displayed significantly higher albumin values than non-compliant patients. No differences were observed for any of the other biochemical factors studied. No age-adjusted differences were observed in BMI. No differences were observed for faecal fat, NI, and spirometric values.

	COMPLIANT Mean (SD)	NON-COMPLIANT Mean (SD)	P
Physiotherapy	9.5 (2)	5 (0.7)	0.000
Respiratory	8.8 (1.5)	6.4 (3)	0.010
Digestive	9.7 (0.7)	7 (1.7)	0.001
Nutritional	8.6 (1.4)	4.3 (3.1)	0.000

Table 4. The importance attached to different therapeutic options by CF patients on a scale from 1 to 10 points.

5.3 Discussion

identified as determinants of adherence to different treatments. At the time of our study, the average number of digestive and respiratory medications to be taken by patients was 3.5 (range 0 to 7) and 4.5 (range 1 to 9) respectively. These medications numbered too many even when compared with other studies, where there are even lists with more than twenty different treatments (Marciel et al., 2010). The explanation for this difference may be that the average age of patients is greater where there is a more prolonged progression of the disease and a possibly more serious illness. Whilst – in our study – the average age of the patients was 14.5 years, the mean time of the evolution of the disease was 12.2 years, and 58.8% of the controlled patients in our unit presented a good global prognostic score according to the Shwachman–Kulczycki scale, and even 26.4% were qualified as excellent.

If these treatments are added to the need for other medications for associated pathologies and daily physiotherapy practice, they can give us an idea of how complicated the treatment was and the time spent on it. Given the long duration and arduous nature of these regimens, the maintenance of good compliance over prolonged periods will be a difficult task for the specialist responsible. Moreover, there are many other factors which may influence a decline in adherence: the perception of the disease which the patient has at any time, their different ways of coping with the disease (which can change throughout life), family, economic or social problems, a lack of trust in the responsible physician, erroneous beliefs about the benefits of different treatments, etc.

As such, the patients who were considered to be particularly compliant could also go through phases of declining adherence. For this reason, it is very important not to relax during the monitoring of these chronic patients and to be alert to any problems that may affect their adherence to their treatment (Duff & Latchford, 2010). During this time, the team of specialists should try to understand and motivate the patient.

Accordingly, there are works that strive to determine not only the degree of compliance of these patients, but also its variation over time and the reasons for this. Using this type of information, it is possible to identify which aspects of the treatment can be improved and to work together with families so as to individualise treatments. For example, a study designed to determine adherence to nebulised antibiotics by monitoring the routine data downloads of an adaptive aerosol delivery nebuliser in children with CF found considerable variation in adherence, both between and within patients, and even over the course of the day (evening adherence was better than morning adherence). Treatment regimens were changed for 8/28 patients, based upon the data on adherence obtained by this study (McNamara et al., 2009).

Treatment adherence in CF cases, as with many other chronic diseases, has been around 50% and has rarely exceeded 80% (Abbott et al., 1996; Conway et al., 1996; Daniels et al., 2011; Kettler et al., 2002; McNamara et al., 2009). According to the data obtained by the questionnaire score, overall treatment compliance with the CF group controlled in our unit was 59%. Also, patients were asked directly as to what their level of compliance was, it was much higher both overall and for each type of treatment. Indeed, half of the patients believe that they comply with the therapeutic indications made by the specialist by at least 90%, a better level of adherence than the indicated by the results obtained by the questionnaire score.

The fact that patients tend to overestimate their adherence to treatment is usually reflected in the literature. By way of contrast, the opinion of health professionals suggests a generally lower level of adherence (Abbott et al., 2001; Conway et al., 1996; Daniels et al., 2011; Modi et al., 2006). Moreover, it is usually the case that the perception of the severity of the disease also differs between physician and patient. A recent study assessed the agreement between rates of adherence to prescribed nebulisers when measured by self-reports, clinician reports and electronic monitoring suitable for long-term use, and differences in adherence were found. Here, median self-reported adherence was 80% whilst median clinician reported adherence was down to 50%-60% (Daniels et al., 2011). This was also observed in our study, as adherence to treatment as assessed by the team of specialists was lower than both the overall and for each type of treatment. So, according to our data, only 70% of those patients who believed themselves to be compliant (according to the questionnaire results) are also considered to be so by their specialised doctors.

However, self-reporting and clinician reporting of adherence does not provide accurate measurement of adherence when compared with more objective measurement methods. In this case, adherence is usually less than as shown in the study mentioned above, where the level of adherence measured by nebuliser downloads was 36% (Daniels et al., 2011).

We are aware that the results of our study are based on subjective data obtained after a personal interview with parents and/or patients, which are then contrasted with the opinions of the clinicians belonging to the CF unit. There are also studies that clearly show that clinical impressions are not accurate enough to determine the real therapeutic adherence of patients, and so it would be also convenient to use a more objective method (Marciel et al., 2010; Modi et al.; 2006; Shemesh et al., 2004). It has been mentioned that the level of adherence could vary according to the subjectivity of the method employed, such as with a personal questionnaire, even if the results are corrected with the opinions of the medical professionals or other objective measures, such as blood-serum levels, the urinary excretion of medications or their metabolites, or the monitoring of adherence with electronic recording devices or the dispensers of medications (Conway et al., 1996; Modi et al., 2006; Rand et al., 1992; Teichman et al., 2000). Nevertheless these methods have their own inconveniences. With regard to the drug levels in serum or urine, we must emphasise that they are invasive methods and they may only represent yet another test for patients, due to the multiple samples needed to check their compliance, in addition to the pharmacokinetic variations of the substance are to be studied. Regarding electronic monitoring, the data obtained only provides information about the use of a medication dispenser, but not about whether the patient is actually taking the medication removed from the dispenser; moreover, this type of monitoring remains too expensive. This could also limit other evaluations concerning such aspects as diet, exercise and physiotherapy (Kettler et al., 2002; Rand et al., 1992).

In addition to finding differences in treatment compliance according to the methods discussed above, there are many works that refer to differences in adherence to the different components of the treatment carried out by patients with CF. Traditionally, it is said that adherence is low – between 40% and 55% – to nutritional supplements and physiotherapy. Meanwhile, treatment compliance to pancreatic enzymes and respiratory antibiotics increases to between 75% and 90% (Abbott et al., 2001; Daniels et al., 2011; Kettler et al., 2002; Modi et al., 2006).

In our study, and with regard to the types of treatment, most patients performed digestive medication (88.2% of patients), followed by respiratory medication (61.8%). Meanwhile 59% of patients were considered compliant with respect to nutritional support whilst only 41.2% were compliant with physiotherapy. In our case, the number of patients who were compliant towards digestive medication is similar to the results shown elsewhere (Abbott et al., 1994, 1996, 2001; Daniels et al., 2011; Modi et al., 2006) as well as the fact that only a third of patients took pancreatic enzymes at every meal, including snacks (Michaud et al., 1991). However, the level of adherence to respiratory medication was less than in others studies, which is perhaps explained by the fact that we did not analyse specific compliance with every aspect of respiratory treatment. If we had taken into consideration the individual's adherence to bronchodilators, antibiotics or inhaled corticosteroids, the adherence to treatment would probably have been greater.

When we asked patients about the importance that they attach to the different types of treatment (on a scale from 1 to 10 points), the highest score was assigned to digestive medication (9.4 points), corresponding with the most valued treatment in terms of compliance and its impact on quality of life. As such, 85.3% of the patients thought that digestive medication significantly improved their quality of life. As described in previous publications, our patients displayed better compliance with those treatments that they believed to be more important (Abbott et al., 2001; Patterson et al., 1993) and to have more repercussions for their quality of life (Conway et al., 1996; Czjkowski et al., 1987).

In accordance with the details above, the two types of treatments that most patients seemed to consider essential were digestive and respiratory medications (94.1% and 70.6% respectively). This idea, coupled with the higher compliance observed in these treatments, is collected in earlier studies and it may reflect the short-term benefits of these and the precocity of the appearance of unpleasant symptoms as a result of non-compliance (Abbott et al., 1994, 1996, 2001; Conway et al., 1996; Kettler et al., 2002). Thus, adherence to pancreatic enzyme typically is high in order to avoid steatorrhea and the main reason for not taking this medication is "forgotten" and only one person says no need to take it despite having malabsorption.

At the opposite end are nutritional supplements and physiotherapy. It is of concern that uniquely 44.1% consider nutritional supplements to be an essential treatment in clear concordance to the main reason given for not taking nutritional supplements: "I don't think I need it". And finally, only 59% of the patients believe physiotherapy is an essential treatment, in clear opposition to what physicians think. In fact, the type of treatment which we found to reflect a greater discrepancy between the opinions of doctors and patients was physiotherapy. This way of thinking agrees with patients' perception of their slight repercussions for their quality of life (half of the CF patients felt that physiotherapy played little or no role in their treatment) and the different degrees of importance attached to physiotherapy by compliant and non-compliant patients (9.5 points vs. 5 points, p<0.001). In this connection, the data of our questionnaire concerning physiotherapy is remarkable since the practise of physiotherapy was particularly deficient with regard to the number of subjects doing it and its frequency; however, this is also found in the literature (Abbott et al., 1996; Bernard & Cohen, 2004; Passero et al., 1981). The number of patients who practised daily physiotherapy only reached 38.2%, similar to other results in CF clinics (Abbott et al., 2001; Oerman et al., 2000), and 20% even say that they never practice physiotherapy.

On the other hand, the beginning of physiotherapy should be instituted at the time of the diagnosis of CF, a finding which is not supported by the average time that our patients have been practising (mean ± SD: 7.6±6.1 years), which is strikingly lower than the average time of the disease (12.2±8.9 years).

Therefore, the main reasons claimed for non-compliance are a lack of time, the erroneous belief that they don't need it or that they can substitute them with other exercise. As such, the perception that there are no beneficial effects with the treatment is wholesale problem for physiotherapy (Bernard & Cohen, 2004; Conway et al., 1996; Czjkowski et al., 1987; Shemesh et al., 2004; Teichman et al., 2001), and it has been published as being substituted with exercise in 20% of cases, just as we found (20.6%).

A particular time when there is a risk of a decrease in adherence occurs, typically, after lung transplantation. Accordingly, we must emphasise that half of our transplanted patients have given up physiotherapy techniques afterwards, giving this hopeful event as the very reason for their lack of adherence. Even if it is known that medical opinions obviously contrast with this attitude, there is a recognised decrease in their therapeutic fulfilment after a lung transplantation which continues over time. It may be that they experience a better sense of wellbeing and so could hypothesise that they didn't need it anymore. At this time, it is essential to provide them with clear information and to take care in following up with adequate supervision so as to reorient and help them eradicate these erroneous beliefs (Foster et al., 2001; Lask, 1994; Kettler et al., 2002; Oerman et al., 2000; Teichman et al., 2000).

Such beliefs about the benefits of and need for each type of treatment significantly influence in the treatment adherence.

In terms of patient satisfaction about their own adherence, it should be noted that is noticeably higher with the digestive intake of medication, such that 70.6% think that they should take this type of medication and only 8.8% think they should take more. At the other extreme is physiotherapy, where only 29.4% of patients believe that they should practise physiotherapy at all and 41% think that they should do it more often. If we compare this data with those described in previous works, it confirms a trend (Abbott et al., 1994). This is to say that patients are more satisfied with their compliance with digestive or respiratory medication than with their practise of physiotherapy. It is a paradoxical result because, although very few are happy with the practise of physiotherapy, there are few who think that they should do it more often.

There are several factors which should be taken into account as possible predictors of adherence in CF cases, with contradictory results: demographic data such as sex, age, level of education, knowledge of sickness, socio-economic status, socio-familial relations and profession, as well as clinical factors such as age at diagnosis, the severity of the CF or the frequency of checkups at CF clinics (Bernard & Cohen 2004; Jaffe & Bush, 2001; Kettler et al., 2002; Oerman et al., 2000; Passero et al., 1981; Zindani et al., 2006). Our study found a statistically significant difference both in terms of the average age of each patient group, (compliant at 10.4 years and non-compliant at 20.5 years) and the time of the evolution of the disease (compliant at 9.5 years and non-compliant at 16.8 years). The fact that adherence to treatment tends to diminish with age has also been mentioned in the earlier studies (Conway et al., 1996; Gudas et al., 1991). In childhood, a high level of compliance is frequently observed, which is probably explained due to the fact that during this period of life the responsibility lies with the parents (Battistini et al., 1998; Foster et al., 2001). Family cohesion and adequate social support have both been associated with better adherence to treatment (Eddy et al., 1998; Foster et al., 2001; Hamutcy et al., 2002; Teichman 20009). In addition, the ways of coping with the disease by the mechanisms of denial and avoidance – which have been described as negative predictors of adherence to treatment – tend to increase with age amongst these chronically ill patients as they facilitate their emotional adjustment into adulthood (Kettler et al., 2002; Lask, 1994).

A special time when compliance with treatment tends to decrease significantly is during adolescence, as was also found in our study, whereby parents release their progeny. This notion is reflected repeatedly in the literature for years (Bernard & Cohen, 2004; Bucks et al., 2009; Conway et al., 1996; Mc Laughlin et al., 2008; Passero et al., 1998). So, in a study done in Montreal University 20 years ago on compliance with treatment amongst adolescents affected by chronic illness, such as CF, it was concluded that there was a global adherence of 50%; nevertheless only 11% of the subjects demonstrated the successful accomplishment of all of the therapeutic components (Michaud et al., 1991). In another study at Michigan University several years later, it has been shown that there is a significant difference between those patients who are less than 12 years old and those who are over twelve year old with regard to the intake of liposoluble vitamins amongst CF patients (Jaffe & Bush, 2001).

Adolescence means that the patients are presented with several other challenges apart from their illness, such that all of a sudden they are supposed to take control of themselves; perhaps they are prone to diminish its importance, or perhaps they display a reluctance to chat with their peers about their 'big' problem, or perhaps, even, they adopt a "hide and run" policy. They apologise, arguing with such reasons as "it interferes with my social life," "I don't want my friends to know that I suffer from CF," as we have confirmed. Another reason in the decrease in self-accomplishment could be the transfer from paediatricians to adult medical staff (McLaughlin et al., 2008; Michaud et al., 1991), since initially it could mean a degree of instability and lack of reliance that is traduced into less adherence.

For all of these reasons, there is often a growing recognition of need for support for their transition into adult-oriented healthcare. There is significant variability in the transitional support provided to young adults with CF (Mc Laughlin et al., 2008; Scal & Ireland; 2005). The first problem is the age of transition, because while in many centres the transfer of care for CF occurs at a median age of 19 years, in other programs it has been reported that the introduction of the concept of transition takes place before the age of 15 years (Anderson 2002). In our CF unit, up until the age of 14 (younger than 15 years) they are controlled by paediatric gastroenterologists and pneumologists, and by an adult specialist from that age onwards. The second problem relates to the different methods of transition that have been used. Few programmes provide educational materials about transition to patients and families, and fewer than half provide a transition time-line or designate a specific team member to be responsible for the key elements of transition (Mc Laughlin et al., 2008; Marciel et al., 2010).

With regard to the severity of the disease, as determined by the score on the Shwachman-Kulczycki scale, significant differences were found between the compliant and non-compliant groups. We have observed that adherence to treatment decreases with the severity of CF. Some authors explain this phenomenon by reasoning to a lack of positive reinforcement whereby patients do not note a beneficial effect with their adherence to treatment (Hamutcy et al., 2002). However, there are also other authors who describe the opposite, with results relating disease severity with adherence to treatment (Oerman et al., 2000; Zindani et al., 2006).

In summary, we can say that there are differences in the degree of compliance by these patients with the various components of the treatment carried out. There is greater adherence to digestive and respiratory medications than to physiotherapy and nutritional supplements. We found a decrease in adherence according to age, the longer the history of the disease and the greater its severity. In addition, the treatments which were evaluated by patients as most important and as having the greatest impact on their quality of life witnessed the most adherence.

6. Conclusion

We can conclude that the global compliance with treatment is similar to that of other works, with a tendency of patients to overestimate their accomplishments as compared with the opinions of clinical staff. There are differences in the level of adherence to the various treatments, and this is realised by these patients.

Of all the treatments that patients carry out, it was felt that the treatment which had the greatest impact on their quality of life, that which most considered to be essential and with which they were personally the most satisfied, involved gastrointestinal medicaments. Nevertheless, the practise of physiotherapy was highly deficient with regard to the number of subjects performing it and the frequency with which they did it, influenced by the general belief that it does not make much difference and that it has little repercussion for their quality of life.

We have confirmed a decrease in therapeutic adherence with age, the longer the duration of evolution and the severity of the illness. There was no influence from the gender of the patients, their nutritional parameters, or from the data on pulmonary function. The treatments mostly appreciated by the patients as most essential were coincident with a higher level of adherence, emphasising the need for careful and continuous information, and the modification of erroneous beliefs.

7. Acknowledgment

We would like to extend our deepest appreciation to the children and their families and the adults with CF of our unit.

8. References

Abbott, J., Dodd, M., Bilton, D. & Webb, A.K. (1994). Treatment compliance in adults with cystic fibrosis, *Thorax* Vol. 49(2): 115-120.

Abbott, J., Dodd, M. & Webb, A.K. (1996). Health perceptions and treatment adherence in adults with cystic fibrosis, *Thorax* Vol. 51(12): 1233-1238.

Abbott, J., Dodd, M., Gee, L. & Webb, A.K. (2001). Ways of coping with cystic fibrosis: implications for treatment adherence, *Disabil Rehabil.* Vol. 23(8): 315-324.

Anderson, D.L, Flume, P.A, Hardy, K.K & Gray, S (2002). Transition programs in cystic fibrosis centres: perceptions of patients, *Pediatr Pulmonol.* Vol.33 (5):327- 331.

Arias-Llorente, R.P; Bousoño, C. & Diaz, J.J. (2008). Treatment compliance in children and adults of cystic fibrosis, *J. Cyst. Fibrosis* Vol. 7: 359-367.

Battistini, A., Grzincich, G.L., Pisi, G., Bocchi, U., Marvasi, R., Costantini, I., et al. (1998) Respiratory physio-Kinesitherapy in cystic fibrosis: the parents' viewpoint, *Pediatr Med. Chir.* Vol. 10 (1): 1-14.

Bernard, R.S. & Cohen, L.L. (2004). Increasing adherence to cystic fibrosis treatment: a systematic review of behaviour techniques, *Pediatr Pulmonol.* Vol.. 37(1): 8-16.

Bucks, R.S., Hawkins, K., Skinner, T.C., Horn, S., Seddon, P & Horne, R. (2009). Adherence to treatment in adolescents with cystic fibrosis: the role of illness perceptions and treatment beliefs, *J. Pediatr Psychol.* Vol. 34(8): 893-902.

Conway, S.P., Pond, M.N., Hamnett, T. & Watson, A. (1996) Compliance with treatment in adult patients with cystic fibrosis, *Thorax* Vol. 51(1): 29-33.

Czajkowski, D. & Koocher, G. (1987) Medical compliance and coping with cystic fibrosis, *J. Child Psychol. Psychiatry* Vol. 23: 311-319.

Daniels, T., Goodacre, L., Sutton, C., Pollard, K., Conway, S. & Peckham, D. (2011). Accurate assessment of adherence: Self and clinical report versus electronic monitoring of nebulisers, *Chest* (Epub ahead of print).

Duff, A.J. & Latchford G.J (2010). Motivational interviewing for adherence problems in cystic fibrosis, *Pediatr Pulmonol* Vol.45(3): 211-220.

Dziuban, E.J., Saab-Abazeed, L. Chaudhry, S.R., Streetman, D.S. & Nasr, S.Z. (2010). Identifying barriers to treatment adherence and related attitudinal patterns in adolescents with cystic fibrosis, *Pediatr Pulmonol.* Vol. 45(5): 450-458.

Eddy, M.E., Carter, B.D., Kronenberger, W.G., Conradsen, S., Eid, N.S., Bourland, S.L. & Adams, G. (1998). Parent relationships and compliance in cystic fibrosis, *J. Pediatr Health Care* Vol. 12(4):196-202.

Foster, C., Eiser, C., Oades, P., Sheldon, C., Tripp, J., Goldman, P., Rice, S. & Trott, J. (2001). Treatment demands and differential treatment of patients with cystic fibrosis and their siblings: patient, parent and sibling accounts, *Child Care Health Dev.* Vol. 27(4): 349-364.

Gudas, L.J., Koocher, G.P. & Wypij, D. (1991) Perceptions of medical compliance in children and adolescent with cystic fibrosis, *J. Dev. Behav Pediatr.* Vol 12(4): 236-242.

Hamutcy, R., Rowland, J.M., Horn, M.V., Kaminsky, C., McLaughlin, E.F., Starnes, V.A. & Woo, M.S. (2002) Clinical Finding and Lung Pathology in children with Cystic Fibrosis, *Am. J. Respir. Crit. Care Med.* Vol. 165: 1172-1175.

Ievers, C.E, Brown, R.T, Drotar, D., Caplan, D., Pishevar, B.S and Lambert, RG. (1999). Knowledge of physician prescriptions and adherence to treatment among children with cystic fibrosis and their mothers. *J Dev Behav Pediatr.* Vol.20(5):335-343.

Jaffe, A. & Bush, A. (2001). Cystic fibrosis: review of the decade, *Monaldi Arch. Chest. Dis.* Vol. 56(3): 240-247.

Kettler, L.J., Sawyer, S.M., Winefield, H.R. & Greville H.W. (2002). Determinants of adherence in adults with cystic fibrosis, *Thorax* Vol. 57: 459-464.

Lask, B. (1994). Non-adherence to treatment in cystic fibrosis, *J. R. Soc. Med.* Vol. 87 (supl 21): 25-27.

Marciel, K.K.,Saiman, L.,Quittell, L.M., Dawkins, K. & Quittner, A.L. (2010). Cell phone intervention to improve adherence: cystic fibrosis care team, patient, and parent perspectives, *Pediatr. Pulmonol.* Vol 45(2):157-164.

McLaughlin, S.E., Diener-West M., Indurkhya, A., Rubin, H., Heckman R. & Boyle M.P. (2008). Improving transition from paediatric to adult cystic fibrosis care: lessons from a national survey of current practices, *Pediatrics* Vol.121(5):1160-1166.

McNamara, P.S., McCormmack, P., McDonald, A.J., Heaf, L. & southern, K.W. (2009). Open adherence monitoring using routine data download from an adaptive aerosol delivery nebuliser in children with cystic fibrosis, *J. Cyst. Fibrosis* Vol. 8(4): 258-263.

Michaud, P.A., Frappier, J.Y. & Pless, I.B. (1991). Compliance in adolescents with chronic disease, *Arch. Fr. Pediatr.* Vol 48(5): 329-336.

Modi, A.C., Lim, C.S., Yu, N., Geller, D., Wagner, M.H. & Quittner, A. (2006). A multimethod assessment of treatment adherence for children with cystic fibrosis, *J. Cyst. Fibros.* Vol. 5(3): 177-185.

Moise, J.R, Drotar, D., Doershuk, C.F. & Stern RC. (1987). Correlates of psychosocial adjustment among young adults with cystic fibrosis, *J. Dev. Behav. Pediatr.* Vol.;8(3):141-148.

Oerman, C.M., Swank, P.R. & Sockrider, M.M. (2000). Validation of an instrument measuring patient satisfaction with chest physiotherapy techniques in cystic fibrosis, *Chest* Vol. 118(1): 92-97.

Passero, M.A., Remor, B. & Salomon, J. (1981). Patient-reported compliance with cystic fibrosis therapy, *Clin. Pediatr.* Vol. 20: 264-268.

Paterson, J.M., Budd, J., Goetz, D. & Warwick, W.J. (1993). Family correlates of a ten year pulmonary health trend in cystic fibrosis, *Pediatrics* Vol. 91: 383-389

Rand, C.S., Wise, R.A., Nides, M., et al. (1992). Metered-dose inhaler adherence in a clinical trial, *Am. Rev. Respir. Dis.* Vol. 146: 1559-1564.

Scal, P. & Ireland, M. (2005).Addressing transition to adult health care for adolescents with special health care needs, *Pediatrics* Vol. 115 (6):1607–1612.

Shemesh, E., Shneider, B.L., Savitzky, J.K., Arnott, L. et al. (2004). Medication adherence in paediatric and adolescent liver transplant recipients, *Pediatrics* Vol. 113(4): 825-832

Smith, B.A., Modi, A.C, Quittner, A.L. & Wood, B.L. (2010). Depressive symptoms in children with cystic fibrosis and parents and its effects on adherence to airway clearance, *Pedriatr Pulmonol.* Vol. 45(8): 756-763.

Teichman, B.J., Burker, E.J., Weiner, M. & Egan, T.M. (2000). Factors associated with adherence to treatment regimens after lung transplantation, *Prog. Transplant.* Vol. 10(2): 113-121.

Zindani, G.N., Streetman, D.D., Streetman, D.S. & Nasr, S.Z. (2006). Adherence to treatment in children and adolescent patients with cystic fibrosis, *J. Adolesc. Health* Vol. 38(1): 13-17.

9

Improving the Likelihood of Success in Trials and the Efficiency of Delivery of Mucolytics and Antibiotics

Carlos F. Lange
Dept. of Mechanical Engineering, University of Alberta
Canada

1. Introduction

The use of models estimating the dosage delivered to a lung region to help design delivery systems for new drugs is well established (e.g. Finlay et al. (1997)). This approach, also called *in silico* testing, however has not yet received regulatory acceptance (Forbes et al. (2011)). A far less common application of lung deposition models is in the estimation of the concentration of the inhaled drug in the liquid layer that coats the human airways, also know as the airway surface liquid (ASL).

One case when the lung concentration of the inhaled drug is more relevant than the total deposited dosage is in the treatment of the effects of cystic fibrosis. To enhance the mucociliary clearance and to promote normal lung function in cystic fibrosis patients, mucolytic agents have been developed for aerosol delivery to the lung. These drug compounds are considered topically active, since their efficacy depends on reaching a proper concentration level, as determined by *in vitro* and *ex vivo* experiments. When designing clinical trials and treatment protocols, the total dosage delivered by inhalation needs to ensure that such concentration levels are reached in the mucus layer in each lung generation.

With the continuing emergence of multiply antibiotic-resistant organisms, the need to develop new, more powerful antibiotics remains evident. For determining an effective dose of a new antibiotic, it is common practise to use a series of clinical trials with different doses of the new drug starting from a small amount and moving to higher amounts gradually. However, resource limitations sometimes constrain the initial trial to a single dose, imposing the condition that this single attempt be effective before additional funds are made available. A requirement for efficacy of antibiotics is that the *in vivo* drug concentration be sustained at a level that ensures minimum inhibitory concentration (MIC), since otherwise resistance may be promoted.

Antibiotics and mucolytics are drugs that exhibit concentration dependence in their efficacy. Therefore, ensuring appropriate concentration of these drugs in the relevant body fluid is important for obtaining the desired therapeutic and physiological result. Until recently there had been no suitable method available to predict the amount of inhaled drug required to ensure efficacious concentration levels in the airway surface liquid (ASL).

Now, the combination of a lung deposition model with a novel model of the ASL layer allow for an estimate of the local average drug concentration in each lung generation k after inhalation

$$C_{k,\text{ASL}} = \frac{m_{k,\text{drug}}}{\left(V_{k,\text{ASL}} + V_{k,\text{aerosol}}\right)} \tag{1}$$

The main focus of this chapter is to present a recently developed model that estimates local concentration of inhaled pharmaceutical aerosols in the ASL and to explain, with examples, how such a model can assist in the development of new inhaled drugs that are topically active, i.e. that depend on reaching proper concentration levels locally in the lung. Examples of recent use of this model are Desai et al. (2003); Sweeney et al. (2005); Wang et al. (2003).

2. Modelling drug deposition in the lung

To estimate the local concentration of a drug in the lung, it is necessary to estimate first the amount of drug deposited in each lung generation.

The modelling of deposition of inhaled aerosols over the years has evolved from simple and limited algebraic models (James et al. (1991)) to more complex and accurate empirical (Martonen et al. (1994)), one-way coupled (Ferron et al. (1988)), and two-way coupled hygroscopic models (Finlay & Stapleton (1995)), based on the Lagrangian approach. All these models treat the lung as unidimensional, calculating deposition on a typical or average aerosol path. While Lagrangian models can well represent the inhalation and deposition from continuous nebulizers, single breath inhalers and smart nebulizers derive their enhanced performance from time dependent effects that can only be accurately captured by Eulerian models. Eulerian deposition models have been available for many years (Egan & Nixon (1985); Roth et al. (2003); Taulbee & Yu (1975)) and recently have also incorporated one-way coupled hygroscopicity (Mitsakou et al. (2005)). However, they have not found widespread use, probably because of the relative complexity of their implementation.

The application of Computational Fluid Dynamics (CFD) to model aerosol deposition in a three-dimensional representation of the airways is relatively recent. Initially, the simulations were constrained to specific stretches of the airway path, such as the trachea and a few generations of the lung, or the alveolar region (Dailey & Ghadiali (2007)). These simulations offer some insight into the local effects of geometry on the flow, such as the tracheal rings, the shape of the carinal ridge or the size change of the alveoli. However, these analyzes are limited by the lack of upstream information about the flow.

Of all components required to predict lung deposition, arguably the most important and most challenging is the correct prediction of extrathoracic losses. These losses, compounded by inhalability losses in the case of infants and small children using masks, define the dosage actually delivered to the lung, assuming the device output is known. As DeHaan & Finlay (2001; 2004) demonstrated with dry powder inhalers, extrathoracic deposition can depart quite significantly from the baseline case of particles inhaled from a smooth, wide, straight tube with approximately constant inhalation rate studied by Stahlhofen et al. (1983). While we now understand much better the flow and deposition mechanisms occurring in the oropharyngeal region following the analysis of Heenan et al. (2004), the large scatter of data caused by intersubject variabilities even during controlled inhalation conditions (Stahlhofen et al. (1983)) would preclude any accurate prediction of extrathoracic losses. Fortunately, a comprehensive study of the effects of intersubject variability by Grgic et al.

(2004) led to the discovery of a universal form of the Stokes parameter allowing for a more accurate prediction of the oropharyngeal deposition in a wide variety of realistic mouth-throat geometries. This mathematical relationship can potentially be used to predict lung dosages from inhalers, instead of the currently used delivered dose.

One-dimensional, dynamical lung deposition models, though heavily simplified with respect to the airway geometry, can incorporate all the fundamental physical processes that affect particle size and deposition at a small fraction of the computational effort of CFD. Naturally, these 1-D models cannot resolve local deposition patterns, such as required by a tumour, but they can be properly tuned to give accurate results for delivery of drugs that target an entire lung region. The treatment of lung diseases associated with cystic fibrosis, such as bacterial infections and mucolytic treatments, are examples of cases that target a single lung region, namely the tracheobronchial region. Advanced one-dimensional models can provide this regional deposition information with high accuracy, as demonstrated by Finlay, Lange, Li & Hoskinson (2000). For these reasons, 1-D models seem better suited for the use in the modelling of local concentration of deposited drugs in the lung.

3. Modelling mucus and the Airway Surface Liquid layer

The model of the Airway Surface Liquid (ASL) layer, developed at the University of Alberta by the author in collaboration with W. Finlay and M. King (Finlay, Lange, King & Speert (2000); Hasan & Lange (2007); Lange et al. (2001)) is the first and, to this date, the only model of its kind. The model approximates the amount of liquid matter present in each lung generation, which, in conjunction with the local dosage provided by the deposition model, allows for the estimate of the local concentration of the inhaled drug.

A previous attempt to estimate concentration of deposited aerosols was performed by Böhm et al. (2003). They used an empirical estimate of lung deposition and a simple assumption of a constant thickness of the ASL layer in a single generation. An approach closer to the one proposed here was employed by Kimmel et al. (2001) to study transient clearance and mucus concentration in rats. But the mucus layer thickness was considered constant throughout the tracheobronchial region.

The ASL model distinguishes two layers with essentially different physical properties: the periciliary liquid layer (PCL), a watery layer (sol) covering the airway epithelium, and the mucus layer, a viscoelastic gel that floats on top of the PCL (see Fig. 1).

The volume of liquid in each layer is modelled separately. The sum of the two gives the total ASL volume in each generation, $V_{k,ASL}$. For the calculation of the volume we assume a continuous annular layer of liquid along each generation. Figure 2 shows a schematic cross-sectional view of an airway.

The dimensions of the airways are obtained from the lung geometry model by Finlay (2001), which has been shown to correlate well with *in vivo* regional deposition experiments (Finlay, Hoskinson & Stapleton (1998)). The geometry assumes a symmetric branching airway system, starting from the extrathoracic region (mouth cavity, pharynx and larynx), followed by the trachea, and branching symmetrically into two main bronchi, then into four lobar bronchi, and so on. Each new branch segment is called a generation, k. The trachea is considered the first generation ($k = 0$), and the main bronchi are $k = 1$, so that the number of airways in each generation is always 2^k.

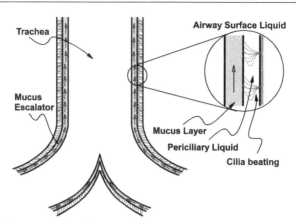

Fig. 1. Schematic of the airways with ASL layer and mucociliary escalator.

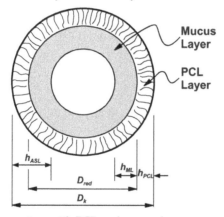

Fig. 2. Airway cross-section with PCL and mucus layers.

In contrast with the classical lung model, Weibel A (Weibel (1963)), which considers generations 0–16 to form the tracheobronchial region, Finlay's model sets the transition between the tracheobronchial region and the more distal alveolar region at the generation 14. This distinction is relevant, because mucociliary transport exists only in the conductive airways, starting at the terminal bronchioles, which are the most distal ciliated airways. While the calculation of the deposited dosage, described above, utilizes the complete lung geometry, the ASL layer is only defined in the tracheobronchial region. The dimensions of the airways in each tracheobronchial generation are reproduced from Finlay (2001) in Table 1.

The ASL model uses the same average airway diameter and length in generation k as the deposition model, D_k and L_k. With these geometric characteristics, the volume of ASL in generation k can be calculated as

$$V_{k,\mathrm{ASL}} = \pi L_k 2^k \left(D_k h_{k,\mathrm{ASL}} - h_{k,\mathrm{ASL}}^2 \right) \tag{2}$$

where the thickness of the ASL layer, $h_{k,\mathrm{ASL}}$, needs to be determined and is defined as

$$h_{k,\mathrm{ASL}} = h_{k,\mathrm{PCL}} + h_{k,\mathrm{ML}} \tag{3}$$

Generation	Length [cm]	Diameter [cm]
0	12.456	1.810
1	3.614	1.414
2	2.862	1.115
3	2.281	.885
4	1.780	.706
5	1.126	.565
6	.897	.454
7	.828	.364
8	.745	.286
9	.653	.218
10	.555	.162
11	.454	.121
12	.357	.092
13	.277	.073
14	.219	.061

Table 1. Airway dimensions in the tracheobronchial tree (from Finlay (2001)).

i.e., it is the sum of $h_{k,\text{PCL}}$ and $h_{k,\text{ML}}$, the thicknesses of the PCL and mucus layers, respectively.

In certain cases, such as in the inhalation of mucolytics, it is the volume of mucus only that is required. In this case, the same assumptions as above give

$$V_{k,\text{ML}} = \pi L_k 2^k \left(D_{k,\text{red}} h_{k,\text{ML}} - h_{k,\text{ML}}^2 \right) \tag{4}$$

where $D_{k,\text{red}}$ is the airway diameter reduced by the PCL layer thickness

$$D_{k,\text{red}} = D_k - 2 h_{k,\text{PCL}} \tag{5}$$

Since the airway geometry follows the deposition model and is known, all that is required to estimate the volumes of mucus and ASL are the layer thicknesses. In the following sections the calculation of the PCL and mucus layer thicknesses is described.

3.1 Thickness of PCL layer

The PCL layer is formed by a watery liquid that facilitates the beating of the cilia and keeps the thicker mucus layer afloat at an exact distance to be reached by the tip of the cilia during their forward beating (Widdicombe (1997)). Although the regulation mechanism of the PCL layer thickness in the airways is still the subject of controversy (Matsui et al. (1998)), it is recognized that this regulated thickness is well approximated by the length of the cilia.

Measurements of cilia lengths in humans were performed by Serafini & Michaelson (1977) and are given in Table 2.

Two curve fits were tested to approximate the Serafini and Michaelson measurements with a smooth curve along the entire tracheobronchial region. The fitted functions that estimate the cilia length at generation k, and by extension the thickness of the PCL layer, are

$$h_{k,\text{PCL}} = 5.911 \, e^{-k/13.4048} \qquad \text{(fit1)} \tag{6}$$

Generation	Length [μm]
0	6.03
3	4.70
5	3.87
6	3.72
7	3.60

Table 2. Human ciliary length in various lung generations from measurements.

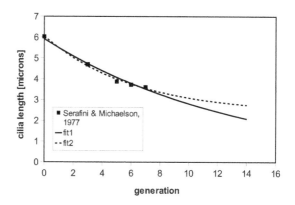

Fig. 3. Experimental and curve fitted values of cilia length in humans.

Generation	$h_{k,\text{PCL}}$ [μm]
0	6.04
1	5.49
2	5.02
3	4.61
4	4.27
5	3.99
6	3.74
7	3.53
8	3.36
9	3.21
10	3.08
11	2.97
12	2.88
13	2.81
14	2.74

Table 3. Human ciliary length and PCL thickness in various lung generations.

$$h_{k,\text{PCL}} = 2.3717 + 3.6724\,e^{-k/6.0837} \qquad \text{(fit2)} \qquad (7)$$

A plot of the raw data and of both curves can be seen in Fig. 3.

Curve fit "fit2" was selected as best fit and the corresponding values of thickness of the PCL layer, based on eq. 7 above, are shown in Table 3.

3.2 Mucus layer thickness

The mucus layer is essentially a gel formed by secretions from goblet cells located in the airway epithelium and also from submucosal glands in the larger airways (Widdicombe (1997)). The thickness of the mucus layer is estimated assuming a continuous layer of constant thickness in each generation, using mass conservation, and modelling the average mucus velocity and production rate for each generation.

The mucus layer is constantly driven by the coordinated beating of airway cilia from the distal generations to the trachea forming the so-called mucus escalator, as illustrated in Fig. 1. The 14th generation is assumed to be the most distal tracheobronchial generation, as described above, where mucus production starts. In reality, as there is no sharp transition from the alveolar region to the tracheobronchial region, the mucus production also does not start always at the 14th generation. In addition, in the more distal generations the mucus layer is not yet fully continuous, but there are probably patches of mucus until the cumulative production ensures full coverage of the airways. For lack of a better alternative, the present model assumes that mucus production starts at generation 14 and forms a continuous annular layer from the onset.

Mucus is actually continuously produced along the conductive airways. The amount produced at a generation k joins the cumulative amount produced at all previous (more distal) generations up to that generation, as the mucus is transported towards the trachea. The amount of mucus that flows through generation k is the accumulated amount produced up to this point, i.e. the sum of all mucus produced by generations $k + 1$ to 14, plus the locally produced amount ($\dot{p}_k$). This local total production is called $\dot{P}_k$.

The flow rate of mucus through all airways of a generation is equal to the product of the annular cross-sectional area of the mucus layer, $A_{k,ML}$, and the mucociliary transport velocity at this generation (clearance velocity), U_k, i.e.

$$\dot{P}_k = A_{k,ML} \, U_k = 2^k \, \pi \left(D_{k,red} \, h_{k,ML} - h_{k,ML}^2 \right) U_k \tag{8}$$

where $D_{k,red}$ is defined in eq. 5, and the cumulative production rate $\dot{P}_k$ at generation k is defined by the recursive formula

$$\dot{P}_k = \dot{p}_k + \dot{P}_{k+1} \tag{9}$$

where $\dot{p}_k$ is the local production rate at generation k. The estimates of $\dot{p}_k$ are described below in section 3.3.

Equation 8 is a quadratic polynomial in terms of $h_{k,ML}$

$$2^k \, \pi \, U_k \, h_{k,ML}^2 - 2^k \, \pi \, U_k \, D_{k,red} \, h_{k,ML} + \dot{P}_k = 0 \tag{10}$$

whose only physical solution is

$$h_{k,ML} = \frac{2^k \, \pi \, U_k \, D_{k,red} - \sqrt{(2^k \, \pi \, U_k \, D_{k,red})^2 - 4 \, (2^k) \, \pi \, U_k \, \dot{P}_k}}{2 \, (2^k) \, \pi \, U_k} \tag{11}$$

Rearranging the terms and defining the reduced airway radius corresponding to $R_{k,red} = D_{k,red}/2$, eq. 11 can be rewritten

$$h_{k,\text{ML}} = R_{k,\text{red}} - \sqrt{R_{k,\text{red}}^2 - \frac{\dot{P}_k}{2^k\,\pi\,U_k}} \tag{12}$$

Hence, the average thickness of the mucus layer in a generation can be determined, if the cumulative production up to that generation ($\dot{P}_k$) and the local clearance velocity (U_k) are known. Their determination in this model is described in the following sections.

Equation 12 provides also a condition to test for airway clogging. If the result from the two terms inside the square root is negative, this means that the clearance velocity is too slow to transport the required mucus flow rate through the whole airway cross-section, which would cause the airways to clog. Although airway clogging actually occurs in severe disease states, the present model is not designed to deal with clogging and parameter sets resulting in clogging should be disregarded.

3.3 Distributed mucus production

For the distribution of the mucus production along the conducting airways there are no human data currently available. As an approximation for the distribution of mucus secretion in humans, the airway surface density of total secretory material measured by Plopper et al. (1989) in various lung generations of the rhesus monkey was adopted. The rhesus monkey is considered in many aspects one of the animals closest to humans, and their similarity in terms of airway surface morphology is well established (Jeffery (1983)).

The volume of total secretory product in the surface epithelium and in submucosal glands per unit airway area measured by Plopper et al. (1989) in specific generations of the monkey's lung was as shown in Table 4.

Generation	Total
0	3.671
3	4.179
6	3.086
11	2.169
13	1.039
15	0.656

Table 4. Distribution of total mucus secretory product in rhesus monkey [$\times 10^{-3}$ mm^3/mm^2] (from Plopper et al. (1989)).

By assuming that the total secretory product per unit airway area is proportional to the amount actually produced per unit area, and by assuming these values scale to humans simply with the airway surface area, i.e. the same rates per unit area apply, these distributed rates were transferred and directly applied to the human lung model. To obtain intermediate values for the missing generations, two straight lines were fit to the data. The first curve fit was a simple interpolation between the first two points. For the second curve fit the value at generation 15 was disregarded. Not only is generation 15 beyond the assumed end of the tracheobronchial region, but also its inclusion would cause the resulting curve fit to end too abruptly at generation 14. With the actual, adjusted values shown in Table 5 the resulting curve tends to zero at generation 16, which agrees better with the adopted lung model (see Fig. 4).

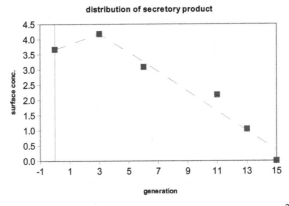

Fig. 4. Distributed mucus production (volumetric surface production [$\times 10^{-3}$ mm^3/mm^2]) and curve fits (eqs. 13 and 14).

Generation	Adjusted Surf. Production
0	3.671
3	4.179
6	3.086
11	2.169
13	1.039
15	0.000

Table 5. Distribution of volumetric mucus production in humans [$\times 10^{-3}$ mm^3/mm^2].

The fitted curves shown in Fig. 4 and used to calculate the distributed local mucus production per unit area $\dot{p}_k''$ correspond to the following functions

$$\text{For generations } 0-3: \qquad \dot{p}_k'' = 0.1693\,k + 3.671 \qquad (13)$$
$$\text{For generations } 3-14: \qquad \dot{p}_k'' = -0.3238\,k + 5.203 \qquad (14)$$

where k is the generation and the result is in $\times 10^{-3}$ mm^3/mm^2. Table 6 shows the corresponding values in each generation.

The distributed local mucus production per unit area $\dot{p}_k''$ is combined with the dimensions of the adopted lung geometry model to result in reference values of average mucus production rates in each generation, according to the following equation

$$\dot{p}_{k,\text{ref}} = \dot{p}_k'' \left(2^k\,\pi\,L_k\,D_k \right) \qquad (15)$$

Equation 15 combined with eq. 9 result in a reference profile of distributed mucus production in the airways, $\dot{P}_{k,\text{ref}}$. Since the production rate of mucus varies from person to person and can also vary with time for the same individual, this reference profile of mucus production is used to scale the actual production profile according to the value of actual total daily production of the subject, $\dot{P}_{\text{tot}}$. A reasonable daily production amount for a healthy, non-smoking adult is 10 ml/day. Typically, a range of values is used in the calculations with 5 ml/day being a reasonable minimum for an adult, and 30 ml/day or greater being considered hypersecretion,

Generation	Surface Production
0	3.67
1	3.84
2	4.01
3	4.18
4	3.91
5	3.58
6	3.26
7	2.94
8	2.61
9	2.29
10	1.97
11	1.64
12	1.32
13	0.99
14	0.67

Table 6. Distribution of volumetric mucus production $\dot{p}_k''$ in humans [$\times 10^{-3}$ mm^3/mm^2].

requiring therapy (Hardy & Anderson (1996)). In fact, patients with severe bronchorrhea have been reported to produce in average more than 60 ml/day (Tamaoki et al. (1994)).

The actual cumulative production values are obtained by modifying the reference values with a scaling factor, namely the ratio between the prescribed total daily production and the cumulative reference production at the trachea (gen. 0)

$$\dot{P}_k = \left(\frac{\dot{P}_{tot}}{\dot{P}_{0,ref}} \right) \dot{P}_{k,ref} \qquad (16)$$

Equation 16 provides the actual cumulative production required in eq. 12.

3.4 Mucus clearance velocity

The airway mucus is a highly viscoelastic fluid that is transported by the lung clearance mechanism (cilia beating) from the terminal bronchioli to the trachea. Due to its viscoelasticity, the mucus forms a continuous layer that flows with almost no mixing. Inhaled particles trapped in this layer are transported smoothly and continuously towards the trachea, where they are swallowed. This mucociliary clearance process can be treated as a series of "escalators" that transport mucus and whatever it is carrying from one generation to the next with constant velocity within each generation.

If a tracer substance is inhaled and its clearance measured, the time to clear the trachea (the first generation to be cleared) would be $\tau_0 = L_0/U_0$, where U_0 is the constant mucus transport velocity at the trachea. The amount of tracer deposited in the main bronchi, the next generation to be cleared, would require the time to travel through the bronchi, $\tau_1 = L_1/U_1$, plus the time to travel through the trachea τ_0 to be cleared. This process is illustrated in Fig. 5. In general, measuring from the time when the first particles deposited in generation k begin

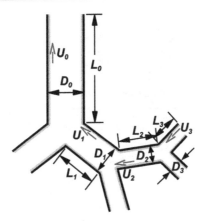

Fig. 5. Schematic of the mucociliary escalator.

to be cleared until the time when the last particles from that generation are cleared results in

$$\sum_{i=0}^{k} \tau_i - \sum_{j=0}^{k-1} \tau_j = \sum_{i=0}^{k} \frac{L_i}{U_i} - \sum_{j=0}^{k-1} \frac{L_j}{U_j} = \frac{L_k}{U_k} = \tau_k \qquad (17)$$

By combining cumulative deposition data from the lung deposition model and the *in vivo* clearance data from Stahlhofen et al. (1980) the time τ_k required to clear each generation was determined. Fig. 6 illustrates this process.

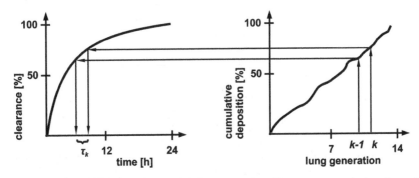

Fig. 6. Time to clear generation k obtained from comparison between cumulative deposition and clearance data.

Four cases measured by Stahlhofen et al. (1980) (breathing pattern A (op. cit., Fig. 8): subject 1 and d_a=9.5 μm, subject 4 and d_a=9.1 μm; breathing pattern B (op. cit., Fig. 9): subject 1 and d_a=7.5 μm, subject 4 and d_a=7.3 μm) were calculated with the 1-D deposition model from Finlay & Stapleton (1995), using the lung geometry dimensions from Finlay (2001). Note that the length of the trachea was shortened by 3 cm, because of the way the tracheobronchial region was imaged in Stahlhofen et al. (1980). The resulting velocity profiles were scaled with a reference clearance velocity at the trachea ($U_{0,ref}$ = 5.5 mm/min) and averaged so that a standard reference clearance velocity profile was generated. This reference profile of mucus transport velocities in each generation ($U_{k,ref}$) is shown in Table 7. Figure 7 shows a comparison of the present reference velocity profile with other similar profiles estimated by Lee et al. (1979), Yu et al. (1986) and Cuddihy & Yeh (1988). All profiles were scaled to a tracheal clearance velocity of 5.5 mm/min.

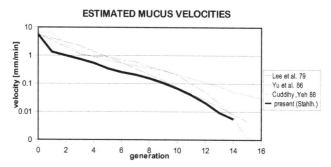

Fig. 7. Comparison of clearance velocity profiles (all profiles scaled to U_0=5.5 mm/min).

Generation	Clearance Velocity
0	5.5000
1	1.3415
2	0.9943
3	0.7439
4	0.5477
5	0.3425
6	0.2551
7	0.2073
8	0.1554
9	0.1063
10	0.0667
11	0.0389
12	0.0206
13	0.0092
14	0.0056

Table 7. Clearance velocity profile ($U_{k,ref}$ in [mm/min], constant in each generation).

Similarly to the variability in the daily mucus production rate, the clearance velocity also shows variation between individuals and for a single individual, depending on their physical activity, for instance. The linear velocity of mucus flow in the trachea in young nonsmokers has been measured by marker particle clearance as typically 10–15 mm/min (Wanner et al. (1996)). CF patients have been assessed with tracheal clearance velocities that range from essentially zero up to these normal values Yeates et al. (1975).

Here again the actual clearance velocities used in the model are obtained by scaling the entire profile with the ratio between the prescribed tracheal velocity $U_{0,set}$ and the reference value $U_{0,ref}$ as follows

$$U_k = \left(\frac{U_{0,set}}{U_{0,ref}} \right) U_{k,ref} \tag{18}$$

Equation 18 provides the actual clearance velocities required in eq. 12.

Using the clearance velocity profiles shown in Fig. 7 and a distributed mucus production based on eqs. 13 and 14, scaled to a total of 10 ml/day, a comparison of estimated mucus layer thicknesses can be calculated. The results are shown in Fig. 8.

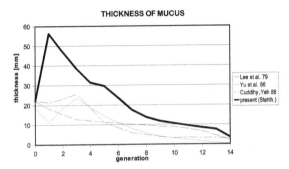

Fig. 8. Comparison of mucus layer thicknesses based on clearance velocities from Fig. 7 and 10 ml/day distributed production.

Combining the thicknesses of the mucus and the PCL layers, the total volume of ASL in each generation can be finally calculated using eq. 2.

4. Modelling local lung concentration of topically active drugs

Once the mass of drug deposited in each generation is obtained with the aerosol deposition model, and the volume of ASL in each generation is obtained with the ASL model, local concentration values can be estimated.

Pharmaceutical aerosols are often an aqueous solution or suspension and the water they carry contributes to the dilution of the drug in the ASL. In addition to knowing the mass of drug deposited in each generation, $m_{k,\text{drug}}$, it is important to also keep track of the mass of water deposited together with the drug, $m_{k,\text{water}}$. If the aerosol is hygroscopic, evaporation may take place in the first few generations and condensation may occur deeper in the more distal airways. The deposition model should account for these changes. We can convert the deposited mass of drug and water to the corresponding volume of deposited aerosol, using

$$V_{k,\text{aerosol}} = \frac{m_{k,\text{drug}}}{\rho_{\text{eff}}} + \frac{m_{k,\text{water}}}{\rho_{\text{water}}} \tag{19}$$

where ρ_{eff} and ρ_{water} are the effective density of the drug formulation and of water, respectively.

All the required information is now available to estimate the average concentration of the drug in the mucus layer, $C_{k,\text{ML}}$, or in the total ASL layer, $C_{k,\text{ASL}}$, in each generation

$$C_{k,\text{ML}} = \frac{m_{k,\text{drug}}}{\left(V_{k,\text{ML}} + V_{k,\text{aerosol}}\right)} \tag{20}$$

$$C_{k,\text{ASL}} = \frac{m_{k,\text{drug}}}{\left(V_{k,\text{ASL}} + V_{k,\text{aerosol}}\right)} \tag{21}$$

To account for inter-subject variability and other uncertainties, ranges of physiological values should be used, resulting in minimum and maximum expected concentration values. Table 8 lists a range of physiological values that can be used.

	unit	Min.	Nominal	Max.
Tracheal Clearance Velocity	mm/min	5	10 to 15	20
Daily Mucus Production	ml/day	5	10	60

Table 8. Range of physiological values of input quantities to the model.

The result of the model is a series of concentration curves for each scenario. These local concentrations are then compared with efficacy levels and toxicity levels of the drug, to verify if they are within those limits. The type of delivery device and the prescribed dosage can be adjusted to optimize the predicted concentration levels, thus increasing the likelihood of a successful outcome.

5. Advances in delivery devices

Recent advances of drug delivery devices have increased substantially their efficiency and their ability to adjust the dose delivered to the lung. From the low cost vented jet nebulizers to the more sophisticated breath-actuated, also known as smart nebulizers, the current generation of inhalers allows for the efficient delivery of large doses with an increasing ability to control the amount delivered. Both aspects are important when delivering antibiotics to the lung. Efficient delivery of a large dose may be required to ensure MIC levels are reached. At the same time, control over the dosage is required to ensure that toxicity levels of the antibiotic are not exceeded.

Despite the development of competing types of devices for drug delivery to the lung, from metered dose inhalers to dry powder inhalers, jet nebulizers have never been completely replaced. They are still capable of delivering the largest dosages to the lung. The ability to contain high volume fills makes them uniquely adapted for this purpose. Many types of continuous output nebulizers are on the market today.   Among them, valved vented (also called breath enhanced) jet nebulizers reduce the amount of drug lost during exhalation by delivering aerosol preferentially during inhalation. Less affordable, but more compact, ultrasonic nebulizers find widespread use in many clinical settings. Finlay, Stapleton & Zuberbuhler (1998) compared various traditional nebulizers and found a large variation in the predicted lung dosage between the devices.

Nebulizers have experienced a revival through the introduction of so-called "smart nebulizers" (Smaldone (2002)). This is a relatively informal classification that includes all the liquid atomizers, which either use or control the breathing pattern for targeted drug delivery. The technologies used for liquid atomization may vary, but these smart nebulizers have in common the attempt to link aerosol generation with the patient inhalation. Examples of smart nebulizers based on jet nebulization are the breath actuated AeroEclipse® (MMC), the Prodose AAD® System (Profile/Respironics), and the AKITA® system (InAMed). Other smart nebulizers or liquid atomizers use different nebulization technologies.   Aerodose® (Aerogen) and eFlow® (Pari) are examples of vibrating orifice based nebulizers, which are capable of more precise dosing. All these new devices incorporate breath actuation and some level of drug delivery control and feedback. Ideally, these monitoring capabilities of the delivered dosage and control of aerosol emission in smart nebulizers could be coupled with an embedded processing unit that estimates the actual deposited dose in the lung, allowing for individually adjusted treatment with the highest probability of successful outcome, as suggested by Lange & Finlay (2006).

This desirable ability to ensure that a prescribed dosage is effectively delivered to the lung is particularly important in the case of antibiotic treatment of lung infections in cystic fibrosis, to reduce the risk of promoting drug resistance through low concentration levels of antimicrobial in the ASL.

6. Applications of the model

The ASL concentration model described above could be in the future incorporated into the control and feedback systems of smart nebulizers, coaching individual patients to inhale the precise dosage required to reach the MIC as estimated by the model.

Currently, the ASL concentration model can be of vital assistance to the design of clinical trials to increase the chances of a positive outcome by ensuring proper concentration levels are achieved in the lung during the tests. An example of how this model can be used to improve the outcome of clinical trials was described by Hasan & Lange (2007). Two antibiotics were compared, using data from the literature. One of the two was tobramycin, an inhaled antibiotic, which is widely used by CF patients. The other example was taurolidine, which was considered for use against *B. cepacia* in CF patients, but failed to produce results in its first clinical trial with delivery by inhalation.

Using the same input parameters described in Hasan & Lange (2007) for the case of tobramycin, corresponding to the study of Ramsey et al. (1999), the estimates of ASL concentration of the antibiotic were recalculated with increased accuracy by taking into account hygroscopic effects in the aerosol size distribution. The new estimates, shown in Fig. 9, result in slightly increased concentrations, which confirm the prediction that concentration levels well exceeded the value of 0.08 mg/mL, or ten times higher than the *in vitro* MIC value, recommended for *in vivo* efficacy against *P. aeruginosa*. These concentration levels were predicted for all 16 scenarios within the range of input parameters studied, while Fig. 9 only shows a few representative cases, including the maximum and minimum curves of the range.

A different outcome befell a clinical trial of taurolidine, a promising drug candidate against *P. aeruginosa* and *B. cepacia* in CF. The outcome of the randomized double-blinded placebo-controlled crossover trial by Ledson et al. (2002), showed no improvement in sputum *B. cepacia* colony counts. As a consequence of this result, development of the inhaled form of this new drug was halted.

Using model input data that matched as closely as possible the study by Ledson et al. (2002), the above-described model estimated ASL concentration levels that in many cases did not exceed the *in vitro* MIC values of 0.4 mg/mL (see Fig. 10), when it is known that *in vivo* concentrations need to be much higher for successful antimicrobial effect.

The higher end of the predictions reached approximately 5 times the *in vitro* MIC, but this scenario (high mucociliary clearance velocity and low mucus production) corresponds more likely to a non-CF patient, such as the single case reported by Ledson et al. (2000). Taking this higher concentration (2 mg/mL) as a new required level, one could use the ASL concentration model to help design a hypothetical trial that would ensure such levels were reached in the

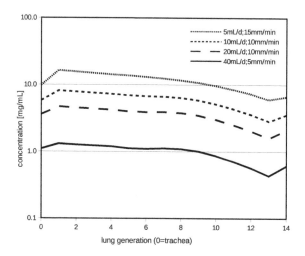

Fig. 9. Estimated ASL concentration of tobramycin in clinical trial.

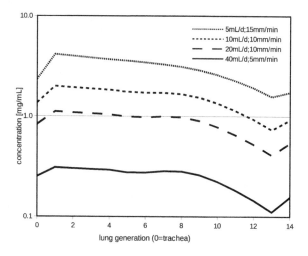

Fig. 10. Estimated ASL concentration of taurolidine in clinical trial.

majority of the cases. Figure 11 demonstrates such a scenario, which could be achieved with a slightly larger nebulizer fill and a significantly larger concentration of taurolidine in the solution.

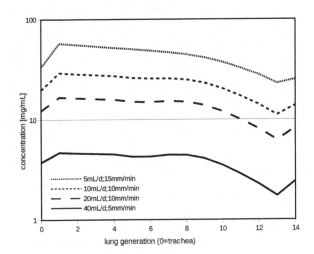

Fig. 11. Estimated ASL concentration of taurolidine in a hypothetical trial that were designed with assistance of the ASL concentration model.

Although a new trial design with higher ASL concentrations would still not be guaranteed to succeed, it would at least stand a better chance of a positive outcome that would allow the continuation of the new drug development.

We conclude that the ASL concentration model is an important tool in the design of clinical trials of inhaled drugs that require a certain concentration level in the lung mucus or the ASL for efficacy.

Similarly, in later stages of the development of a new inhaled drug, the ASL concentration model can greatly assist in the selection of the most appropriate drug delivery device and in establishing the most adequate treatment protocols.

7. Acknowledgements

The mucus and ASL models were developed by the author under the supervision of W. Finlay and in close collaboration with M. King. Their contribution is gratefully acknowledged.

8. References

Böhm, R., Nikodemova, D. & Holy, K. (2003). Use of various microdosimetric models for the prediction of radon induced damage in human lungs, *Radiat. Prot. Dosim.* 104(2): 127–137.

Cuddihy, R. G. & Yeh, H. C. (1988). *Respiratory tract clearance of particles and substances dissociated from particles*, Springer, Berlin, chapter 11, pp. 169–193.

Dailey, H. L. & Ghadiali, S. N. (2007). Fluid-structure analysis of microparticle transport in deformable pulmonary alveoli, *J. Aerosol Sci.* 38: 269–288.

DeHaan, W. H. & Finlay, W. H. (2001). *In vitro* monodisperse aerosol deposition in a mouth and throat with six different inhalation devices, *J. Aerosol Med.* 14(3): 361–367.

DeHaan, W. H. & Finlay, W. H. (2004). Prediciting estrathoracic deposition from dry powder inhalers, *J. Aerosol Sci.* 35(3): 309–331.

Desai, T. R., Tyrrell, G. J., Ng, T. & Finlay, W. H. (2003). In vitro evaluation of nebulization properties, antimicrobial activity and regional airway surface liquid concentration of liposomal polymyxin B sulfate, *Pharm. Res.* 20: 442–447.

Egan, M. J. & Nixon, W. (1985). A model of aerosol deposition in the lung for use in inhalation dose assessments, *Radiation Protection Dosimetry* 11(1): 5–17.

Ferron, G. A., Kreyling, W. G. & Haider, B. (1988). Inhalation of salt aerosol particles – II. Growth and deposition in the respiratory tract, *J. Aerosol Sci.* 19(5): 611–631.

Finlay, W. H. (2001). *The Mechanics of Inhaled Pharmaceutical Aerosols: An Introduction*, Academic Press, London.

Finlay, W. H., Hoskinson, M. & Stapleton, K. W. (1998). Can models be trusted to subdivide lung deposition into alveolar and tracheobronchial fractions?, *Respiratory Drug Delivery VI*, Interpharm Press, Buffalo Grove, IL, USA, pp. 235–242.

Finlay, W. H., Lange, C. F., King, M. & Speert, D. P. (2000). Lung delivery of aerosolized dextran, *Am. J. Respir. Crit. Care Med.* 161: 91–97.

Finlay, W. H., Lange, C. F., Li, W.-I. & Hoskinson, M. (2000). Validating deposition models in disease: what is needed?, *J. Aerosol Med.* 13: 381–385.

Finlay, W. H. & Stapleton, K. W. (1995). The effect on regional lung deposition of coupled heat and mass transfer between hygroscopic droplets and their surrounding phase, *J. Aerosol Sci.* 26(4): 655–670.

Finlay, W. H., Stapleton, K. W. & Zuberbuhler, P. (1997). Predicting regional lung dosages of a nebulized suspension: Pulmicort® (budesonide), *Part. Sci. Technol.* 15: 243–251.

Finlay, W. H., Stapleton, K. W. & Zuberbuhler, P. (1998). Variations in predicted regional lung deposition of salbutamol sulphate between 19 nebulizer models, *J. Aerosol Med.* 11: 65–80.

Forbes, B., Asgharian, B., Dailey, L. A., Ferguson, D., Gerde, P., Gumbleton, M., Gustavsson, L., Hardy, C., Hassall, D., Jones, R., Lock, R., Maas, J., McGovern, T., Pitcairn, G. R., Somers, G. & Wolff, R. K. (2011). Challenges in inhaled product development and opportunities for open innovation, *Adv. Drug Deliv. Rev.* 63: 69–87.

Grgic, B., Finlay, W. H., Burnell, P. K. P. & Heenan, A. F. (2004). *In vitro* intersubject and intrasubject deposition measurements in realistic mouth-throat geometries, *J. Aerosol Sci.* 35(1): 1025–1040.

Hardy, K. A. & Anderson, B. D. (1996). Noninvasive clearance of airway secretions, *Respir. Care Clin. N. Am.* 2: 323–345.

Hasan, M. A. & Lange, C. F. (2007). Estimating *in vivo* airway surface liquid concentration in trials of inhaled antibiotics, *J. Aerosol Med.* 20(3): 282–293.

Heenan, A. F., Finlay, W. H., Grgic, B., Pollard, A. & Burnell, P. K. P. (2004). An investigation of the relationship between the flow field and regional deposition in realistic extra-thoracic airways, *J. Aerosol Sci.* 35: 1013–1023.

James, A. C., Stahlhofen, W., Rudolf, G., Egan, M. J., Nixon, W., Gehr, P. & Briant, J. K. (1991). The respiratory tract deposition model proposed by the ICRP task group, *Radiation Protection Dosimetry* 38(1): 159–165.

Jeffery, P. K. (1983). Morphologic features of airway surface epithelial cells and glands, *Am. Rev. Respir. Dis.* 128: S14–S20.

Kimmel, E. C., Reboulet, J. E. & Carpenter, R. L. (2001). A typical path model of tracheobronchial clearance of inhaled particles in rats, *Toxicol. Ind. Health* 17: 277–284.

Lange, C. F. & Finlay, W. H. (2006). Liquid atomising: nebulizing and other methods of producing aerosols, *J. Aerosol Med.* 19(1): 28–35.

Lange, C. F., Hancock, R. E. W., Samuel, J. & Finlay, W. H. (2001). *In vitro* aerosol delivery and regional airway surface liquid concentration of a liposomal cationic peptide, *J. Pharm. Sci.* 90(10): 1647–1657.

Ledson, M. J., Cowperthwaite, C., Walshaw, M. J., Gallagher, M. J., Williets, T. & Hart, C. A. (2000). Nebulized taurolidine and *B. cepacia* bronchiectasis, *Thorax* 55: 91–93.

Ledson, M. J., Gallagher, M. J., Robinson, M., Cowperthwaite, C., Williets, T., Hart, C. A. & Walshaw, M. J. (2002). A randomized double-blinded placebo-controlled crossover trial of nebulized taurolidine in adult cystic fibrosis patients infected with *Burkholderia cepacia*, *J. Aerosol Med.* 15(1): 51–57.

Lee, P. S., Gerrity, T. R., Hass, F. J. & Lourenco, R. V. (1979). A model for tracheobronchial clearance of inhaled particles in man and a comparison with data, *IEEE Trans. Biomed. Eng.* BME-26(11): 624–629.

Martonen, T. B., Yang, Y. & Hwang, D. (1994). Hygroscopic behaviour of secondary cigarette smoke in human nasal passages, *S.T.P. Pharma Sciences* 4: 69–76.

Matsui, H., Randell, S. H., Peretti, S. W., Davis, C. W. & Boucher, R. C. (1998). Coordinated clearance of periciliary liquid and mucus from airway surfaces, *J. Clin. Invest.* 102(6): 1125–1131.

Mitsakou, C., Helmis, C. & Housiadas, C. (2005). Eulerian modelling of lung deposition with sectional representation of aerosol dynamics, *J. Aerosol Sci.* 36: 75–94.

Plopper, C. G., Heidsiek, J. G., Weir, A. J., St. George, J. A. & Hyde, D. M. (1989). Tracheobronchial epithelium in the adult rhesus monkey: a quantitative histochemical and ultrastructural study, *Am. J. Anat.* 184: 31–40.

Ramsey, B. W., Pepe, M. S., Quan, J. M., Otto, K. L., Montgomery, A. B., Warren, J. W., Vasilijev, K. M., Borowitz, D., Bowman, C. M., Marshall, B. C., Marshall, S. & Smith, A. L. (1999). Intermittent administration of inhaled tobramycin in patients with cystic fibrosis, *New Eng. J. Med.* 340(1): 23–30.

Roth, A. P., Lange, C. F. & Finlay, W. H. (2003). The effect of breathing pattern on nebulizer drug delivery, *J. Aerosol Med.* 16(3): 325–339.

Serafini, S. M. & Michaelson, E. D. (1977). Length and distribution of cilia in human and canine airways, *Bull. Europ. Physiopath. Resp.* 13: 551–559.

Smaldone, G. C. (2002). Smart nebulizers, *Respir. Care* 47: 1434–1441.

Stahlhofen, W., Gebhart, J. & Heyder, J. (1980). Experimental determination of the regional deposition of aerosol particles in the human respiratory tract, *Am. Ind. Hyg. Assoc. J.* 41(6): 385–398a.

Stahlhofen, W., Gebhart, J., Heyder, J. & Scheuch, G. (1983). New regional deposition data of the human respiratory tract, *J. Aerosol Sci.* 14: 186–188.

Sweeney, L. G., Wang, Z., Loebenberg, R., Wong, J. P., Lange, C. F. & Finlay, W. H. (2005). Spray-freeze-dried liposomal ciprofloxacin powder for inhaled aerosol drug delivery, *Int. J. Pharm.* 305: 180–185.

Tamaoki, J., Chiyotani, A., Tagaya, E., Sakai, N. & Konno, K. (1994). Effect of long term treatment with oxitropium bromide on airway secretion in chronic brochitis and diffuse panbronchiolitis, *Thorax* 49: 545–548.

Taulbee, D. B. & Yu, C. P. (1975). A theory of aerosol deposition in the human respiratory tract, *J. Appl. Physiol.* 38(1): 77–85.

Wang, Z., Cheng, H. T., Roa, W. & Finlay, W. H. (2003). Farnesol for aerosol inhalation: nebulization and activity against human lung cancer cells, *J. Pharm. Sci.* 6: 95–100.

Wanner, A., Salathé, M. & O'Riordan, T. G. (1996). Mucociliary clearance in the airways, *Am. J. Respir. Crit. Care Med.* 154: 1868–1902.

Weibel, E. R. (1963). *Morphology of the human lung*, Acedemic Publishers, New York.

Widdicombe, J. G. (1997). Airway surface liquid: concepts and measurements, *in* D. F. Rogers & M. I. Lethem (eds), *Airway Mucus: Basic Mechanisms and Clinical Perspectives*, Birkhäuser, Basel, chapter 1, pp. 1–17.

Yeates, D. B., Sturgess, J. M., Kahi, S. R., Levison, H. & Aspin, N. (1975). Mucociliary transport in trachea of patients with cystic fibrosis, *Arch. Dis. Childhood* 51: 28–33.

Yu, C. P., Hu, J. P., Yen, B. M., Spektor, D. M. & Lippmann, M. (1986). *Models for mucociliary particle clearance in lung airways*, Lewis, Chelsea, Michigan, chapter 39, pp. 569–578.

10

Exercise Performance and Breathing Patterns in Cystic Fibrosis

Georgia Perpati

Adult Cystic Fibrosis Unit, Athens Hospital of Chest Diseases,
Greece

1. Introduction

Cystic fibrosis (CF) patients often experience exercise limitations. Although exercise capacity in CF patients has been extensively investigated over the past 15 years, factors contributing to exercise limitation in such patients have not been fully characterized.

The prognostic value of various exercise indices is considered in numerous clinical studies. However, whether exercise rehabilitation programs will improve the long term prognosis for CF patients remains controversial.

2. Cardiopulmonary exercise testing (CPET): Physiology of exercise

Ventilation, pulmonary gas transfer, cardiac output and peripheral blood flow, all increase in response to the metabolic demands of working muscles.

The pattern of breathing can be described by the following equation:

$$V_E = V_T \times f_b \tag{1}$$

where V_E is pulmonary ventilation, V_T the tidal volume (the volume of air inhaled and exhaled during one respiratory cycle) and f_b the frequency of breathing. In normal subjects during exercise the increase in V_E is achieved by increases in V_T at low and moderate work load, up to 50-60% of vital capacity (Jones and Rebuck , 1979). This is achieved by gradual increases in end inspiratory lung volume to about 80% of total lung capacity (TLC) and reductions in end expiratory volume to about 40% of TLC (Cotes, 1979).

At higher exercise intensity the increase of ventilation is achieved through rise in frequency of breathing. Obviously, in smaller lung volumes, like in children, the f_b commonly seen is at higher levels , not rare up to 60 br/min.

Furthermore, the breathing pattern during exercise includes additional variables, as inspiratory flow (V_I) and the duty cycle (T_i / T_{tot}). In these terms, the above mentioned equation could be written as:

$$V_E = V_I \times T_i / T_{tot} \times 60/f_b \tag{2}$$

Also, the V_D / V_T ratio (physiological dead space) normally is 25 to 35% at rest and in exercise falls to 5 to 20%, due to V_T increase (Jones et al., 1966).

Oxygen consumption depends on work rate levels. The characteristics of oxygen uptake kinetics (VO_2) differ with exercise intensity (Webb and Dodd, 1995). When exercise is performed at a given work rate below lactate threshold (LT) there is a linear dynamic relationship between VO_2 and the work rate. When exercise is performed at work rate above LT, the VO_2 kinetics become more complex and there is an additional slow component either drives to the max VO_2 levels (VO_2 max) or delay steady state VO_2 (then the highest VO_2 value is characterized as VO_2 peak) (Xu and Rhodes, 1999).

Also, in healthy population, cardiac output (Q) during exercise is linearly related to oxygen uptake (Smith et al., 1988, Wasseman et al., 1997). It is important to note that at low exercise intensity (up to 30% of VO_2 max) approximately 50% of energy demands covered by carbohydrates as the other 50% use lipids as source of energy (Borsheim and Bahr, 2003). At higher exercise levels, the energy sources used remain under investigation.

The anaerobic threshold (AT) is the point reached during exercise of increasing intensity, at which aerobic processes give way to anaerobic processes. At this point oxygen intake is unable to meet energy needs and for additional work the energy provided by anaerobic glycolysis. There are various methods have been used to estimate the AT, like measurement of lactate production in plasma accompanies increase in ventilation or measurements of carbon dioxide output and ventilation as indicators of blood lactate increases (Wasserman, 1987, 1994, Zoladz et al 1998).

VO_2 t / slope is an index expresses the oxygen debt and used to describe the early phase of recovery after exercise. VO_2 t / slope has been evaluated in congestive heart failure, chronic obstructive pulmonary disease, cystic fibrosis, beta thalassaemia etc. (Nanas, 1999,2009, Vogiatzis 2005, Pouliou 2001, Koike, 1995). In healthy subjects all these changes during exercise, express their ability for a normal response to exercise. However, in this adaptive capacity should be taken into account some factors affect it like gender, age and physical activity.

CPET is an important tool for evaluation of exercise performance in healthy individuals and additionally utilized in clinical practice to assess a patient's level of intolerance to exercise and the possible underlying causes for this.

During the test, patients are subjected to symptom-limited incremental exercise and breath by breath monitoring of cardiopulmonary variables mentioned above (VO_2, V_E, VCO_2, f b, VO_2 t / slope, HR, Q etc). Moreover they undergo assessment of perceptional responses (eg dyspnea, leg fatigue), measurements of arterial oxygen desaturation, lung volumes and muscle pressures. The incremental exercise period should last 10 – 12 minutes. The measures are reproducible and useful for diagnostic and prognostic purposes (Jones, 1997).

3. Ventilatory response and oxygen kinetics during maximal exercise and early recovery in patients with cystic fibrosis (CF)

One of the earliest observed abnormalities of pulmonary function in CF is an increase in the physiological dead space related to disease severity (Godfrey et al., 1971). This high resting ratio increases further with exercise due to a limited V_T and severe mismatching of ventilation and perfusion (Cerny et al 1982). Ventilation is higher for a given workload.

When Forced Expiratory Volume in first second (FEV_1) is > 60%, the CF patients can exercise almost as the healthy population, while patients with severe disease have limited capacity to increase their tidal volume during exercise and in order to maintain alveolar ventilation they heighten f_b.

As airways obstruction progresses the tidal expiratory flow limitation (EFL), accompanied by decreased inspiratory time (T_i) and lower inspiratory time to total respiratory cycle time (T_i / T_{tot}), leads to raised f_b and essentially to air trapping. EFL has been associated with chronic dynamic hyperinflation during tidal breathing where end-expiratory lung volume is greater than the relaxation volume of the respiratory system.

This dynamic hyperinflation affects the function of respiratory muscles by diaphragm flattening and shortening of the auxiliary and intercostals muscles. Inspiratory muscles overworked on large volumes become unable to pay off the oxygen debt and with exercise progress will fatigue prematurely (Hirsch et al., 1989, Coates et al., 1988).

Oxygen uptake kinetics are slowed in cystic fibrosis. During exercise, ventilation rises in a linear fashion until oxygen consumption reaches a level of 60-70% of VO_2 max, but in CF patients the VO_2 max usually is not reached and at earlier point the oxygen supply becomes inadequate to meet demand and begins anaerobic metabolism and lactic acid accumulation. The recovery is also slower, as it expressed by increased VO_2 t / slope (Webb and Dodd, 1995, Pouliou et al, 2001, Perpati et al., 2010).

The mechanisms causing prolonged oxygen kinetics on early phase of exercise recovery, has not been fully understood although has been observed in deconditioning, heart failure, COPD and CF. A possible cause is a slow recovery of energy stores of the peripheral skeletal muscles (Harris et al., 1976). In the muscles of patients with chronic respiratory impairment the oxidative phosphorylation impaired and there is an early activation of anaerobic glycolysis. Another mechanism that should be considered in the prolonged VO_2 recovery is the oxygen cost of breathing. In CF patients there is a basic physiologic defect leading to enlarged dead space and it is present even in the most mildly affected patients. Progressive airway obstruction reduces vital capacity resulting in VT limitation. In compensation, decreased inspiratory time and increased end-expiratory volume are observed in order to preserve adequate inspiratory and expiratory flow rates. Airway obstruction causes prolongation of expiratory flow rate and in association with the increased breathing frequency results in air trapping. The work and oxygen cost of breathing are increased at high lung volumes and finally exercise is discontinued.

Studies to assess cardiac output in CF patients during steady state exercise found that cardiac function did not influence exercise performance. Although a limitation in diastolic reserve has been observed and there is a rapid rise in the heart rate, the cardiovascular responses are relatively normal for a given workload. However there are some recent data conclude that in CF patients with severe disease, CF related diabetes and older CF patients there is abnormal haemodynamic response to exercise (Hull et al., 2011). As for gas exchange abnormalities, it has been demonstrated that in patients with mild to moderate disease oxygen desaturation is not present during exercise.

The first time that exercise limitation in CF patients had been correlated with pulmonary mechanics rather than circulatory factors and hypoxia was in 1971 (Godfrey et al). Later, Browning et al. investigating 11 adult patients with CF showed that there was a correlation between disease severity and respiratory rate during exercise (Browning et al., 1990). Coates et al also found that there is decreased V_T and T_i, don't lead necessary to respiratory failure although there is a carbon dioxide rise at the onset (Coates et al., 1988). Lands et al. in a study with 14 patients found VE max and VO_2 max decreased during exercise without V_E/VO_2 and V_E/VCO_2 difference between patients and healthy controls. In the same study VO_2 max correlated with FEV_1 (Lands et al., 1992). Nixon and Webb confirmed that VO_2 max was statistically significant prognostic index for disease severity and survival (Nixon et al., 1995). Pouliou et al. describe prolonged oxygen kinetics at early recovery in adult patients with CF (Pouliou et al., 2001). Perpati et al. described breathing pattern in CF patients during maximal CPET and evaluated the correlation between resting respiratory variables and exercise capacity in CF participants (Perpati et al., 2010). They investigated 18 adult patients and 11 healthy subjects who underwent pulmonary function test at rest and symptom-limited treadmill CPET. The main ventilatory response indices at rest, peak exercise and recovery, for each group, are presented at Table 1. Patient's ability to increase V_T and V_E was limited in comparison with healthy subjects. CF patients showed similar ability to increase f_b from rest to peak exercise in comparison with healthy subjects, however they exhibited a prolonged rapid breathing after exercise along with shortened inspiratory time. VO_2 peak was lower in patients and in the same group recovery was longer, as it is expressed by lower VO_2 /t slope.

	Patients			Healthy subjects		
	Rest	Peak	Recovery	Rest	Peak	Recovery
V_E (lt/min)	12.5 ± 2.4	57.2 ± 19	14.4 ± 6.7	11.3 ± 2	81.3 ± 13.2	20.5 ± 5.8
V_T (lt)	0.56 ± 0.1	1.53 ± 0.6	0.72 ± 0.3	0.57 ± 0.2	1.88 ± 0.4	1.2 ± 0.3
f_b (breaths/min)	23 ± 6	38 ± 9	32 ± 8	19 ± 4	44 ± 8	22 ± 5
T_i (s)	1.2 ± 0.3	0.8 ± 0.2	0.9 ± 0.2	1.5 ± 0.3	0.7 ± 0.1	1 ± 0.2
V_T/T_i (lt/s)	0.5 ± 0.2	1.9 ± 0.6	0.8 ± 0.3	0.4 ± 0.1	2.7 ± 0.4	1.2 ± 0.3
VO_2	4.93 ± 1.8	29.12 ± 7	5.77 ± 3.3	4.03 ± 1.1	35.54 ± 7.3	4.82 ± 1.9
V_D/V_T	0.35 ± 0.2	0.16 ± 0.02	0.19 ± 0.04	0.36 ± 0.2	0.10 ± 0.02	0.16 ± 0.04
V_E/VO_2		25.65 ± 5.5			19.9 ± 5.88	
V_E/VCO_2		28.51 ± 5.3			26.62 ± 3.14	
VO_2/t-slope		0.59 ± 0.25			0.95 ± 0.18	

Table 1. CPET indices at rest, peak exercise and recovery for patients with cystic fibrosis and healthy subjects

4. Factors limiting maximal exercise performance in cystic fibrosis: The role of resting lung function, nutrition and disease severity

As mentioned above, it appears that the role of pulmonary mechanics is crucial to exercise limitation. The resting lung function and thus the disease severity have been associated with exercise performance as it is expressed by VO_2 max and VO_2 t / slope.

In serial studies there is a significant correlation between these variables and   FEV1 (Moorcroft et al., 1997, Nixon et al., 1992, Pouliou et al., 2001). Moreover, recent data confirm that oxygen uptake at maximal exercise and early recovery are correlated to resting respiratory variables including inspiratory capacity (IC) and explore its role as predictor of exercise capacity (Perpati et al., 2010). The significant correlations of VO_2 peak and VO_2/t-slope to resting lung function are listed in Table 2. In a multivariate stepwise regression analysis, using peak VO_2 as the dependent variable and the pulmonary function test measurements as independent variables respectively, the only significant predictor emerged was IC. VO_2/t-slope was also lower in CF patients and showed significant correlation with IC. In a final stepwise regression analysis including all independent variables of the resting pulmonary function tests, the only predictor selected for VO_2 peak and VO_2/t-slope was IC (Figure 2).

Parameters	VO_2 peak		VO_2/t-slope	
	r	p value	r	p value
FEV_1, % pred	0.575	0.013	0.774	0.0001
FVC, % pred	0.602	0.008	0.663	0.003
FEV_1/FVC, %	0.513	0.029	0.678	0.002
IC, ml	0.608	0.007	0.859	0.0001

Table 2. Significant correlations of VO_2 peak and VO_2/t-slope to various resting respiratory parameters.

Although pulmonary disease correlates with exercise tolerance, especially in those CF patients with an FEV_1 less than 50% of predicted, nutritional status and muscle function may also play an important role for maintaining anaerobic and aerobic exercise. Several studies with mild or moderate pulmonary disease reported increases in lactate levels and early occurrence of the lactate threshold during incremental exercise, indicating an increase in muscle metabolism and suggesting that peak exercise is not limited by ventilation, but rather by non pulmonary factors that lead to leg fatigue (Moorcroft et al., 2005, Mc Loughlin et al., 1997, Nikolaizik et al., 1998)

In a study included 104 CF who performed progressive cycle ergometry to a symptom limited maximum, the conclusion was that the main factor limiting exercise in mild to moderate disease is peripheral muscle effort (Moorcroft et al., 2005). Reduced muscle performance may be due to poor nutritional status or reduced habitual activity. There are some data to support the hypothesis that the cause is an intrinsic muscle defect.

However, clearly there is a strong relationship between nutrition and muscle function (Elkin et al., 2000). In patients with CF and advanced lung disease, nutritional status plays a significant role in determining exercise capacity but poor nutrition is not correlated with pulmonary function and resting O_2 partial pressure (PaO_2). Malnutrition leads initially to loss of body fat and then to lean tissue wasting and can have adverse metabolic and structural effects on skeletal muscles. Leading to loss of leg muscle mass and decreased respiratory muscle strength, malnutrition can impair exercise performance.

The data of studies exploring the effect of nutritional supplementation on exercise tolerance are controversial. This fact support the hypothesis that exercise limitation in CF patients is the result of multiple combined effects of airways obstruction, nutritional status and metabolic processes.

5. The prognostic value of exercise testing in patients with cystic fibrosis

FEV_1, maximum oxygen consumption (VO_2 peak) during CPET and the Schwachman score (SS) are commonly used to assess functional capacity and disease severity in CF patients. Pouliou et al. explored the relationship between oxygen kinetics during early recovery after maximal CPET and the severity of the disease. They showed that VO_2 t / slope is closely correlated to FEV_1 and SS (Figure 1).

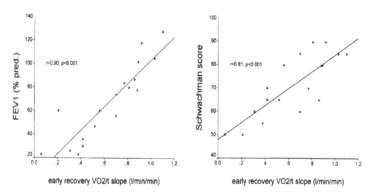

Fig. 1. Correlation between VO_2 t / slope and disease severity.

To the knowledge that resting respiratory variables have a significant correlation to VO_2 peak and to VO_2 t/slope, recent data have been reported about the potential role of IC as of independent predictor of exercise capacity (Perpati et al., 2010).

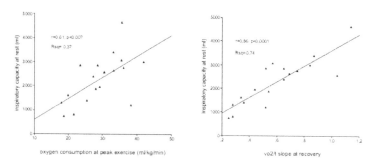

Fig. 2. Correlation between inspiratory capacity and oxygen kinetics at peak exercise and early recovery.

In studies designed to determine the prognostic value of CPET in CF patients higher levels of aerobic fitness are associated with a significantly lower risk of dying. Better aerobic fitness may simply be a marker for less severe illness, however measurement of VO_2 peak appeared to be valuable for predicting prognosis. A multicenter retrospective study analysed 3-year outcomes indicated that there is higher risk of death in patients with lower FEV_1, BMI, diabetes mellitus and higher alveolar arterial gradient for oxygen at peak exercise. Prospective studies needed to confirm the prognostic value of CPET in long term survival and compare its prognostic value with that of FEV_1, especially in patients with mild to moderate disease.

5.1 Submaximal cardiopulmonary exercise testing in cystic fibrosis patients

Submaximal exercise testing is considered a promising exercise capacity testing, especially in patients with limited performance because of fatigue due to disease severity. Submaximal CPET is more tolerable for CF patients as the test is terminated when oxygen uptake approached 75 % of the VO_2 peak. There are a few data showing that VO_2 kinetics during submaximal CPET are a more sensitive index of beneficial effects of exercise training than VO_2 peak and AT in healthy subjects. However, the experience with submaximal CPET in CF patients is generally limited (Hebestreit et al., 2005, Braggion et al., 1989).

In contrast there is a large experience over time with 6 min walk test (6MWT) as a useful tool assessed exercise capacity in patients with CF, mainly for severe disease and children (Gulmans et al., 1996, Nixon et al, 1996, Upton et al., 1988, Butland et al., 1982). The 6MWT is a practical, simple test that measures the maximal distance that a patient can walk at his or her own pace in six minutes. This self paced test is performed in an indoor corridor (or alternatively on a treadmill). The walking course should be 30 m long. The 6MWT provides a global assessment of functional capacity and although it doesn't give specific information and therefore has limited diagnostic capacity, it can be an excellent tool for severe ill patients as it resembles to everyday life activities. Many lung transplant centers use it at the time of assessment prior to transplantation, to determine baseline at start of program, at 6 weeks and every 3 months or to reflect functional changes and after transplantation at 6 weeks, 3 months and formal assessments. This is used in processes of patients referral for transplantation, training protocol design and rehabilitation potential estimation, as severe exercise intolerance could also be a factor precluding transplantation.

6. Perspectives in clinical practice: Rehabilitation programs

CF lung disease is often associated with physical inactivity and deconditioning. The effectiveness of exercise training program in CF patients has been studied in randomized controlled trials. The objective change in exercise capacity was reported as an improvement in VO_2 peak in two studies. Also there are studies reported change in peak heart rate, desaturation during exercise and annual decline in FVC at three years. Controversially, there are studies showing no significant differences in peak minute ventilation or annual decline of FEV_1, although there is a trend for FEV_1 improvement. If exercise training including anaerobic exercises can improve muscle strength and muscle size resulting in weight gain remains also under consideration. Further, in terms of quality of life, positive effects towards perceived feasibility have been noted (Turchetta eta l., 2004, Selvadurai et al., 2002, Schneiderman-Walker et al., 2000, Orenstein et al., 1981).

In a recent systematic Cohrane review of trials investigating the effect of exercise training programs on exercise endurance in patients with CF, the authors conclude that there is limited evidence that regular exercise training is associated with improved aerobic and anaerobic capacity, higher pulmonary function and enhanced airway mucus clearance (Bradley, Moran., 2008). Further research is needed to assess relative benefits of rehabilitation program for these patients.

In another review, Williams et al. present general exercise and training recommendations for children and adolescents with CF including cycling, walking, gymnastics and day to day activities for about 30 min, 3-5 times per week intermittently (Williams et al., 2010). For patients with mild to moderate disease they add activities like swimming, tennis and climbing. In all cases is suggested to avoid activities like bungee-jumping, high diving, scuba diving and hiking in high altitude. The potential risks is associated with more intensive exercise includes dehydration, hypoxemia, hemoptysis, pneumothorax, arrhythmias and fractures in presence of CF related bone disease (Goldbeck et al., 2011).

However, improvements in exercise endurance require individual dosages of training stimuli and vary among individuals.

Prior to transplantation, an individualized pulmonary rehabilitation program is prescribed in order to increase or maintaining mobility and functional capacity, decrease dyspnea and hospitalizations, monitoring oxygen saturation and maintaining morale. Postoperative rehabilitation's goals is safe discharge of functional patients and accelerate recovery in outpatients setting. The training focuses on shoulder range of motion, stretching, strengthening and aerobics to increase endurance (Helm D., 2007).

7. Conclusions

Exercise testing is an important outcome variable in CF patients, correlated with disease severity and survival, exploring the ventilator and cardiac responses to progressively increasing workload and indentifying factors related to this ability for exercise. As there is no perfect test for that, is suggested (Orenstein, 1998) each Cystic Fibrosis Center to adopt the most appropriate for its patients needs and use it consistently.

Looking at pulmonary rehabilitation as a program of medical practice implies methods of improvement the patient's functional ability, in terms of medical, mental, emotional and social potential, we will have to explore further the effect of an individualized approach in designed exercise training protocols and encourage physical training as a part of multimodality treatment of CF.

8. References

Børsheim E, Bahr R. Effect of exercise intensity, duration and mode on post-exercise oxygen consumption. Sports Med. 2003;33(14):1037-60.

Bradley J and Moran F. Physical Training for Cystic Fibrosis. Cochrane Database of Systematic Reviews, no 1, Article ID CD002768, 2008.

Braggion C, Cornacchia M, Miano A, et al. Exercise tolerance and effects of training in young patients with cystic fibrosis and mild airway obstruction. Pediatr Pulmonol. 1989;7(3):145-52.

Browning B, D'Alonso GE, Tobin MJ. Importance of respiratory rate as an indicator of respiratory dysfunction in patients with cystic fibrosis. Chest June 1990;97(6):1317e21.

Butland RJ, Pang J, Gross ER, et al. Two-, six-, and 12-minute walking tests in respiratory disease. Br Med J (Clin Res Ed). 1982 May 29;284(6329):1607-8.

Coates AL, Canny G, Zinman R, et al. The effects of chronic airflow limitation, increased dead space, and the pattern of ventilation on gas exchange during maximal exercise in advanced cystic fibrosis. Am Rev Respir Dis 1988; 138:1524 –1531

Elkin SL, Williams L, Moore M, et al. Relationship of skeletal muscle mass, muscle strength and bone mineral density in adults with cystic fibrosis. Clin Sci (Lond). 2000 Oct;99(4):309-14.

Godfrey S, Mearns M. Pulmonary function and response to exercise in cystic fibrosis. Arch Dis Child 1971; 46:144-151.

Goldbeck L, Holling I., Schlack R. et al. The impact of an inpatient family-oriented rehabilitation program on parent-reported psychological symptoms of chronically ill children. Klin Paediatr.2011; 223 (2): 79-84

Gulmans VA, van Veldhoven NH, de Meer K, Helders PJ. The six-minute walking test in children with cystic fibrosis: reliability and validity. Pediatr Pulmonol. 1996 Aug;22(2):85-9.

Harris RC, Edwards RHT, Hultman E, et al. The time course of phosphoryl-creatine resynthesis during recovery of the quadriceps muscle in man. Pflugers Arch 1976; 367:137-142

Hebestreit H, Hebestreit A, Trusen A, Hughson RL. Oxygen uptake kinetics are slowed in cystic fibrosis. Med Sci Sports Exerc. 2005 Jan;37(1):10-7.

Hirsch JA, Zhang SP, Rudnick MP, et al. Resting oxygen consumption and ventilation in cystic fibrosis. Pediatr Pulmonol. 1989;6(1):19-26.

Helm D. Physiotherapy. Lung Transplantation Manual, UHN, 2007: Chapter 10; 80-84.

Hodson and Geddes, Saunders 2nd edition, 2000.

Jones NL, McHardy GJR et al. Physiological dead space and alveolar-arterial gas pressure differences during exercise. . Clin Sci 1966; 31:19-29

Jones NL, Rebuck AS. Tidal volume during exercise in patients with diffuse fibrosing alveolitis. Bull Eur Physiopathol Respir 1979;15: 321-327

Jones NL. Clinical Exercise Testing. 4th edition, 1997.

Koike A, Yajima T, Adachi H, et al. Evaluation of exercise capacity using submaximal exercise at a constant work rate in patients with cardiovascular disease. Circulation. 1995 Mar 15;91(6):1719-24.

Lands LC, Heigenhauser GJ, Jones NL. Analysis of factors limiting maximal exercise performance in cystic fibrosis. Clin Sci 1992;83:391e7.

Mc Loughlin P, McKeogh D., Byrne P. et al. Assessment of fitness in patients with cystic fibrosis and mild lung disease. Thorax 1997; 52: 425-430.

Moorcroft J, Dodd ME, Webb AK. Exercise testing and prognosis in adult cystic fibrosis. Thorax 1997;52:291e3.

Moorcroft J, Dodd ME, Morris J, Webb AK. Symptoms, lactate and exercise limitation at peak cycle ergometry in adults with cystic fibrosis. Eur Respir J 2005; 25: 1050-1056.

Nanas S, Nanas J, Kassiotis CH, et al. Respiratory muscles performance is related to oxygen kinetics during maximal exercise and early recovery in patients with congestive heart failure. Circulation 1999; 100:503-508

Nanas S, Vasileiadis I, Dimopoulos S, et al. New insights into the exercise intolerance of beta-thalassemia major patients. Scand J Med Sci Sports. 2009 Feb;19(1):96-102.

Nikolaizik, Knopfli, Leister et al. The anaerobic threshold in cystic fibrosis: comparison of V-slope method, lactate turn points and Conconi test. Pediatr. Pulmonol.1998; 25: 147-153.

Nixon PA, Orenstein DM, Kelsey SF, et al. The prognostic value of exercise testing in patients with cystic fibrosis. NEJM 1992; 327:1785e8.

Nixon P, Joswiak M, Fricker F. A six minute walk test for assessing exercise tolerance in severely ill children. J Paediatr. 1996; 129: 362-366

Orenstein DM, Franklin BA, Doershuk CF et al. Exercise conditioning and cardiopulmonary fitness in cystic fibrosis. The effects of a three-month supervised running program. . Chest. 1981 Oct;80(4):392-8.

Orenstein DM. Exercise Testing in Cystic Fibrosis. Editorial. Pediatric Pulmonology, 1998; 25: 223-225.

Perpati G., S. Nanas, E. Pouliou et al. Resting respiratory variables and exercise capacity in adult patients with cystic fibrosis. Respiratory Medicine 2010 (104) 1444 -1449.

Pouliou E, Nanas S, Papamichalopoulos A, et al. Prolonged oxygen kinetics during early recovery from maximal exercise in adult patients with cystic fibrosis. Chest 2001 Apr;119(4): 1073e8.

Selvadurai, Blimkie, Meyers et al. Randomized controlled study of in-hospital exercise training programs in children with cystic fibrosis, Pediatric Pulmonology, 2002: vol.33, no3, pp194-200.

Smith SA, Russell AE, West MJ et al Automated non-invasive measurement of cardiac output: comparison of electrical bioimpedance and carbon dioxide rebreathing techniques. Br Heart J. 1988 Mar;59(3):292-8.

Schneiderman-Walker, Pollock, Corey at al. A randomized controlled trial of a 3-year home exercise program in cystic fibrosis. Journal of Pediatrics, 2000: vol.136, no3: 304-310.

Turschetta A., Salerno T., Lucidi V., et al. Usefulness of a program of hospital supervised physical training in patients with cystic fibrosis. Pediatric Pulmonology, 2004:vol.38, no2, pp115-118.

Upton CJ, Tyrrell JC, Hiller EJ. Two minute walking distance in cystic fibrosis. Arch Dis Child. 1988 Dec;63(12):1444-8.

Vogiatzis I., Georgiadou O., Golemati S. et al. Patterns of dynamic hyperinflation during exercise and recovery in patients with severe chronic obstructive pulmonary disease. Thorax. 2005 Sep;60(9):723-9.

Wasserman K. Determinants and detection of anaerobic threshold and consequences of exercise above it. Circulation. 1987 Dec;76(6 Pt 2):VI29-39. Review.

Wasserman K. et al. Dynamics of oxygen uptake for submaximal exercise and recovery in patients with chronic heart failure. Chest. 1994 Jun;105(6):1693-700

Wasserman K. et al. Cardiac output estimated noninvasively from oxygen uptake during exercise. J Appl Physiol. 1997 Mar;82(3):908-12.

Webb AK, Dodd ME. Exercise and cystic fibrosis. J R Soc Med 1995; 88(suppl 25):30–36

Williams CA, Benden C, Stevens D, Radtke T. Exercise training in children and adolescents with cystic fibrosis: theory into practice. Int J Pediatr. 2010;2010. pii: 670640. Epub 2010 Sep 19.

Xu F, Rhodes EC. Oxygen Uptake kinetics during exercise. Sports Med 1999; 27(5): 313-27.

Zoladz JA, Duda K, Majerczak J. VO2/power output relationship and the slow component of oxygen uptake kinetics during cycling at different pedaling rates: relationship to venous lactate accumulation and blood acid-base balance. Physiol Res. 1998;47(6):427-38.

11

Airways Clearance Techniques in Cystic Fibrosis: Physiology, Devices and the Future

Adrian H. Kendrick

Department of Respiratory Medicine, University Hospitals, Bristol
England

1. Introduction

The appearance of the lungs of a cystic fibrosis (CF) patient at post mortem is typically one of consolidation, with areas of bronchiectasis filled with mucopurulent material and of mucus plugging of the small airways (Yankaskas et al., 2004). The airways of the upper respiratory tract have increased secretion production, whilst in the lower respiratory tract there is increased mucus production and an increase in sputum. This sputum is usually thick and tenacious, becoming thicker and more abundant during an exacerbation and leading to progressive lung damage. It is therefore essential that in patients with CF the process of airway clearance is enhanced, where needed, to attempt to reduce these long-term effects.

The purpose of this chapter is to outline 1) the normal structure and function of the airways, 2) the process of mucus clearance in normal airways, 3) the effects that CF has on both the physiology and mucus clearance, 4) the current understanding of airway clearance device in terms of how they work and their application and finally 6) to look towards the future.

2. Structure and function in normal airways

The structure of the airways, and hence the function of the airways is affected by disease (Ranga & Kleinerman, 1978). Understanding the structure of the normal airways and how CF changes the airway function is essential in understanding the potential application of airway clearance techniques in clinical practice.

2.1 Normal airway structure

The airways start at the trachea and terminate at the alveolar sacks where gas exchange takes place (Fig 1).

There are about 23 branches of the airways from trachea to alveoli. The first 15 generations do not play a role in gas exchange and constitute the anatomical dead space (~150 ml). Gas exchange commences from generation 15 onwards, with alveolar ducts appearing at generations 19 – 22. Generation 23 is the last generation of the airways, constituting the alveolar sacs. The total number of alveoli ranges from 200 to 600 million (mean 300 million), the number correlating with the standing height of the subject (Angus & Thurlbeck, 1972).

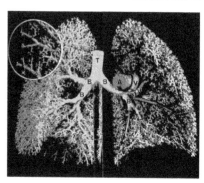

Fig. 1. Resin cast of a human lung showing the branching pattern of the bronchial tree (B) which originates from the trachea (T). In the left lung, the pulmonary arteries (A) and veins (V) are marked. The inset shows the peripheral airway branching at higher power. Reproduced with permission from Wiebel ER, The Pathway for Oxygen: Structure and Function in the Mammalian Respiratory System. Harvard University Press, London, England, 1984

The bronchi contain cartilage which maintains airway patency, whilst the bronchioli have no cartilage (Fig 2). Histologically, the airway epithelium becomes thinner towards the alveoli, where the distance between the air in the alveoli and blood in the pulmonary capillaries is about 0.2 μm.

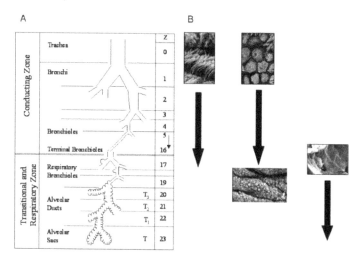

Fig. 2. A) Organization of the airway tree, divided into conducting zones, the transitional and respiratory zones where alveolar begin to appear before leading to the alveolar ducts and sacs. Based on Weibel ER. Morphometry of the human Lung. Heidelberg: Springer. New York Academic, 1963. B) Ciliated epithelia cells and goblet cells occur in the larger airways, decreasing towards the smaller airways. Goblet cells are replaced in the transitional and conducting zones by Clara cells. Pores of Kohn appear in the alveolar walls and are important in terms of collateral ventilation.

Ciliated epithelial cells decrease in number and shape from the large airways towards the small airways. Goblet cells abound in the larger airways, with around 6000 mucus secreting cells.mm^{-2}, and are responsible, along with the submucosal secretory cells, for producing the thick layer of mucus that lines all but the smallest of conducting airways. Mucin is rapidly released from the mucus-secreting cells in response to a range of stimuli including direct chemical irritation, inflammatory cytokines and neural activity (Rogers, 1994). The number of Goblet cells and their secretions increases significantly in CF.

In the smaller airways, Goblet cells are replaced by Clara cells which constitute about 80% of the cell population. Clara cells may play a role in the *Cystic Fibrosis transmembrane conductance regulator* (CFTR) gene-dependant regulation of epithelial electrolyte and water secretion in addition to their roles of surfactant production, protection against oxidative stress and suppression of inflammation (Kulaksiz et al, 2002). CFTR expression is significantly greater in the respiratory and terminal bronchioles compared to the proximal airways and alveoli (Engelhardt et al, 1994). Smooth muscle in the airway wall gradually increases so that in the terminal bronchioles it constitutes around 20% of the wall thickness.

2.2 Normal function

The normal lung maintains sterility below the first bronchial division despite breathing in 450 l.h^{-1} at rest of air contaminated with viruses and bacteria. To move this volume of gas, the ventilatory pump must create negative and positive pressures within the thorax for air to enter and leave, respectively. In addition, the pump must provide a system of distributing the inhaled gas to the alveoli, where blood supplied to the alveoli by the pulmonary circulation will come into contact with the alveolar gas. Hence, for gas exchange to take place 1) the lungs must be ventilated, 2) the pulmonary circulation must be perfused, and 3) the ventilation and perfusion must be matched.

The airways present a major challenge to the movement of air from the atmosphere to the alveoli. The airways narrow with each branching, decreasing from about 18 mm in the trachea, to 0.7 mm at generation 14 and 0.3 mm at the alveolar ducts. Hence, there is a significant increase in the surface area for gas exchange, which may be as great as 143 m^2 in the average male (Weibel, 1984).

As the airways narrow, the resistance (pressure ÷ flow) to airflow increases along a single airway. In reality though, the highest resistance is found in the large central airways, whilst the resistance in the peripheral airways accounts for only 20% of the total resistance due to the increased cross-sectional area of the millions of peripheral airways in parallel. In the large airways, where air moves by bulk flow, a turbulent airflow pattern predominates, thus increasing resistance, whilst in the peripheral airways, diffusion is the predominant means for moving gas (Fig 3).

As the respiratory bronchioles and alveolar ducts contribute little to the overall resistance of the lungs as a whole, the distribution of gas within these units is determined principally by the compliance of the lungs (C$_L$)—a measure of stiffness or floppiness of the object (C$_L$ =Δvolume ÷ Δpressure). In normal lungs, the pressure-volume relationship is such that each tidal breath occurs at the steep part of the relationship, where compliance is high (Fig 4).

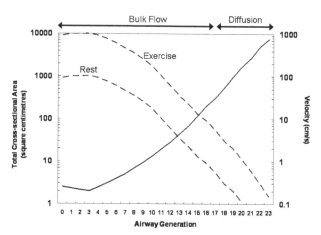

Fig. 3. The relationship of airway cross-sectional area and airflow velocity to airway generation in the human lung. As the airways branch, the total cross-sectional area increases from 2.5 cm² in the trachea, to around 13 cm² at the tenth generation (1024 airways) with a final cross-sectional area of around 300 cm² in the acinar region. The airflow velocity falls by more than 100-fold from the trachea down to the acinus (1 m.s^{-1} to 1 cm.s^{-1}). In exercise, the airflow velocity may be up to ten times greater and so greater airflow is observed within the acinus. Data from various sources.

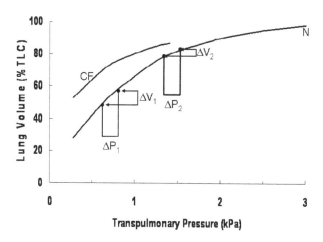

Fig. 4. Schematic of pressure volumes curves in normal subjects (N) and in patients with CF. In normal subjects, for the change in pressure ($\Delta P_1 = \Delta P_2$) there is a greater change in volume at ΔP_1 than for ΔP_2 demonstrating that the compliance of the lungs is greater at ΔP_1 than at ΔP_2. Normal tidal breathing occurs on the steeper portion of the pressure-volume curve. In CF, the pressure volume curve is altered – there is normal compliance of the lungs over the normal tidal volume range, but reduced compliance at high lung volumes (summary data from Mansell et al, 1974)

When we breathe in close to maximum, the pressure-volume relationship is much flatter (more pressure needed to increase a given volume) and so it is much harder to breathe, making the work of breathing greater. On the other hand, when we breathe fully out, the pressure-volume curve is much steeper, indicating that full exhalation is not limited by lung compliance. One key point on this curve is the end-expiratory lung volume (EELV) or functional residual capacity (FRC). This is the equilibrium point in the relationship between the outward pull of the chest wall and the inward collapse of the lungs, where the relative magnitudes are equal, but opposite.

If we apply this observation to an individual alveolus, then the larger it is at the start of tidal inhalation, the stiffer (less compliant) it is and so less air enters the alveoli. This is observed by looking at the distribution of inspired air, which goes preferentially to the more complaint lung bases. In addition to the compliance, ventilation is further distributed within the alveolar units by the pores of Kohn, which connect the alveoli within a lobe; this is referred to as collateral ventilation. (Desplechain et al, 1983). This should permit equilibrium of gas pressures in different lung regions, but this only appears to apply in diseased lungs, as in normal lungs the flow resistance of the collateral pathways is high, and so movement of gas via this route is minimal. (Macklem, 1971). These pores allow transfer of gas between alveoli and function to minimize the collapse of lung units if a more central airway becomes blocked. (Hogg et al, 1969).

One aspect of ventilation that is affected by respiratory disease is the work of breathing. (Campbell et al, 1957; Milic-Emili, 1991). During the passive expiration of a normal resting tidal breath, the work of breathing is performed entirely by the inspiratory muscles. Approximately 50% of the work during inspiration is dissipated as heat in overcoming the frictional forces that oppose inspiration. The remaining 50% is stored as potential energy in the deformed elastic tissues of the lungs and chest wall, as they are at a point above the EELV and hence are not in equilibrium. This potential energy is available for expiration and is dissipated as heat in overcoming the frictional forces that resist expiration.

Energy that is stored in the deformed elastic tissue allows the work of expiration to be transferred to the inspiratory muscles. The actual work performed by the respiratory muscles is very small ($\sim$ 3 ml.min^{-1} O$_2$), compared to the average resting oxygen uptake of 250 ml.min^{-1}, and so accounts for only about 1 – 2% of the resting metabolic rate.

The work of breathing overcomes two main problems—the elastic recoil of the lungs and chest wall, and the airway resistance to gas flow. The total work of breathing is the sum of the elastic and resistive work and may be related to lung volume or breathing frequency (Fig 5). It is likely that each individual selects the most appropriate breathing frequency in order to minimize the work of breathing.

3. Mucus clearance mechanisms

When the lungs are ventilated they are exposed to a vast range of particulate matter, bacteria and viruses. The main defence mechanism against these is the viscous mucus layer, which provides a physical protective barrier to chemical damage of the epithelium (Foster, 2002; Rubin, 2002).

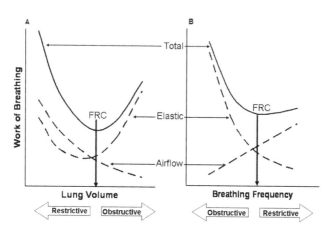

Fig. 5. Schematic diagram of the relationships of work of breathing against lung volume (A) and breathing frequency (B). The total work of breathing is the summation of the elastic properties of lungs and chest wall and airway resistance components. In normal subjects, there will be an optimal lung volume and optimal breathing frequency which is probably set for each individual. The effects of obstructive and restrictive lung disorders are shown for both relationships.

Airway mucus is a complex substance that lines the respiratory tract. Bacteria and other airborne particles become trapped in this sticky mucus and then are swept upwards and outwards by the tiny hair-like structures - cilia. The interaction between normal mucus, cilia and associated structures make up the mucociliary clearance system (MC).

Many inhaled irritants simply dissolve in the mucus, whilst inhaled particles are deposited in the airways either by impaction or sedimentation. These particles are then degraded by the proteases in the mucus or removed intact by the mucus. In the smaller airways sedimentation occurs due to the low airflow, so the particles are deposited and removed by macrophages.

For bacteria and viruses, the first line of defence is the physical removal by the mucus. Within the mucus, humoral defences include immunoglobulins, protease inhibitors and endogenous antibiotics. The airway provides numerous defence mechanisms to prevent microbial colonization by the large numbers of bacteria and viruses present in ambient air. Important components of this defence are the antimicrobial peptides and proteins present in the airway surface fluid—the mucin-rich fluid covering the respiratory epithelium (Rose & Voynow, 2006; Voynow & Rubin, 2009). Recently, evidence has indicated that within the airways of normal subjects is an endogenous antibiotic—human defensins, which is believed to play an important role as part of the airway defence mechanisms (Schneider et al, 2005). Human β-defensin gene (*HBD-2*) represents the first human defence that is produced following stimulation of epithelial cells by contact with micro-organisms, such as *Pseudomonas aeruginosa*, or cytokines, such as tumour necrosis factor-α (*TNF-α*) and Interleukin-1β (*IL-1β*) (Laube et al, 2006). Cellular immunity is also in evidence throughout the epithelium with macrophages, neutrophils and lymphocytes commonly occurring during infections in the normal lung.

Respiratory health is dependent on consistent clearance of airway secretions (Wanner et al, 1996; Houtmeyers et al, 1999). A healthy MC moves respiratory secretions to central airways, with the final clearance achieved by a combination of coughing and swallowing.

3.1 Cough and expiratory flow

Cough may be increased in respiratory infection and assists in clearing the airways from generations 7 - 8 upwards, augmenting the MC when overwhelmed by copious secretions.

Cough is a normal reflex mechanism that commences with a brief rapid inspiration usually greater than the resting tidal volume, this volume being sufficient for expiratory activity. (Ross et al, 1955; Bennett et al, 1990; Bennett & Zeman, 1994). The glottis closes for about 200 ms. There is an associated sharp rise in both pleural and abdominal pressure to between 6.6 to 13.3 kPa, resulting from expiratory muscle and diaphragmatic contraction; lung volume is held constant. Glottal closure limits expiratory muscle shortening, so promoting the isometric contraction of the expiratory muscles. This allows the expiratory muscles to maintain a much more advantageous force-length relationship, resulting in the generation of greater positive intra-abdominal and intrathoracic pressures, which may be up to 40 kPa.

Once the glottis is opened, the expiratory phase of cough occurs. The high intrathoracic pressures developed during the compressive phase promote high expiratory flow rates. Initially, there is a very brief blast of turbulent flow. This initial peak of expiratory flow lasts for between 20 ms to 50 ms and the cough Peak Expiratory Flow (cPEF) may exceed 720 l.min^{-1} (Fig 6). This burst of air is due to the additive effects of the gas expired from the distal parenchymal units and the gas displaced by the more central airways, which are compressed by the high intrathoracic pressures. (Knudson et al, 1974). Although glottal closure enhances this phase of cough, it is not essential for an effective cough. (Von Leden & Isshiki, 1965). After the initial explosive burst of air, a period of between 200 to 500 ms occurs with much lower expiratory flows of between 180 to 240 l.min^{-1}. During this period, lung volume, transpulmonary pressure and cough expiratory flows all decrease.

As expiratory flow rate decreases, the airflow velocity changes—the relationship being dependent on the cross-sectional area of the airways (velocity = flow ÷ cross-sectional area). As shown in Fig 3, the peripheral airways have the largest cross-sectional area, whilst the larger bronchi and trachea have a much lower cross-sectional area. Hence as the cross-sectional area of the airways decreases, the velocity of air increases for a given expiratory flow rate. In other words, the velocity of the gas increases as the air moves from the peripheral to the central airways.

Gas velocity may be further enhanced in the central airways due to dynamic airway compression, where the airway narrows due to the pressure surrounding it being greater than the pressure within it. Narrowing the airway reduces the cross-sectional area, and so velocity increases for a given flow rate.

In normal airways, and during resting tidal breathing, the velocity of air is around 500 cm.s^{-1} down to the airway generations 7 to 8 (Fig 3). At the peak of cough the velocity of air may exceed 16,000 cm.s^{-1}. The cough lasts for approximately 0.5s: up to 1 litre of air may be expelled and the cough is ended either by glottal closure or respiratory muscle relaxation, with a consequent fall in pleural pressure (Fig 6). Often there are further small coughs, which diminish in intensity as lung volume declines towards residual volume.

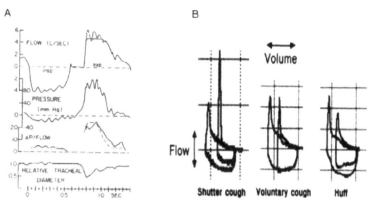

Fig. 6. A) Measurements taken during a cough and the preceding inspiration of a healthy male subject. From top to bottom: volume flow of air; oesophageal pressure; resistance to airflow (ΔP/flow). The inspiratory phase lasts about 0.65 seconds and resulted in an intake of about 2.5 litres of air. Following a short period of glottal closure (about 0.2 sec.) about the same volume of air was expelled within 0.5 sec. During inspiration, the change in intrapleural pressure measured using the oesophageal balloon rarely exceeded - 20 mmHg but, during expiration, the change reached between +100 to 140 mmHg. Maximum inspiratory flow rates were 3 - 4 l.s⁻¹ and expiratory flow rates reached maxima of 5 - 6.5 l.s⁻¹. (From Ross et al, 1955 with permission). B) Coughs performed by a subject, either voluntary, shutter, or huff, was recorded by having the subject cough into a rolling seal spirometer. On average an airway pressure of +70 cmH₂O was required. Finally, the partial forced expiration or huff was performed in the same manner but without glottal closure. These manoeuvres are superimposed upon the subject's normal flow volume curve (From Bennett & Zeman, 1990 with permission)

In relation to mucous clearance, the actual velocity of airflow through the airways alters the kinetic energy (KE) available. As KE = mv² ÷ 2, ($\therefore$ KE $\propto$ v²), where m is the mass of the object and v the velocity, a doubling of the velocity will result in a fourfold increase in the KE. So, the effects of dynamic compression are such that a narrowing of the airways results in an increase in velocity, which in turn results in increases in kinetic energy, thus enhancing the removal of mucus adhering to the airway wall. Zahm et al (1991), using a simulated cough device, found that the displacement of artificial mucus following a simulated cough was greater at smaller airway diameters. Hasani et al (1994) observed that during expiratory flow, mucus transport was more efficient in the central rather than the peripheral airways.

In order to understand how airway clearance devices may be used to assist in the removal of these secretions, we need to understand how cough works in reality. Cough is effective in removing mucus and particulates if the secretions lining the airways are dispersed into the expiratory gas. The high velocity of airflow interacts with the bronchial secretions, resulting in 'two-phase air-liquid flow' by which energy is transferred from the air to the liquid, resulting in a shearing effect on the liquid secretions, thus aiding the expectoration of sputum (Clarke et al, 1970; Kim et al, 1986). At velocities of between 1000 – 2500 cm.s⁻¹ an annular type of two-phase flow occurs, whilst at a velocity of > 2500 cm.s⁻¹ a mist flow with aerosol formation occurs (Fig 7).

A number of factors may be observed -

1. Airways are collapsible structures and so may vibrate and their walls may approximate each other, further aiding the loosening of mucus and promoting clearance (McCool & Leith, 1987);
2. Shearing and expectoration are affected by the viscosity, elasticity and surface tension of the bronchial secretions in a highly complex manner. (Scherer, 1981).
3. Waves of mucus have been observed in the range of airflow occurring during a cough (King et al, 1985) which may further enhance particle clearance (Kim et al, 1983);
4. The physical properties of mucus also affect cough efficiency. Mucus clearance is directly proportional to the depth of the mucus, and is inversely proportional to its viscosity and elasticity (King et al, 1985; King, 1987; King et al 1989; King et al, 1990; Albers et al, 1996)
5. Through use of radiographic methods to measure flow and tracheal cross-section during coughing, an index of 'scrubbing action' has been derived (Harris & Lawson, 1968). In healthy subjects during the first cough, around 59% of the scrubbing action occurs, with only 26% and 16% for the second and third coughs in a sequence of coughs.
6. During a forced expiration, high expiratory flow develops within about 100 ms and results in a high shear rate. Mucus transport varies inversely with shear rate, referred to as pseudoplastic flow or shear thinning. This observed decrease in viscosity can be explained by a temporary realignment of macromolecular glycoproteins due to the applied force (Lopez-Vidriero, 1981). Therefore, repeated forced expirations with short time intervals between each forced expiration may result in a reduction of the mucus viscosity and hence improve mucus transport (Zahm et al, 1991).

In healthy individuals, the rate of mucus secretion is carefully balanced with mucus clearance. The consistency of mucus is maintained such that it is thick enough to trap bacteria and other inhaled particles but thin enough to be moved easily by cilia. When airways are kept free of bacteria, other particles and excess mucus, airways remain open and permit normal gas exchange.

When mucus secretion and mucus clearance are not in balance, excessive airway mucus can cause serious problems. Excess, often sticky mucus may accumulate in the airways, resulting in an increase in the work of breathing. Regardless of the causes, the consequences for the patients are the same—a vicious cycle of recurrent, worsening episodes of inflammation, pulmonary infection, increased production of excess mucus, and airway obstruction, lung damage and respiratory failure.

The consequences of uncleared airway secretions in the airways are a clear link between mucus hypersecretion/secretion retention, exacerbation of illness, hospitalization, a sharply declining one second forced expiratory volume (FEV_1) and death (Annesi & Kauffmann, 1986; Lange et al, 1990; Prescott et al, 1995; Vestbo et al, 1996). The recognition of the clinical significance of excessive, abnormal, or retained airway secretions provides the rationale for improving mucociliary clearance as a logical treatment goal in order to avoid mucus retention and to prevent or break the life-destroying cycle of recurrent infection and progressive pulmonary deterioration.

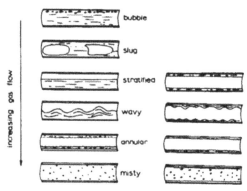

Fig. 7. Effects of gas flow rates on a mixture of gas and liquid flowing through a horizontal tube. At low flows, bubbles of gas may be dispersed in the liquid (bubble flow). As the gas flow rate increases, the bubbles become larger and fill most of the tube cross section; these gas 'slugs' alternate with volumes of liquid and are displaced toward the top of the tube (slug flow). At higher flows the gas slugs merge randomly, leading to the liquid occupy the lower part of the tube with a fairly smooth surface (stratified flow), which as the flow-rate increases further lead to marked surface roll waves appear (wavy flow). With continued increases in flow rates the film of liquid is covered by a dense array of small waves and the surface may appear smoother although there is extreme agitation of the liquid (annular flow). At extreme flow rates, the liquid waves are entrained and blow through the tube in the form of droplets (mist flow). (From Clarke et al, 1970 with permission).

4. Cystic fibrosis

There are a number of significant changes that occur in patients with CF in terms of the respiratory physiology and the mucociliary clearance mechanisms.

4.1 Respiratory physiological changes in CF

The changes that occur to the normal physiology are principally airflow obstruction, which worsens as the disease progresses. In patients with virtually normal spirometry, evidence of mild airways disease is observed by changes in airflow within the small airways, as measured by the Maximal Expiratory Flow (MEF) with 25% of the Forced Vital Capacity (FVC) remaining[1]. This is known as the $MEF_{25\%FVC}$ (Zapatal et al, 1971). In terms of gas exchange function there is widening of the alveolar-arterial PO_2 ($AaPO_2$) and an increased dead space to tidal volume ratio (V_D/V_T) (Lamarre et al, 1972). Whilst the total lung capacity (TLC) is often normal (Reis et al, 1988), the static pressure-volume curve (compliance) shows a loss of recoil pressures at low lung volumes with normal recoil pressures at high lung volumes. (Mansell et al, 1974). This results in a normal compliance of the lungs over the normal tidal volume range, but reduced compliance at high lung volumes (Fig 4).

---

[1]The $MEF_{25\%FVC}$ is obtained from a maximal expiratory flow volume curve. The subject inhales fully and then forcibly exhales. The volume of air exhaled in total is the forced vital capacity (FVC). With 25% of the FVC remaining, the flow rate at this point can be obtained and hence is the $MEF_{25\%FVC}$. In the US this is referred to as the forced expiratory flow (FEF) after 75% of the FVC has been exhaled ($FEF_{75\%FVC}$).

Despite malnutrition being common in CF patients, respiratory muscle weakness is not common, and, if present, is generally mild. (Mier et al, 1990). This is important as cough is common in CF with median rates being 21.2 coughs.h^{-1} (interquartile range [IQR] 14 – 34.9) at the time of exacerbation, but reducing to a median of 9.0 coughs.h^{-1} (IQR 5.8–12.8). (Smith et al, 2006) The other major abnormality of note is that exercise capacity is often limited by the combined effects of airflow obstruction and muscle wasting due to malnutrition. (Lands et al, 1992). As indicated above, the small airways may have reduced function ($\downarrow$MEF$_{25\%FVC}$).

The causes of this small airways disease are possibly the result of significant increases in the inner wall and the smooth muscle areas of the peripheral airways. (Tiddens HA, et al, 2000) Changes in the airway dimensions of CF patients compared to chronic obstructive lung disease (COPD) patients showed that, for airways of 1.9 mm diameter (12th generation), there was an approximately fivefold increase in the smooth muscle area and a threefold increase in the inner wall area without epithelium. In the larger airways (35 mm diameter) there was a ~1.5 increase in smooth muscle area with an almost identical inner wall area without epithelium. These changes may also be related to age (Soboya & Tausig, 1986). Finally, the work of breathing is increased, although the increase is not solely explained by changes in lung function and lung mechanics (Fig 8), but also by the effects of TNF-α and CFTR (Bell et al, 1996).

These pathological studies demonstrate the variability of the destructive processes in the lungs of CF patients. Airway wall thickening is a marked feature of CF and is likely to extend into the small airways and be associated with airways inflammation and obstruction.

4.2 Mucus and mucociliary clearance in CF

In CF, there is increased mucus retention and bacterial colonization, due to the viscous nature of the mucus. However, there is inhibition of antimicrobial peptide activity or gene expression can result in an increased susceptibility to infections where the CF phenotype leads to reduced antimicrobial capacity of peptides in the airway. (Goldman et al, 1997; Rosenstein & Zeitlin, 1998). Thus in CF, bacterial colonization and mucus hypersecretion occur as a consequence, leading to progressive lung damage (Tiddens et al, 2000)

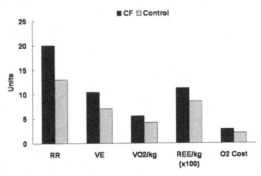

Fig. 8. Summary data on resting energy expenditure and oxygen cost of breathing in control subjects and patients with CF. The data shown (means only) shows that CF patients have a significantly higher respiratory rate (RR; breaths.min^{-1}: p<0.05), minute ventilation (VE; l.min^{-1}: p<0.001); oxygen uptake/kg (VO$_2$/kg; l.min^{-1}.kg^{-1}: p<0.001) and resting energy expenditure/kg (REE; kJ.min^{-1}.kg^{-1}: p<0.001) and O$_2$ cost (ml.l^{-1} VE). (From Bell et al, 1996).

Patients with CF have impaired airway clearance due to the following problems:

1. **Ineffective ciliary clearance:** Normal cilia beat in a coordinated unidirectional fashion to mobilize mucus and clear particulate matter from the airways. Damaged cilia perform this function inadequately or not at all;
2. **Excessive or abnormal mucus production:** CF results in excess mucus production and the mucus is abnormally thick and sticky. Large quantities of mucus, or mucus with altered physical properties, may overwhelm the mucociliary apparatus, inhibiting normal airway clearance (Rose & Voynow, 2005; Voynow & Rubin, 2009);
3. **Ineffective cough:** Cough function may be weak or ineffective if the muscles have become weak or fatigued;
4. **Obstructive lung disease:** The airway size is decreased as a result of structural changes, bronchospasm and excess mucus, limiting the ability to exhale. These effects result in much slower clearance of mucus than in normal subjects, (Regnis et al, 1994; Matthys & Kohler, 1986; Yeates et al, 1976; Wood et al, 1975) with a correlation between the lung function and mucociliary clearance (Robinson et al, 2000; Fig 9).

Because at-risk individuals are prone to recurrent episodes of respiratory inflammation, infection and, eventually, irreversible lung damage, improvement of MC is an essential goal of any treatment plan. Importantly, it is a goal that can be achieved by the individual and must include effective airway clearance therapy.

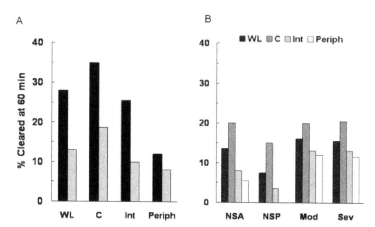

Fig. 9. Percentage of radioactivity cleared from different regions of the right lung at 60 minutes in normal subjects (black columns) and in patients with CF (grey columns). In A), the differences are observed for the whole lung (WL), Central (C), Intermediate (Int) and peripheral (Periph) airways. In B), the same regions as in A) are shown in relation to the degree of airway dysfunction in CF patients – normal small airway function (NSA; $FEV_1 \geq$ 80%pred and $FEF_{25-75} \geq$ 80%pred)[2], normal spirometry (NSP; $FEV_1 \geq$ 80%pred and $FEF_{25-75} <$ 80%pred), moderate (Mod; 40% $\leq FEV_1 <$ 80%pred) and severe (Sev; $FEV_1 <$ 40% pred) lung disease. There is no data for NSP – peripheral. Redrawn from Robinson et al, 2000)

---

[2]The FEF25-75% is the flow rate during a maximal forced exhalation and represents the averaged flow rates between 75% and 25% of the FVC.

5. Airway clearance devices

A number of adjunctive techniques and devices have been used to assist those who are unable, for whatever reason, to clear pulmonary secretions effectively and have been extensively reviewed (Cystic Fibrosis Trust, 2003; Yankaskas et al 2004; Kendrick, 2007; van der Schans, 2007; Bott et al, 2009; Flume et al, 2009; Daniels, 2010).

5.1 Criteria for airway clearance devices

The key to any device used to clear secretions is that it meets a number or criteria, based on the physiology. These criteria are:

1. Increase absolute peak expiratory flow (PEF) to move secretions towards the oropharynx;
2. Use of two-phase gas–liquid flow, both in closed and open airways. In the latter, mucus transport can be achieved by expiratory airflow during forced expiration, as well as tidal breathing. The peak expiratory flow/peak inspiratory flow ratio (PEF/PIF) needs to be > 1.1 to achieve this (Kim et al, 1986; Kim et al, 1986a; Kim et al, 1987) and the frequency of oscillation needs to be between 3 – 17 Hz, with the ideal frequency being around 13 Hz (Gross et al, 1985)
3. Decrease the mucus visco-elasticity in the airway, and hence improve mucus transport (App et al, 1998)
4. Elicit spontaneous coughs by mechanical stimulation of the airways to remove mucus from the trachea, inner and intermediate regions of the lungs (Laube et al, 2006; Hasani et al 1994)
5. Increase expectorated mucus volume (Konstan et al, 1994).

However, what all of these are dependent upon is the mechanical properties of the lungs of CF patients, which may deteriorate with disease progression (Arora & Gal, 1981; van der Schans, 1997). This might mean alternative approaches have to be adopted, and although these above criteria are the "ideal" criteria, there are alternative approaches which use different criteria and which may work as well or better. What is important is that we understand the criteria that each device achieves, how it may be adapted to an individual patient's needs and that changing the device as the disease progresses should always be an option worth considering.

5.2 Physiological aspects of airway clearance devices

Perhaps surprisingly, there are virtually no studies that have investigated exactly how these devices work from the physiological viewpoint and hence our understanding of how we are applying these devices into clinical practice is limited. Recently, McCarren et al (2006a, b, c) have provided evidence of how a variety of techniques work physiologically. These three studies conclude:

1. Chest wall circumference changed by 0.8 cm, the frequency of vibration was 5.5 Hz, the PEF was 58.2 l.min^{-1} and the PEF/PIF ratio was 0.75, all of which are well below the ideal criteria for removing mucus (McCarren et al 2006a). What this study demonstrated was that the PEF during vibration was 50% greater than from a relaxed TLC manoeuvre and was composed of the flow rate due to a) elastic recoil, b) chest wall compression and c) chest wall oscillation. When summed, these three contributors

equated to the PEF observed during vibration, the proportional contributions being 67%, 15% and 14%, respectively;
2. There were clear relationships between the external chest wall force applied, chest wall circumference, intrapleural pressure (Fig 10) and expiratory flow (McCarren 2006b). Similar to the previous reference (McCarren et al 2006a), the intrapleural pressure observed was composed of the sum of the lung recoil, compression and oscillation components, the proportional contributions being 75%, 13% and 12%, respectively.

These two studies (McCarren et al 2006a; McCarren et al 2006b) have demonstrated some important relationships between the mechanics of the lung and the potential to remove sputum. The flow rates generated by vibration would be insufficient to augment secretion clearance by annular flow, since the PEF/PIF ratio was 0.75 and needs to exceed 1.1 (Kim et al, 1987). Why the inspiratory flow bias occurred is unclear, but may be related to the way in which physiotherapists ask the patient to take a deep breath. The frequency of vibration is also much lower than the ideal of between 11–15 Hz (Gross et al, 1985). It is currently unknown whether this vibration frequency would have a significant influence on the sputum rheology, but any decrease that may occur is likely to enhance the ability of cilia to move mucus (Wanner et al, 1996).

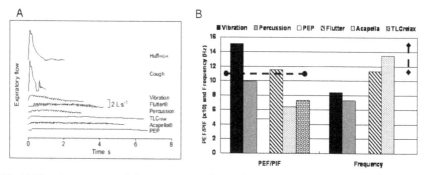

Fig. 10. A) The time course of the expiratory flow of the interventions in one subject. The eight traces have been separated vertically for clarity. Huff$_{HIGH}$: huff from high lung volumes; TLC$_{relax}$: total lung capacity passive expiration; PEP: positive expiratory pressure. B) Summary of data comparing measured data for PEF/PIF ratio and frequency of oscillation in various methods of airway clearance. The vertical dashed line is the ideal frequency range for the methods, whilst the horizontal dashed line is the minimum ideal PEF/PIF ratio. From McCarren et al, 2006b, with permission.

In normal subjects, expiratory flows are enhanced by lung recoil due to the additional forces applied to the chest wall during vibration by manual compression and oscillation. Where there is increased mucus and more viscous secretions, the airways will have a reduced airway radius and airway resistance will be increased.

Physiologically, these observations can be explained using Poiseuille's Equations (Resistance $\propto$ 1/airway radius^4 and Flow $\propto$ radius^4). If the airway narrows (smaller radius), there will be an increase in the resistance to airflow, and a reduction in airflow. Furthermore, Poiseuille's Equation includes a term for viscosity (η) on the denominator, and therefore changes in the viscosity of the mucus will potentially further alter the resistance and flow rates of air.

The third study in CF patients, (McCarren et al, 2006c) investigated vibration, percussion, PEP device, flutter, VRP valve and Acapella PEP. In addition, forced expiratory manoeuvres were voluntary cough and huff from high lung volumes (huff$_{HIGH}$). The important new measurements were inspiratory and expiratory flow rates recorded during the manoeuvres and the oscillation frequency determined by frequency spectral analysis. The key findings of this study were –

1. The PEF of vibration (1.58 ± 0.73 l.s⁻¹) was greater by 1.4 (flutter: 1.13 ± 0.3 l.s⁻¹) to 3.6 times (PEP: 0.44 ± 0.15 l.s⁻¹), but cough PEF was 4.67 ± 1.19 l.s⁻¹and huff$_{HIGH}$ PEF was 5.04 ± 2.3 l.s⁻¹;
2. The frequency of oscillation ranged 6.5–18.3 Hz, with flutter and Acapella devices having the higher oscillation frequencies (Fig 10).

None of these devices achieved the ideal combination. Vibration did not achieve the critical PEF/PIF of > 1.1, nor the critical optimal frequency (8.4 Hz). PEF was reduced due to the added resistance presented to expiration. However, the added resistance may result in stabilization of collapsible airways and allow for collateral ventilation to occur between alveoli via the Pores of Kohn, resulting in an increase in gas volume behind the mucus and hence aiding the movement of the secretions (Fink, 2002; Delaunois, 1989). As with the devices assessed, cough and huff$_{HIGH}$ do not achieve the ideal intervention status, as they do not oscillate airflow; increasing cilia beat frequency and/or decrease mucus viscosity.

Previous studies looking at the oscillation frequency using bench testing have noted that, for the Acapella and Flutter devices, the frequencies range from 8 – 25 Hz (Acapella blue), 13 – 30 Hz Acapella green) and 15 - 29 Hz (Flutter) (Volsko et al, 2003). More recently, Alves et al (2008) has demonstrated that the angle of use of the Flutter VRP1 may influence the outcome and treatment application.

With the limited physiological studies, the remaining question that has been answered to some extent is whether or not these devices alter sputum rheology (App et al, 1998). Using the flutter device and comparing changes in the characteristics of sputum, this study showed that the elastic properties of CF sputum samples were affected significantly by application of oscillations generated by the flutter at 15 and 30 min (Fig 11). The median frequency of the flutter-generated oscillations was 19 Hz.

These findings suggest that applied oscillations are capable of decreasing mucus visco-elasticity within the airways at frequencies and amplitudes achievable with the flutter device, and provide direct evidence of changes in the visco-elasticity of sputum.

Whilst the ideal frequency may be around 13 Hz, there is new evidence that suggests that a combination of 1) a higher frequency causing the airways to vibrate, resulting in the loosening (shearing) of the mucus from the airways, and 2) applying minimal positive pressure (+ 1 cmH$_2$O) via the Pores of Kohn and hence through the use of collateral ventilation, aids mucus clearance (Clini, 2009). This is clearly demonstrated in Fig 12 using lung ventilation scintography (Fazzi et al, 2009)

One of the other ways of removing excess sputum from the airways is by increasing airflow along the airways. During normal tidal breathing the airflow can be artificially increased by applying a venturi effect within a breathing circuit, and this increase in the velocity of the air can enhance the movement of sputum. This is achieved because the movement of air above a layer of mucus develops a shearing force over the surface of this liquid layer. When the shearing force exceeds the surface tension in the mucous layer, the mucus starts to move in the direction of the air flow (Kim et al, 1987). As the mucus moves up the bronchial tree, it will eventually be swallowed. Importantly, this effect can be achieved with minimal discomfort and without the need to cough. Where a patient's clinical condition is deteriorating and they have fatigued muscles, the cough PEF may well be reduced to the extent that clearing secretions is inhibited significantly. A device that removes excessive airway secretions only under tidal breathing conditions would obviate the need for cough.

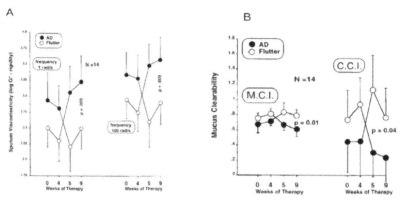

Fig. 11. Studies using Autogenic Drainage (AD) and Flutter therapy after an acute session at the start and end of 4 weeks of therapy, followed by a crossover to 4 weeks of treatment with the other therapy. A) Changes in sputum visco-elasticity and B) Mucus clearability indices, where the mucociliary clearance index (M.C.I.) and cough clearability index (C.C.I.) were calculated from sputum viscoelastic data. From App et al, 1998, with permission.

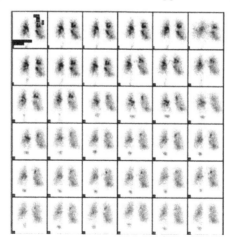

Fig. 12. Dynamic ventilation obtained using lung ventilation scintography (anterior scan) over 30 min during Temporary Positive Expiratory pressure (TPEP) therapy in a patient with COPD. Note how the central deposition of mucus plugs (dark areas) progressively clears over time. From Fazzi et al, 2008.

5.3 Do airway clearance techniques work in reality? (Cochrane reviews)

The range of techniques has recently been evaluated in six Cochrane reviews (Van der Schans, et al, 2000; Elkins et al, 2004; Main et al, 2005; Moran et al, 2009; Morrison & Agnew, 2009; Robinson et al, 2010). The conclusions from these Cochrane reviews are that: -

1. Airway clearance is important in the short term for patients with CF, but the long-term effects of no airway clearance is unknown;
2. Conventional chest physiotherapy is as effective as other forms of airway clearance;
3. Patients like their independence, and therefore any technique which they themselves can use is preferred;
4. Oscillation devices were no more or no less effective than other forms of physiotherapy;
5. There is not enough evidence to conclude, one way or the other, that Active Cycle of Breathing Techniques (ACBT) are any better or worse than any other technique.
6. Non-Invasive Ventilation (NIV) appears to help patients clear sputum more easily than other airway clearance techniques, and particularly in those patients who have difficulty in expectorating sputum.

What is somewhat disheartening in all of these reviews is the almost complete lack of really good quality research, and it is important to ensure data is collected appropriately and the primary and secondary outcome measures are available in order to fully understand the effects of any intervention.

These findings are confirmed in the review by McCool and Rosen (2006) where much of the level of evidence for airway clearance devices is fair to low and the benefits were intermediate to conflicting.

What is consistent in these studies is that, regardless of the device used, or the way in which the trial was conducted, there appears to be little change in the observed primary, and in many cases secondary, outcome measures. However, what makes these studies difficult to compare is the complete lack of commonality between recruitment, methodology, primary and secondary outcome measures, severity of disease, etc. This makes setting evidence-based practice guidelines interesting and limited in their conclusiveness.

5.4 Mathematical modelling

Whilst considerable work has been undertaken with studies on patients, other work has looked at bench testing and modelling some of the airway clearance techniques.

High Frequency Chest Compression (HFCC) has been investigated in such a way. Milla et al. (2004) investigated the actual waveform used in HFCC, which previously had been a sine wave. Changing to a triangular waveform significantly increased sputum production (4%–41%, mean 20%). From this small study of eight patients, the authors concluded that further investigation in patients using the sine and triangular waveform should be undertaken to determine the best frequencies for each waveform, disease and patient. They also pointed out that the original, and now neglected, square wave should be reassessed.

In a subsequent study (Milla et al, 2006), they investigated which frequency was appropriate to use for HFCC in order to 'tune' the device with the patient. In 100 patients, they found that the highest airflows for the sine waveform occurred between 13 – 20 Hz, with the largest volumes occurring between 6 – 10 Hz. For the square waveform, the highest flows and volumes occurred between 6 – 14 Hz. The authors provided a 'tuning' protocol for prescribing frequencies with the various HFCC machines, because they are different from one another.

Sohn et al (2005) used a computational model to investigate the non-linear effects of airway resistance, lung capacitance, and inertness of air on respiratory airflow, with airways resistance contributing the greatest effect.

Bench testing of other devices has been limited to oscillating Positive Expiratory Pressure (PEP) devices (Volsko et al, 2003) and HFCC (Lee et al, 2008). In the study of Volsko et al (2003), there was a statistically significant difference, but probably not a clinically significant difference between mean pressure, pressure amplitude and frequency over a range of experimental conditions. At medium flows, there were similar pressure waveforms, and hence overall similar performance characteristics.

Lee et al (2008) investigated the effects of different frequency and pressure waveforms using three different HFCC devices, bench tested using a mannequin. They concluded that a better understanding of the differences in frequency and pressure amplitude when applying devices to patients would allow clinicians and patients to optimize the efficacy of HFCC.

5.5 Which device to use?

Whatever technique is used to aid airway clearance, its application to a given patient must be such that we achieve a balance between the treatment demands and the patient's lifestyle. It is known that there are adherence issues as a result of the increasing time and effort required by patient self-management strategies, particularly when adults have to try and balance family, work, education etc with managing a chronic disease (Boyle, 2003). Whilst adherence to antibiotic treatment is high (80% - 95%), adherence to physiotherapy is low (40% - 55%; Kettler et al, 2002: 30%; Myers & Horn, 2006). Of note, airway clearance techniques, in adult CF patients, are perceived as a higher treatment burden with only 49% of patients performing airway clearance (Sawicki et al, 2009).

In selecting which airway clearance technique or combination of techniques to use, there are a number of key questions that should be taken into consideration –

1. Is the technique appropriate for the patient's clinical state and environment?
2. Is the technique compatible with the patient's lifestyle?
3. What does the patient like and dislike about each technique appropriate for use at that stage of their clinical status?
4. Does the patient perceive that the technique actually works?
5. What is the balance between the cost of the technique and the benefits, efficacy and preference of the technique?

Taking all of these questions into account and listening to the patient and their needs and preferences should allow the most appropriate airway clearance technique to be used, with or without the addition of behavioural techniques that increase adherence (Bernard & Cohen, 2004).

6. The future

Parents of children and adult patients want treatments that will help them achieve optimal health and quality of life goals. To make appropriate choices, they require accurate information, including a clear description of the theory and technique of available airway clearance methods. Additionally, they need information to allow them rule out treatments that are likely to be unsuitable based on particular physical or mental limitations and upon the psychological, social and economic circumstances of the entire family. Useful decision making criteria may include: -

1. What the patient and medical team want to achieve;
2. The clinical effectiveness of the technique;
3. Medical contraindications;
4. The ease of teaching/learning the technique by the patients and/or by the carer;
5. The likely acceptability and hence adherence with the technique;
6. The likely effort/work required by the technique compared to its likely benefit;
7. The patient's age, motivation, cognitive ability, concentration level and caregiver situation;
8. The degree of independence that a given technique gives the patient from the carer or the medical teams.

Airway clearance techniques are an essential part of the management of patients with CF. However, our understanding of how these devices work from bench testing and from physiological studies is limited to a very small number of studies. The studies themselves have used different populations (adults, children, mixed), with a range of disease severity and in general used the FEV_1 as the primary outcome measure. Whilst the FEV_1 is useful for assessing the respiratory well-being of patients, it presents only a limited picture of airway function. The $FEF_{25\%-75\%}$ has been used, and is thought to be sensitive to abnormalities in the small airway (McFadden & Linden, 1972; Landau et al, 1973). This, however, is only true when both the elastic recoil of the lungs and airways resistance are normal (Woolcock, 1998).

This may not be the case in CF, and is probably overlooked when interpreting results. The other key point about the $FEF_{25\%-75\%}$ is that it is very dependent on a true FVC being achieved on every occasion, which in itself may also be a significant variable. Furthermore, if the FVC increases or decreases then interpretation of this index becomes difficult. An alternative is to use the $MEF_{25\%FVC}$ which is similarly believed to be sensitive to small airway abnormalities. Again, however, if the FVC changes, the $MEF_{25\%FVC}$ cannot be compared post intervention to pre-intervention. Both these indices need careful analysis pre-to-post intervention and this can be achieved by using the iso-volume method of assessment (Boggs et al, 1982a; Boggs et al, 1982b).

Assessing the inhomogeneity of ventilation can be assessed either by nitrogen washout (Paiva & Engel, 1981) or by the use of the Lung Clearance Index (LCI) and the mixing ratio using the inert gas sulphur hexafluoride (SF6). The second method has been shown to be a more sensitive index than spirometry, (Gustafsson et al, 2003) does not require the respiratory gymnastics needed for forced expiratory manoeuvres and also appears to be age independent (Aurora et al, 2004), thereby making it highly useful for longitudinal studies. It is being increasingly used in both adult and paediatric CF patients (Horsley et al, 2008; Horsley, 2009; Kieninger et al (2011).

Whilst these physiological measurements are important guides to the course of disease, they do not present the whole picture. As stated above, what matters to the patient is how much independence they have and how much they themselves can actually do. Techniques which give the patient greater independence in the management of their own disease may well improve adherence to treatment and therapies. Including in studies, measures of patient adherence and patient acceptability are equally important.

Few studies have investigated health-related quality-of life measures, the number of exacerbations or hospital days per year, the costs or harm associated with intervention, or mortality rates. These need to be included along with the appropriate physiological measurements in any properly randomized control trial of airway clearance techniques to ensure that we fully understand how these techniques benefit or otherwise patients with CF. Furthermore, in our increasingly cost sensitive society, there needs to be a cost-benefit analysis included.

There are new techniques emerging and modifications of existing techniques which will improve the already difficult lives of patients with CF. As observed in all of the Cochrane reviews there is a clear need for properly controlled randomized trials and sensible and carefully selected primary and secondary outcomes that present the whole picture, provide the much needed evidence-based information needed to understand and apply these techniques. It is therefore incumbent on all researchers and clinicians working with CF patients to ensure that this good quality research is undertaken and published.

7. References

Albers GM, Tomkiewicz RP, May MK, et al (1996). Ring distraction technique for measuring surface tension of sputum: relationship to sputum clearability. *J Appl Physiol*, 81, 2690 – 2695.

Alves L, Pitta F, Brunetto AF (2008). Performance analysis of the Flutter VRP1 under different flows and angles. *Respir Care*, 53, 316 – 323.

Angus GE, Thurlbeck WM (1972). Number of alveoli in the human lung. *J Appl Physiol*, 32, 483 – 485.

Annesi I, Kauffmann F (1986). Is respiratory mucus hypersecretion really an innocent disorder? A 22-year mortality survey of 1,061 working men. *Am Rev Respir Dis*, 134, 688 – 693.

App EA, Kieselmann R, Reinhardt D, et al (1998). Sputum rheology changes in cystic fibrosis lung disease following two different types of physiotherapy. *Chest*, 114, 171 – 177.

Arora NS, Gal TJ (1981). Cough dynamics during progressive expiratory muscle weakness in healthy curanized subjects. *J Appl Physiol*, 51, 494 – 498

Aurora P, Gustafsson PM, Bush A, et al (2004). Multiple breath inert gas washout as a measure of ventilation distribution in children with cystic fibrosis. *Thorax*, 59, 1068 – 1073.

Bell SC, Saunders MJ, Elborn JS, Shale DJ (1996). Resting energy expenditure and oxygen cost of breathing in patients with cystic fibrosis. *Thorax*, 51, 126 – 131

Bennett WD, Foster WM, Chapman WF (1990). Cough-enhanced mucus clearance in the normal lung. *J Appl Physiol*, 69, 1670 – 1675

Bennett, WD, Zeman KL (1994). Effect of enhanced supra-maximal flows on cough clearance. *J Appl Physiol*, 77, 1577 – 1583

Bernard RS, Cohen LL (2004). Increasing adherence to cystic fibrosis treatment: a systematic review of behavioural techniques. *Pediatr Pulmonol*, 37, 8 – 16.

Boggs PB, Bhat KD, Vekovius WA, Debo MS (1982). Volume-adjusted maximal mid-expiratory flow (Iso-volume $FEF_{25-75\%}$): definition of "Significant" responsiveness in healthy, normal subjects. *Ann Allergy*, 48, 137 - 138

Boggs PB, Bhat KD, Vekovius WA, Debo MS (1982). The clinical significance of volume-adjusted maximal mid-expiratory flow (Iso-volume $FEF_{25-75\%}$) in assessing airway responsiveness to inhaled bronchodilator in asthmatics. *Ann Allergy*, 48, 139 - 142.

Bott J, Blumenthal S, Buxton M, et al (2009). Guidelines for the physiotherapy management of the adult, medical, spontaneously breathing patient. Joint BTS/ACPRC Guideline. *Thorax*, 64, Suppl 1, 1 – 52.

Boyle MP (2003). So many drugs, so little time: the future challenge of cystic fibrosis care. *Chest*, 123, 3 – 5.

Campbell EJM, Westlake EK, Cherniack RM (1957). Simple methods of estimating oxygen consumption and the efficiency of the muscles of breathing. *J Appl Physiol*, 11, 303 – 308.

Clarke S, Jones JG, Oliver DR (1970). Resistance to two-phase gas-liquid flow in airways. *J Appl Physiol*, 29, 464 – 471.

Clini E (2009). Positive expiratory pressure techniques in respiratory patients: old evidence and new insights. *Breathe*, 6, 153 – 159.

Cystic Fibrosis Trust (2003). Association of Chartered Physiotherapists in Cystic Fibrosis. Clinical Guidelines for the Physiotherapy Management of Cystic Fibrosis. Kent: Cystic Fibrosis Trust.

Daniels T (2010). Physiotherapeutic management strategies for the treatment of cystic fibrosis in adults. *Journal of Multidisciplinary Healthcare*, 3, 201 – 212.

Delaunois L (1989). Anatomy and physiology of collateral respiratory airways. *Eur Respir J*, 2, 893 – 904

Desplechain C, Foliguet B, Barrat E, et al (1983). The Pores of Kohn in pulmonary alveoli. *Bull Eur Physiopathol Respir*, 19, 59 – 68.

Elkins M, Jones A, van der Schans CP (2004). Positive expiratory pressure physiotherapy for airway clearance in people with cystic fibrosis. Cochrane Database of Systematic Reviews, Issue 2. Art. No.: CD003147. DOI: 10.1002/14651858.CD003147.pub3.

Engelhardt JF, Zepada M, Cohn JA, Yankaskas JR, Wilson JM (1994). Expression of cystic fibrosis gene in adult human lung. *J Clin Invest*, 93, 737 - 749.

Fazzi P, Girolami G, Albertelli R, et al (2008). IPPB with temporary expiratory (TPEP) in surgical patients with COPD. *Eur Respir J*, 32, Suppl 52, 577s

Fazzi P, Albertelli R, Grana M, Paggiaro PL (2009). Lung ventilation scintography in the assessment of obstructive lung diseases. *Breathe*, 5, 252 – 262.

Fink JB (2002). Positive pressure techniques for airway clearance. Respir Care, 47, 786 – 796

Flume PA, Robinson KA, O'Sullivan BP, et al (2009). Cystic Fibrosis pulmonary guidelines: airway clearance therapies. *Respir Care*, 54, 522 – 537.

Foster WM (2002). Mucociliary transport and cough in humans. *Pulm Pharmacol Ther*, 15, 277 - 282.

Goldman MJ, Anderson GM, Stolzenberg ED, et al (1997). Human *β-defensin-1* is a salt-sensitive antibiotic in the lung that is inactivated in cystic fibrosis. *Cell*, 88, 553 - 560.

Gross D, Zidulka A, O'Brien C, et al (1985). Peripheral mucociliary clearance with high-frequency chest wall compression. *J Appl Physiol*, 58, 1157 - 1163.

Gustafsson PM, Aurora P, Linblad A (2003). Evaluation of ventilation maldistribution as an early indicator of lung disease in children with cystic fibrosis. *Eur Respir J*, 22, 972 - 979.

Harris RS, Lawson TV (1968). The relative mechanical effectiveness and efficiency of successive voluntary coughs in healthy young adults. *Clin Sci*, 34, 569 - 577

Hasani A, Pavia D, Agnew JE, Clarke SW (1994). Regional lung clearance during cough and forced expiration technique (FET): effects of flow and viscoelasticity. *Thorax* 49, 557 - 561.

Hogg JC, Macklem PT, Thurlbeck WM (1969). The resistance of collateral channels in excised human lungs. *J Clin Invest*, 48, 421 - 431

Horsley AR, Macleod KA, Robson AG, et al (2008). Effects of cystic fibrosis lung disease on gas mixing indices derived from alveolar slope analysis. *Respir Physiol*, 162, 197 - 203.

Horsley A (2009). Lung clearance index in the assessment of airways disease. *Respir Med*, 103, 793 - 799.

Houtmeyers E, Gosselink R, Gayan-Ramirez G, Decramer M (1999). Regulation of mucociliary clearance in health and disease. *Eur Respir J*, 13, 1177 - 1188.

Kendrick AH. (2007). Airway clearance techniques in cystic fibrosis: physiology, devices and the future. *J R Soc Med*, 100, Suppl 47, 3 - 23.

Kettler LJ, Sawyer SM, Winfield HR, Greville HW. (2002). Determinants of adherence in adult cystic fibrosis. *Thorax*, 57, 459 - 464.

Kieninger E, Singer F, Fuchs O, et al (2011). Long-term course of lung clearance index between infancy and school-age in cystic fibrosis subjects *J Cyst Fibros*, 10, 487 - 490.

King M, Brock G, Lundell C. (1985). Clearance of mucus by simulated cough. *J Appl Physiol*, 58, 1776 - 1785.

King M. (1987). The role of mucus viscoelasticity in cough clearance. *Biorheology*, 24, 89 - 97.

King M, Zahm JM, Pierrot D, Vaquez-Girod S, Puchelle E (1989). The role of mucus gel viscosity spinnability and adhesive properties in clearance by simulated cough. *Biorheology*, 26, 747 - 752.

King M, Zidulka A, Phillips DM, Wight D, Gross D, Chang HK (1990). Tracheal mucus clearance in high-frequency oscillation: effect of peak flow rate bias. *Eur Respir J*, 3, 6 - 13.

Kim CS, Brown LK, Lewars GG, Sackner MA (1983). Deposition of aerosol particles and flow resistance in mathematical and experimental airway models. *J Appl Physiol*, 55, 154 - 163.

Kim CS, Rodriguez CR, Eldridge MA, Sackner MA (1986) Criteria for mucus transport in the airways by two-phase gas-liquid flow mechanism. *J Appl Physiol*, 60, 901 - 907.

Kim CS, Greene MA, Sankaran S, Sackner MA (1986a). Mucus transport in the airways by two-phase gas-liquid flow mechanism: continuous flow model. *J Appl Physiol*, 60, 908 – 917.

Kim CS, Iglesias AJ, Sackner MA (1987). Mucus clearance by two-phase gas-liquid flow mechanism: asymmetric periodic flow model. *J Appl Physiol*, 62, 959 – 971.

Knudson RJ, Mead J, Knudson DE (1974). Contribution of airway collapse to supramaximal expiratory flows. *J Appl Physiol*, 36, 653 – 667.

Konstan MW, Stern RC, Doershuk CF (1994). Efficacy of the Flutter device for airway mucus clearance in patients with cystic fibrosis. *J Pediatr*, 124, 689 – 693.

Kulaksiz H, Schmid A, Hanschied M, Ramaswamy A, Cetin Y (2002). Clara cells impact in air-side activation of CFTR in small airways. *Proc Natl Acad Sci*, 99, 6796 – 6801.

Lamarre A, Reilly BJ, Bryan AC, Levison H (1972). Early detection of pulmonary function abnormalities in cystic fibrosis. *Pediatrics*, 50, 291 – 298.

Landau LI, Hill DJ, Phelan PD (1973). Factors determining the shape of maximum expiratory flow-volume curves in childhood asthma. *Aust N Z J Med*, 3, 557 – 564

Lands LC, Heigenhauser GJF, Jones NL (1992). Analysis of factors limiting maximal exercise performance in advanced cystic fibrosis. *Clin Sci*, 83, 391 – 397.

Lange P, Nyboe J, Appleyard M, Jensen G, Schnohr P. (1990). Relation of ventilatory impairment and of chronic mucus hypersecretion to mortality from obstructive lung disease and from all causes. *Thorax*, 45, 579 – 585

Laube DM, Yim S, Ryan LK, Kisich KO, Diamond G (2006). Antimicrobial peptides in the airway. *Curr Top Microbiol Immunol*, 306, 153 – 182.

Lee YW, Lee J, Warwick WJ (2008). The comparison of three high-frequency chest compression devices. *Biomed Instrum Technol*, 42, 68 – 75.

Lopez-Vidriero MT (1981). Airway mucus; production and composition. *Chest*, 80 (Suppl), 799 – 804.

Macklem PT (1971). Airway obstruction and collateral ventilation. *Physiol Rev*, 51, 368 – 436.

Main E, Prasad A, van der Schans CP (2005). Conventional chest physiotherapy compared to other airway clearance techniques for cystic fibrosis. Cochrane Database of Systematic Reviews, Issue 1. Art. No.: CD002011. DOI: 10.1002/14651858.CD002011.pub2.

Mansell A, Dubrawsky C, Levison H, Bryan AC, Crozier DN (1974). Lung elastic recoil in cystic fibrosis. *Am Rev Respir Dis*, 109, 190 – 197.

Matthys H, Kohler D (1986). Bronchial clearance in cystic fibrosis. *Eur J Respir Dis*, 146, 311 – 318.

McCarren B, Alison JA, Herbert RD (2006a). Vibration and its effect on the respiratory system. *Aust J Physiother*, 52, 39 – 43

McCarren B, Alison JA, Herbert RD (2006b). Manual vibration increases expiratory flow rate via increased intrapleural pressure in healthy adults: and experimental study. *Aust J Physiother*, 52, 267 – 271

McCarren B, Alison JA (2006c). Physiological effects of vibration in subjects with cystic fibrosis. *Eur Respir J*, 27, 1204 – 1209.

McCool FD, Leith DE. (1987). Pathophysiology of cough. *Clin Chest Med*, 2, 189 – 195.

McCool FD, Rosen MJ. (2006). Non-pharmacologic airway clearance therapies: ACCP evidence-based clinical practical guidelines. *Chest*, 129, 250S – 259S

McFadden ER, Linden DA. (1972). A reduction in maximum mid-expiratory flow rate. A spirographic manifestation of small airway disease. *Am J Med*, 52, 725 – 737

Mier A, Ridington A, Brophy C, Hudson M, Green M (1990). Respiratory muscle function in cystic fibrosis. *Thorax*, 45, 750 – 752.

Milic-Emili J (1991). Work of breathing. In: Crystal RG, West JB, Eds. The Lung: Scientific Foundations. New York: Raven, 1065 – 1075.

Milla CE, Hansen LG, Weber A, Warwick WJ (2004). High-frequency chest compression: effect of the third generation compression waveform. *Biomed Instrum Technol*, 38, 322 – 328.

Milla CE, Hansen LG, Warwick WJ (2006). Different frequencies should be prescribed for different high frequency chest compression machines. *Biomed Instrum Technol*, 40, 319 – 324

Moran F, Bradley JM, Piper AJ (2009). Non-invasive ventilation for cystic fibrosis. Cochrane Database of Systematic Reviews, Issue 1. Art. No.: CD002769. DOI: 10.1002/14651858.CD002769.pub3.

Morrison L, Agnew J (2009). Oscillating devices for airway clearance in people with cystic fibrosis. Cochrane Database of Systematic Reviews, Issue 1. Art. No.: CD006842. DOI: 10.1002/14651858.CD006842.pub2.

Myers LB, Horn SA (2006). Adherence to chest physiotherapy in adults with cystic fibrosis. *J Health Psychol*, 11, 915 – 926.

Paiva M, Engel LA (1981). The anatomical basis for the sloping N_2 plateau. *Respir Physiol*, 44, 325 – 337

Prescott E, Lange P, Vestbo J (1995). Chronic mucus hypersecretion in COPD and death from pulmonary infection. *Eur Respir J*, 8, 1333 – 1338.

Ranga V, Kleinerman J (1978). Structure and function of small airways in health and disease. *Arch Pathol Lab Med*, 102, 609 – 617.

Regnis JA, Robinson M, Bailey DL, et al (1994). Mucociliary clearance in patients with cystic fibrosis and in normal subjects. *Am J Respir Crit Care Med*, 150, 66 – 71.

Reis AL, Sosa G, Prewitt L, Friedman PJ, Harwood IR (1988). Restricted pulmonary function in cystic fibrosis. *Chest*, 94, 575 – 579.

Robinson KA, Mckoy N, Saldanha I, Odelola OA (2010). Active cycle of breathing technique for cystic fibrosis. Cochrane Database of Systematic Reviews, Issue 11. Art. No.: CD007862. DOI: 10.1002/14651858.CD007862.pub2.

Robinson M, Eberl S, Tomlinson C, Daviskas E, Regnis JA, Bailey DL, Torzillo PJ, Menache M, Bye PT (2000). Regional mucociliary clearance in patients with cystic fibrosis. *J Aerosol Med*, 13, 73 - 86.

Rogers DF (1994). Airway goblet cells: responsive and adaptable frontline defenders. *Eur Respir J*, 7, 1690 – 1706.

Rose MC, Voynow JA (2006). Respiratory Tract Mucin Genes and Mucin Glycoproteins in health and Disease. *Physiol Rev*, 86, 245 – 278.

Rosenstein BJ, Zeitlin PL (1998). Cystic Fibrosis. *Lancet*, 351, 277 – 282

Ross BB, Gramiak R, Rahn H. (1955). Physical dynamics of the cough mechanism. *J Appl Physiol*, 8, 264 – 268.

Rubin BK (2002). Physiology of airway mucus clearance. *Respir Care*, 47, 761 – 768.

Sawicki GS, Seller DE, Robinson WM (2009). High treatment burden in adults with Cystic Fibrosis: Challenges to Disease Self-Management. *J Cyst Fibros*, 8, 91 – 96.

Scherer PW (1981). Mucus transport by cough. *Chest*, 805, 830 – 833.

Schneider JJ, Unholzer A, Schaller M, Schäfer-Korting M, Korting HC (2005). Human Defensins. *J Mol Med (Berl)*, 83, 587 – 585.

Smith JA, Owen EC, Jones AM, Dodd ME, Webb AK, Woodcock A (2006). Objective measurement of cough during pulmonary exacerbations in adults with cystic fibrosis. *Thorax*, 61, 425 – 429.

Soboya RE, Tausig LM. (1986). Quantitative aspects of lung pathology in cystic fibrosis. *Am Rev Respir Dis*, 134, 290 – 295

Sohn K, WJ Warwick, Lee YW, Lee J, Holte JE (2005). Investigation of non-uniform airflow signal oscillation during high frequency chest compression. *Biomed Eng Online* 2005 [http://www.biomedicalengineering-online.com/content/4/1/34]

Tiddens HA, Koopman LP, et al (2000). Cartilaginous airway wall dimensions and airway resistance in cystic fibrosis. *Eur Resp J*, 15, 735 – 742.

van der Schans CP (1997). Forced expiratory manoeuvres to increase transport of the bronchial mucus: a mechanistic approach. *Monaldi Arch Chest Dis*, 52, 367 – 370.

van der Schans CP, Prasad A, Main E (2000). Chest physiotherapy compared to no chest physiotherapy for cystic fibrosis. Cochrane Database of Systematic Reviews, Issue 2. Art. No.: CD001401. DOI: 10.1002/14651858.CD001401

van der Schans CP (2007). Conventional chest physical therapy for Obstructive Lung Disease. *Respir Care*, 52, 1198 – 1206.

Vestbo J, Prescott E, Lange P (1996). Association of chronic mucus hypersecretion with FEV_1 decline and chronic obstructive pulmonary disease morbidity. Copenhagen City Heart Study Group. *Am J Respir Crit Care Med*, 153, 1530 – 1535

Volsko TA, DiFiore JM, Chatburn RL (2003). Performance comparison of two oscillating positive expiratory pressure devices: Acapella versus Flutter. *Respir Care*, 48, 124 – 130.

Von Leden H, Isshiki N (1965). An analysis of cough at the level of the larynx. *Arch Otolaryngol*, 81, 616 – 625.

Voynow JA, Rubin BK. (2009). Mucins, mucus and sputum. *Chest*, 135, 505 – 512.

Wanner A, Salathe' M, O'Riordan TG (1996). Mucociliary clearance in the airways. *Am J Respir Crit Care Med* 154, 1868 – 1902

Weibel ER (1984). The Pathway of Oxygen. Cambridge, Mass: Harvard University Press.

Wood RE, Wanner A, Hirsch J, Di Sant'Agnese (1975). Tracheal mucociliary transport in patients with cystic fibrosis and its stimulation by terbutaline. *Am Rev Respir Dis*, 111, 733 – 738.

Woolcock AJ (1998). Effects of drugs on small airways. *Am J Respir Crit Care Med*, 157 (Suppl 5), S203 – S207

Yankaskas JR, Marshall BC, Sufian B, Simon RH, Rodman D (2004). Cystic fibrosis adult care: consensus conference report. *Chest*, 125, 1 (Suppl), 1S - 39S.

Yeates DB, Sturgess JM, Kahn SR, Levison H, Aspin N. (1976). Mucociliary transport in trachea of patients with cystic fibrosis. *Arch Dis Child*, 51, 28 – 33.

Zahm JM, King M, Duvivier C, Pierrot D, Girod S, Puchelle E. (1991). Role of simulated repetitive coughing in mucus clearance. *Eur Respir J*, 4, 311 – 315.

Zapatal A, Motoyama EK, Gibson LE, Bouhuys A. (1971). Pulmonary mechanics in asthma and cystic fibrosis. *Pediatrics*, 48, 64 – 72.

12

The Physiotherapist's Use of Exercise in the Management of Young People with Cystic Fibrosis

Allison Mandrusiak and Pauline Watter

The University of Queensland, Division of Physiotherapy
Australia

1. Introduction

The aim of this chapter is to provide an overview of how physiotherapists (physical therapists) can use exercise in their management of young people with cystic fibrosis (CF), assisting the multidisciplinary team to optimise outcomes for this population. While many resources provide management information about the CF health condition, the focus is often on medical management. However, physiotherapists play an integral role in the multidisciplinary team being at the coalface of daily intervention for this population. Consequently, their role - supported by contemporary evidence - must be considered in the holistic approach to management. In this chapter we will briefly discuss the physiotherapists' general management of people with CF, with the focus directed towards the role of exercise in this management regimen.

This chapter explores the benefits of exercise to this population, and considers the factors limiting exercise performance in young people. A review of the previous studies of exercise intervention programs for people with CF in inpatient and outpatient settings will be provided, and issues affecting adherence and clinical applicability will be discussed. A novel exercise program the *Cystic Fibrosis Fitness Challenge* was developed by Mandrusiak & Watter et al. (2009c) and was specifically designed to address the limitations described in the literature. Aspects of this program and its accompanying *FitKit*TM will be presented in this chapter, with an exploration of how the International Classification of Function, Disability and Health – Children and Youth (ICF-CY) (World Health Organization, 2007) was used to frame the selection of performance measures and program elements. Relationships between exercise and other physiotherapy measures commonly reported for this population will also be considered, since applying the ICF framework, we can expect to find relationships between measures within and between domains. For example, impaired cardiorespiratory function may relate to reduced exercise tolerance, which then may be associated with limited activity and restricted participation. However, weak muscles due to decreased activity may also contribute to limited activity, suggesting that management needs to consider impairment, limitations and restrictions holistically rather than as separate issues.

1.1 The ICF framework for describing performance in young people with cystic fibrosis: A basis of design for exercise intervention

This chapter is scoped within the framework of the International Classification of Functioning, Disability and Health – Children and Youth (ICF-CY) (World Health Organization, 2007) which is an extension of the original framework developed in 2001 (World Health Organization, 2001). Because CF is a multifactorial health condition and usually utilizes a team management approach, the ICF-CY provides an excellent framework for a holistic description of assessments, to direct intervention and identify overlaps and gaps in management. In conjunction with family- or client-centred practice, this contemporary approach considers the client with the health condition of CF and their family as the center of management. Of specific interest to physiotherapists in their management of those with CF, relevant *body structures and functions* would include respiratory function, muscle strength and range of motion, *activities* would include motor skills and functional capacity, and *participation* would include activities of daily life at school, home and in leisure pursuits. Further, *contextual factors* include environmental and personal factors (for example, age, gender, inpatient/outpatient status and attitudes towards exercise) and are also considered within this framework. The theoretical underpinnings of the ICF framework state that performance on measures *within* a domain may be related, and further that relationships may exist in measures of performance *between* domains. This implies that changes in respiratory function (*body structures and functions* domain) may be associated with changes in muscle strength (*body structures and functions* domain). Such associations will guide selection of both assessment measures and interventions. As a between-domain example, improvements in respiratory function are expected to relate to improvements in distance walked in the six-minute walk test (*activities* domain) or sports played at school (*participations* domain). Overall, it is proposed that these interactions will provide an important foundation for comprehensive investigation of the performance of young people with CF, and for exploring the impact of contextual factors on their function (Mandrusiak et al., 2009b). Understanding these relationships will provide a strong evidence-base to direct physiotherapy.

2. The focus of the physiotherapist in the management of individuals with cystic fibrosis

The physiotherapist is considered a cornerstone member of the CF multidisciplinary team, and conventionally their management aims to reduce the respiratory impairments related to this health condition by clearing thick, tenacious secretions from the airways (Farbotko et al., 2005). To achieve this, physiotherapy has traditionally focused on airway clearance techniques, and more recently, attention has been given to the integral role of exercise to enhance management and achieve better outcomes across the now extended lifespan of those with CF. In addition, now that we understand the range of impairments that include musculoskeletal issues such as impaired strength (de Meer et al., 1999; de Jong et al., 2001; Hussey et al., 2002) and range of motion (Mandrusiak et al., 2010) , which limit activity and restrict participation in those with CF, physiotherapists are better placed to provide broad based intervention at all levels of the ICF to facilitate optimal outcomes and reduce barriers to participation by these affected children.

The theoretical basis for airway clearance techniques is included elsewhere in this text and will not be considered here. 'Passive' techniques of postural drainage, percussion and vibration, were traditionally the mainstay of respiratory physiotherapy management. These applications were "done to" the individual with CF, and while these techniques continue to play an important role, more active techniques are now available such as the active cycle of breathing technique and positive expiratory pressure devices, as well as inhalation therapy and thoracic mobility exercises (McIlwaine, 2007). This now emphasizes the role of the individual with CF and the family (especially in the case of the young person) in being an active member of the management team and proactively participating in their own treatment, using a "done with the client" or "selected by the client" philosophy. With this trend to encompass more dynamic techniques as a consequence of emerging evidence, physiotherapy now emphasizes the importance of physical exercise as an adjunct to traditional airway clearance techniques. In CF, exercise has other benefits addressing the unique complications which are emerging as longevity improves, such as impairments in posture and bone mineral density. A diagram of the ICF-CY representing the physiotherapists' perspective of possible interventions relevant to the young person with CF is provided below (Figure 1).

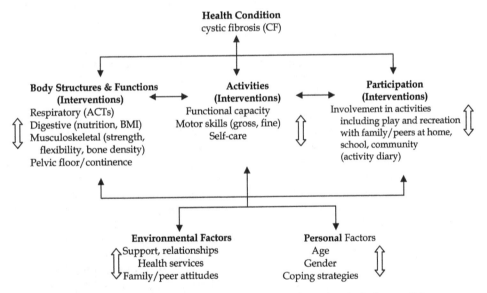

Fig. 1. The ICF-CY (World Health Organisation, 2007): adapted to include possible interventions relevant to the young person with CF.

2.1 Benefits of exercise for people with cystic fibrosis

On the most basic level, exercise is regarded as a natural daily activity for young people, and allows participation in the typical play activities of childhood as well as life-long leisure activities. Ideally, those with CF would be able to partake in exercise with its attendant benefits, and consequently engagement in exercise should be an expectation or goal as well as part of their management. Beyond this basic premise, research and evaluation in the clinical setting has earned exercise its place in the routine management of people with CF (Dodd & Prasad, 2005). Exercise has long been promoted as an essential element of the care for people with CF because exercise intolerance has always been a trait of disease progression (Orenstein and Higgins, 2005). It is therefore crucial to recognize that participation in regular physical activity is a positive prognostic factor in this population (Nixon et al., 1992). Consequently, promoting exercise for people with CF has become an integral aspect of practice, and its prescription must be based on best evidence.

Cooper (1998 p143) believes the physiological influences of exercise suggest its *"profound and important role as therapy"* for people with CF, and exercise programs show potential to be *"an elegant and natural way to stimulate and/or promote the expression of beneficial genes"*. More globally, the psychosocial changes from exercise validate its *"multidimensional impact for people with CF"* (Klijn et al., 2004 p1303). Thus the possibility of potentially modifying the clinical course of the CF health condition by an *"intervention as simple, cheap, safe and enjoyable as exercise remains appealing"* (Barker et al., 2004 p351).

A recent overview of Cochrane systematic reviews performed by Bradley and Moran (2008) summarised the evidence for physical training (exercise) for people with CF. Seven trials using randomised parallel-group design were included, with a total of 231 participants including children and adults. Three studies included children only (Selvadurai et al., 2002; Klijn et al., 2004; Turchetta et al., 2004), and two notable studies included adults and children (Cerny, 1989; Schneiderman-Walker et al., 2000). Overall, these trials showed some evidence of benefits of short- and long-term physical training for people with CF, and this was also the conclusion provided by other reviews in the field (Smidt et al., 2005; Bradley et al., 2006; Shoemaker and Hurt, 2008).

While the effectiveness of exercise intervention programs for this population has traditionally been determined by reduced impairment in body structures and functions (particularly respiratory function) and reduced activity limitations (such as greater six-minute walk distance), the role of exercise for promoting more holistic changes in function is increasingly being recognised. With increased longevity of people with CF, the prevalence of secondary musculoskeletal complications is increasing (Massery, 2005) and must be considered as part of their presentation. This supports the important role of physiotherapy beyond affecting airway clearance, and strengthens the need for an holistic approach which incorporates exercise for prevention or management of secondary musculoskeletal changes (Dodd & Prasad, 2005; Lannefors, 2004; Massery, 2005) to enhance client outcomes. This approach would include addressing range of motion, muscle strength, power and endurance, as well as strong promotion of physical activity. The ICF-CY provides a framework against which such parameters and relationships can be considered.

Further, improving a child's activity and participation are recognized as important goals of exercise intervention for this population, to maintain fitness and thus curtail the cycle of deconditioning associated with this health condition (Stanghelle, 1988; Stevens and Williams, 2007). Importantly, participation in regular physical activity is associated with many holistic benefits, such as improved quality of life and wellbeing (Boas, Danduran, & McColley, 1999; Orenstein, Nixon, Ross, & Kaplan, 1989; Selvadurai et al., 2002). The ICF-CY model facilitates exploration of the impact of exercise intervention on these wider aspects of functioning.

2.2 Providing exercise opportunities across inpatient and outpatient settings: Research supporting advances in practice

Although the performance of exercise is now an integral component of the management of young people with CF, the most effective style of exercise program across inpatient and outpatient settings is yet to be established. During hospitalization, young people with CF are often segregated to minimize cross-infection of respiratory pathogens (Cystic Fibrosis Trust, 2001; Koch et al., 2003), and this presents practical challenges for physiotherapy exercise intervention (Hind et al., 2008). In consequence, it is clear that physiotherapy exercise programs must be adaptable to the limited space at the hospital bedside for performance by individuals in isolation who cannot participate in group exercise sessions or share exercise equipment in the gym. Development of tailored programs which provide a variety of physical activities has been identified as an important aspect to enhance adherence to exercise in this population (Holzer et al., 1984; Blomquist et al., 1986; Stanghelle, 1988; Salh et al., 1989; Abbott et al., 1996; Britto et al., 2000; Schneiderman-Walker et al., 2000; Moorcroft et al., 2004; Turchetta et al., 2004), and such programs must be evidence-based to target issues characteristic of young people with CF.

Developing attractive and efficacious inpatient programs is a challenge in itself, but as highlighted by Moorcroft, Dodd, Morris and Webb (2004) and Dodd and Prasad (2005), transferring exercise programs to the outpatient setting and sustaining them in the long term is also a challenge in the CF population. Physical activity and prescribed exercises are a permanent part of living for those with CF and compliance leading to optimal outcomes is difficult to sustain. Despite these challenges, a range of literature supports the incorporation of outpatient exercise programs in the management of young people with CF. As CF is a lifelong health condition, and the benefits of exercise are well established, strategies to enhance exercise performance across the lifespan are imperative. However, the impact on health resources and clients' distances from established hospital centres make it difficult to facilitate long term supervised hospital-based outpatient exercise programs (Schneiderman-Walker et al., 2000), and sustainable programs based outside of the hospital are needed (Moorcroft et al., 2004).

During outpatient periods, there is support for home-based exercise programs rather than hospital-based programs (Bar-Or, 2000; Bernard & Cohen, 2004; Moorcroft et al., 2004; Schneiderman-Walker et al., 2000; Turchetta et al., 2004). These need to be engaging for the young person with CF, especially if s/he is to continue with these activities as an outpatient once discharged from hospital acute care. Further, it is believed that exercise programs in hospital are not attractive for young people, and that home-based programs are more acceptable (Turchetta et al., 2004). Physical activity should be enjoyable and natural, rather than bear the stigma of therapy, and this may be better achieved in the home environment (Bar-Or, 2000). Further, it is likely that home-based exercise programs save the family time and expense (Bar-Or, 2000) and are more feasible (Bernard and Cohen, 2004). Therefore, research is warranted to establish effective home-based outpatient exercise programs, and facilitate client transition into these programs from the inpatient setting.

2.2.1 Recommendations for exercise programs for young people with cystic fibrosis: Linkages to development of a novel exercise program

A summary of systematic reviews of exercise across a range of populations (Smidt et al., 2005) indicated that targeted and individualized exercise programs were more beneficial than standardized programs. In a Position Statement published by the *Australian Physiotherapy Association* (Taylor et al., 2006) the important skills of the physiotherapist for prescribing exercise are highlighted as three major dimensions: management of disorders of movement, knowledge of exercise regimens and dosages, and clinical reasoning skills to ensure that exercises are optimal for the individual. Specifically for young people with CF, exercise programs should be tailored to individual needs, as there is considerable variability in terms of disease severity, fitness, enthusiasm and preference for types of activities (Webb & Dodd, 1999; Prasad and Cerny, 2002).

To address the aforementioned needs, the *Cystic Fibrosis Fitness Challenge* (CFFC) developed by Mandrusiak & Watter et al. (2009c) is a targeted exercise program for use in inpatient and outpatient settings, based on recommendations from the field. Part of this innovative exercise program is a portable exercise tool (*FitKit*™) that is adaptable to limited space environments such as at the hospital bedside in the inpatient setting. The design aspects of this novel program and tools are presented in Section 2.3.

Although specific guidelines are not currently reported, it is recommended that all people with CF should be encouraged to exercise 'several times per week' (Yankaskas et al., 2004), and across the lifespan (Thoracic Society of Australia and New Zealand 2007). Specifically, exercise for *young people* with CF should be viewed as fun as well as therapy and its role should be regarded equally from the young person's point of view as well as a clinical mandate from the multidisciplinary team (Webb & Dodd, 1999). Exercises must be stimulating, age-appropriate and enjoyable, and varied to avoid monotony as well as to avoid overuse injuries (Stanghelle, 1988). Further, prescription of exercise programs should be timely, and appropriate for different settings including within the hospital and the home (Lannefors, 2004). The exercise program must be realistic and allow for the treatment demand and time pressures faced by young people with CF and their families each day, and thus the program must integrate into their lifestyle (Moorcroft et al., 2004). Enthusiasm from the multidisciplinary team members towards exercise and a flexible approach to encouraging physical activities should not be underestimated (Moorcroft et al., 2004).

Educational dialogue is also recommended, as knowledge of the CF health condition and reasons for treatment are associated with increased adherence (Gardner, 2004; Hinton et al., 2002; Prasad & Cerny, 2002). Educational resources must be age-appropriate and thus attractive and colourful (Hinton et al., 2002; Gardner, 2004). These recommendations were integrated into the design of the resources and delivery of the *CFFC* described in Section 2.3.

The ideal elements of exercise programs for this population are presented in the literature, and include: endurance and strength training for the upper and lower limbs; aerobic and anaerobic activities; interval training; weight bearing activities; and flexibility exercises (Webb & Dodd, 2000; Selvadurai et al., 2002; Klijn et al., 2004; Dodd & Prasad, 2005; Bradley et al., 2006; Sahlberg, 2008). As well as addressing the function across these multiple areas, providing a variety of activity types makes it possible to individually tailor the program according to the young person's preferences, thereby improving exercise participation (Klijn et al., 2004). These elements were considered and incorporated into the CFFC program.

As recommended by Rogers, Prasad and Doull (2003), intensity of exercise performance should be derived from results of exercise testing. The *"Clinical Guidelines for the Physiotherapy Management of Cystic Fibrosis: Recommendations of a Working Group"* (Cystic Fibrosis Trust, 2002) recognize that no specific information exists for exercise program intensity and duration for people with CF, and that general recommendations for the 'normal' population are used. These include an intensity of 70-85% of peak heart rate (Orenstein et al., 1981), starting with a duration of exercise classified as 'tolerable' and progressing to 20 to 30 minutes, three- to four-days per week. However, these *Clinical Guidelines* also highlight the differences between children and adults, in relation to exercise ability, indicating that prescriptions for adults may not be appropriate for young people. These differences include: differences in growth, muscle and fat; higher respiratory rate and heart rate; inferior cooling mechanisms; increased energy expenditure and increased reliance on fat metabolism (Cystic Fibrosis Trust, 2002). In young people, strength training must be properly performed, planned and not over-strenuous, as growing bones are sensitive to stress (especially repetitive loading) and the epiphysial plate is susceptible to injury before full growth is complete (Behm et al., 2008). To further minimize these risks it is important to provide a variety of activities to ensure joints are not subjected to repetitive stress (Stanghelle, 1988). Therefore, exercise programs for young people with CF should be specifically designed for this age group, and not just based on those designed for adults.

The health condition of CF affects quality of life in adults mainly due to dyspnea and limitations in exercise capacity which lead to limitations in physical functioning (de Jong et al., 1997). Thus, programs which aim to improve exercise capacity and thus reduce dyspnea may impact positively on quality of life, and it is important to incorporate these strategies into programs for younger people with CF to optimise quality of life across the lifespan.

2.2.2 Fostering adherence to exercise programs in young people with cystic fibrosis

While maintaining adherence to medications and dietary schedules is difficult in the young person with CF and considered elsewhere in this text, our focus as physiotherapists is on fostering adherence to respiratory physiotherapy programs and exercise programs especially as the child with CF enters adolescence and may expect to experience greater autonomy. Overall, people with CF prefer exercise to other components of therapy (Abbott, Dodd, Bilton, & Webb, 1994; Moorcroft et al., 2004; Moorcroft, Dodd, & Webb, 1998), regarding it as a socially acceptable 'normal activity'(Prasad and Cerny, 2002; Orenstein and Higgins, 2005), and an area over which they have control (Abbott et al., 1996). Importantly, adherence to exercise is higher than adherence to respiratory physiotherapy (Schneiderman-Walker et al., 2000). Thus, the integral role of exercise for people with CF is strengthened by its positive perception, which is important to maintaining interest and adherence across the lifespan.

Despite this reported positive perception towards exercise as therapy, the issue of treatment adherence is a growing concern for multidisciplinary CF teams (Kettler et al., 2002). This discrepancy represents a missing link between viewing exercise positively, and adhering to exercise programs. Adherence is a complex and multidimensional issue (Hobbs et al., 2003) and a detailed review is beyond the scope of this chapter. Instead, key literature in the field of adherence to exercise in young people with CF is presented, to provide strategies for the intervention exercise programs presented here.

Non-adherence to exercise programs may lead to wasted resources, reduced quality of life, missed days at school/work, and higher health care costs (Ireland, 2003; Modi and Quittner, 2003) and thus focusing attention on increasing exercise adherence in this population is critical (Bernard and Cohen, 2004). As children progress into adolescence, the desire to have more control over their lives and a tendency to rebel against authority often result in problems with adherence (Gudas et al., 1991). While strategies to improve adherence in adolescents with CF are integral, it is critical to instill knowledge about exercise during early childhood to enhance adherence into later life stages (Bernard and Cohen, 2004). People tend to look to the short- rather than the long-term benefits of treatment to decide whether to continue (Abbott et al., 1994), so strategies that track progress and improvement in exercise performance, such as log books, pedometry and field tests, may enhance perception of the short-term benefits, and thus enhance adherence.

The multidisciplinary CF team should provide universal support, continued encouragement and education to reinforce the message to the young person and their family that exercise is an important part of treatment (Boas et al., 1999; Dodd & Prasad, 2005; Prasad & Cerny, 2002). Specifically, the role of the physiotherapist for people with CF has been described as that of educator, clinician, researcher and manager (Ireland 2003). The role of educator is particularly important, as empowering patients through education positively affects adherence to treatment and thus health outcomes (Gudas et al., 1991; Hinton et al., 2002; Prasad and Cerny, 2002; Ireland, 2003; Gardner, 2004). Patients are influenced by their own internal belief system; any information or required action needs to make sense and be justifiable to them (Carr et al., 1996). To this end, there is an increasing focus on informing patients and involving them in healthcare decisions (Hinton et al., 2002), and patients should be 'fully involved in any decision-making process during treatment planning' (Chartered Society of Physiotherapy 2000: 8.1). Therefore, using exercise programs that include educational strategies and incorporate the individual in tailoring the exercise program are essential for the physiotherapist to enhance adherence across the lifespan.

An older study by Carr et al. (1996) found that many people with CF (>16 years) did not perceive physiotherapists as having a role in tailoring exercise programs for them. Further, it is reported that exercise prescriptions are often presented in a general manner, without clear specifications of parameters such as frequency and duration (Hobbs et al., 2003). Lannefors (2004) advised that recommending patients to be "physically active" is not enough, and that more active guidance and continuing encouragement is needed. These important findings and the developing evidence base suggest now that physiotherapists need to take a more active involvement in promoting exercise, and in individualizing and monitoring the effects of these programs to strengthen their role in management. Currently, best practice physiotherapy would enhance knowledge of the young person and their family to facilitate ongoing compliance.

The role of parents in influencing their child's participation in exercise is well documented. Lack of parental support towards physical activity may lead to a reduction in regular exercise (Boas et al., 1999), and considering the established relationship between fitness and prognosis (Nixon et al., 1992; Pianosi et al., 2005), this issue of parent education is of particular relevance. Attitudes toward exercise may be acquired as part of life experience and social support, and with parental encouragement to participate are especially important factors (Baker and Wideman, 2006). Further, parents with an ethos of active personal lifestyle facilitate the young person to be active (Dodd & Prasad, 2005). Education of the family is paramount: a study by Boas et al. (1999) reported that parents of young people with CF perceived fewer benefits of, and greater barriers to exercise than parents of healthy young people, and that less than half of parents in the CF group understood the long term benefits of exercise or knew that exercise performance was related to long term prognosis. However, this education may be improving, as a recent questionnaire provided to 50 young people with CF (8-18 years) and their parents showed they had "substantial exercise knowledge" (Higgins et al., 2007). Overall, there is a need for ongoing comprehensive education of the young person and their family regarding the role of exercise, to achieve optimal outcomes of intervention.

Behavioural strategies to increase adherence to exercise in young people with CF have shown some promise (Bernard & Cohen, 2004; Tuzin et al., 1998). These strategies include self-monitoring, exercising with a partner, behavioural contracting, goal-setting, contingency management, and praise and differential attention. Some of these strategies were incorporated to optimise adherence to the CFFC exercise program described in Section 2.3.

As outlined in a review by Dodd and Prasad (2005), there are several perceived barriers to exercise, including unsupportive parental attitudes towards exercise (Boas et al., 1999) and unacceptability of rigid training programs (Gulmans et al., 1999). Further, the daily treatment burden and fatigue associated with the CF health condition make adherence to recommended exercise programs more difficult (Prasad and Cerny, 2002), and this population receives relatively little positive reinforcement for efforts to adhere to treatment (Kettler et al., 2002). This is a driver for physiotherapists when individualizing exercise programs for this population, to ensure integration of physical activity into daily life instead of imposing 'extra' treatment, and to provide appropriate positive reinforcement for participation in exercise. As per the ICF-CY, parents have best impact when facilitatory behaviours towards exercise are displayed.

Specific recommendations for optimising adherence to exercise programs developed for young people with CF are presented in the literature. It is recognised that young people participate more consistently in programs that include a variety of activities, recreational elements and fun (Blomquist et al., 1986), particularly individualized programs which employ activities based on personal preference and perceived competence (Abbott et al., 1996; Britto, Garrett, Konrad, Majure, & Leigh, 2000; Holzer et al., 1984; Moorcroft et al., 2004; Salh et al., 1989; Schneiderman-Walker et al., 2000; Turchetta et al., 2004). In contrast, when the program is regimented, prescribed at an incorrect intensity or not age-appropriate, adherence tends to be poor (Gulmans et al, 1999). Further, programs delivered with specific information about optimal frequency and duration will enhance adherence (Hobbs et al., 2003). An individualised program will facilitate incorporation of regular exercise into their daily life and an already demanding treatment routine (Klijn et al., 2004; Moorcroft et al., 2004). These suggestions to enhance adherence were considered in the development of the exercise program presented later in this chapter.

In summary, addressing adherence issues is paramount to the effectiveness of exercise programs, particularly in a population already burdened by many daily treatments. The multidisciplinary CF team, particularly physiotherapists, must provide support and enthusiasm to promote exercise performance. Educational dialogue is paramount, and should be targeted at the level of the young person with CF and their family. Individualized exercise programs that provide a variety of activities based on the young person's preference and competence, and that allow tracking of personal progress, are more likely to succeed. Overall, this highlights the importance of promoting effective and tailored exercise regimes for young people with CF, and it is vital to include strategies aimed at improving and encouraging adherence.

2.3 A novel approach to facilitating exercise for young people with cystic fibrosis

As outlined above, exercise is a central feature of management in youth with CF due to its positive effects in reducing impairments in cardiorespiratory and musculoskeletal structures and functions, increasing activity and facilitating participation, acknowledging that individual contextual factors may also impact. In response to current clinical challenges and to recommendations in the literature, we developed a novel program (the *Cystic Fibrosis Fitness Challenge* (*CFFC*), and accompanying *FitKit*TM) to facilitate performance of exercise integrated into daily life for young people with CF, and design aspects of this program are presented in this section.

The *FitKit*TM (Figure 2) was developed as a portable, tailored resource designed to facilitate exercise performance in a variety of settings - the bedside, gym, inpatient and outpatient - representing an effective tool for physiotherapists working with young people with CF. The portable design of the *FitKit*TM and overall *CFFC* is particularly appropriate in the hospital setting, to support exercise performance where space issues are increasingly common due to segregation of patients for infection control. A variety of exercise elements was included in this program, supported by previous studies in the field, and by findings from earlier studies by Mandrusiak and Watter et al. (2009c) into the presentation of young people with CF in the context of the ICF-CY. A pool of 100 activities presented on colour-coded Activity Cards was developed to address each of the exercise components of aerobic, anaerobic, strength and flexibility. The program facilitator pre-selected the Activity Cards suitable for each participant, and then worked with the participant to select those that they enjoyed, at the same time achieving the therapeutic goals. The *CFFC* involved a 30-60 minute session each weekday over the course of a usual 10-14 day inpatient period, and independently 3-5 days per week at home (outpatient period). Clear guidelines were developed to guide the program facilitators to achieve optimal implementation of the *CFFC*.

A Physical Activity Log (PAL) was designed for participants to record activities performed in each session, during inpatient and outpatient phases of management. Demonstrations for completing the PAL during the inpatient period were provided by the program facilitator, progressing towards self-completion prior to discharge. Information documented in the PAL included exercise type, intensity (for example, heart rate, level of perceived exertion or breathlessness), duration / repetitions, enjoyment level of the activity, limiting factors, pedometry score, and quality and quantity of the sputum expectorated. A sticker system was integrated whereby participants received a gold star for vigorous intensity activities, and a coloured star for moderate intensity activities. This system provided visual feedback and positive reinforcement regarding the intensity and appropriateness of activities performed, and encouraged participants to monitor and progress performance. Also, the PAL provided visual reminders to the participant to ensure adequate hydration during each session. Educational strategies were incorporated into the resources in the *FitKit*™ to increase awareness within this population about the role of exercise (Gudas et al., 1991; Hinton et al., 2002; Prasad and Cerny, 2002; Ireland, 2003; Gardner, 2004) during inpatient and outpatient periods, with emphasis on monitoring exercise intensity (heart rate, and to be aware of exertion and breathlessness levels) to ensure inclusion of activities of vigorous intensity. Overall, the *FitKit*™ is feasible, utilizing inexpensive and readily available resources and equipment (Figure 2), which has significant clinical implications (Orenstein & Higgins, 2005).

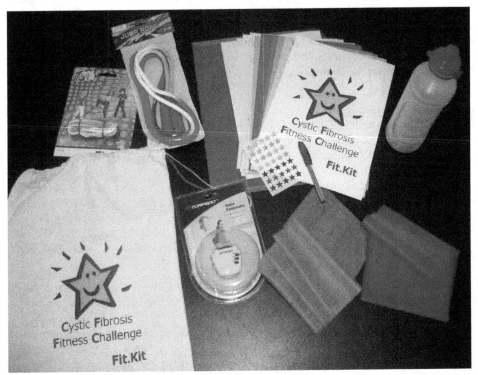

Fig. 2. The portable *FitKit*™ used in the *Cystic Fibrosis Fitness Challenge* program

The *CFFC* program provides an evidence–based novel approach to facilitating performance of physiotherapy exercise programs, across both inpatient and outpatient settings. A randomised controlled trial (Mandrusiak & Watter et al., 2009c) showed the effectiveness of this program during inpatient (10-14 days) and outpatient (8-12 weeks) phases of management in a group of young people with CF 7-17 years of age (n=31).

To summarize the recommendations that have been integrated into the design and delivery of this program, the *CFFC* provided a variety of age-appropriate activities that can be tailored to individual preferences across inpatient and outpatient (home) settings, incorporating education, communication and behavior modification strategies. The overall aim is to enhance integration of physical activity into daily life, and thus achieve long term adherence and optimal outcomes. Individualized exercise programs that provide a variety of activities based on the young person's preference and competence, and that allow tracking of personal progress, are more likely to succeed, and these elements were embedded into the design of the CFFC and FitKit™.

2.4 Overview of the role of exercise testing for young people with cystic fibrosis: What do physiotherapists measure?

A holistic range of measures which map to all of the ICF domains described above are provided by various professionals in the team managing those with CF, including measures of respiratory function, diet, medication, musculoskeletal function, as well as activity and quality of life. The physiotherapist is not necessarily involved in collecting them all, but is most likely to collect data about body structures and functions such as respiratory function tests and musculoskeletal measures, activity and functional exercise capacity. The focus of this section is on exercise testing.

Exercise testing is the global assessment of the response to exercise, and is an important parameter that is inadequately reflected by resting respiratory function tests (Baraldi and Carraro, 2006). It is an important outcome measure (Stevens and Williams, 2007) which may be more sensitive to disease progression and survival than respiratory function tests (McIlwaine, 2007), and specifically, aerobic fitness is a reliable indicator of disease status and prognosis (Nixon et al., 1992). For young people with CF, measures of activity performance and exercise testing can provide valuable information about the impact of the disease, functional limitations and trends over time (Rogers et al., 2003; Barker et al., 2004), and it is employed as an outcome variable in some intervention studies (Orenstein and Higgins, 2005). Further, Rogers et al. (2003) suggest that regular exercise testing accentuates the value of exercise to young people with CF and their families, which may encourage active lifestyles.

The guidelines for the *Association of Chartered Physiotherapists in Cystic Fibrosis* (in Rogers et al., 2003) recommend that all young people with CF should have annual exercise testing. Measurements of exercise capacity should provide the foundation for any prescription and adaptation of exercise programs (Rogers et al., 2003). Currently, exercise capacity is assessed using a range of laboratory- and clinically-based tools including cycle ergometry, walk tests, step tests and shuttle tests. Debate remains as to the most effective way of determining exercise capacity (Rogers et al., 2003), and some of the most commonly used measures are discussed below.

2.4.1 Maximal and submaximal tests of capacity

Maximum oxygen consumption (VO_2max) is the best index of aerobic capacity, and is significantly correlated with subsequent survival in people with CF (Pianosi et al., 2005). VO_2max is the "gold standard" measure of cardiorespiratory fitness, and maximal tests are performed in a laboratory using cycle ergometry or treadmills (Bruce, 1971). However, a number of factors limit the application of maximal tests to young people. Firstly, most daily activities are not performed at maximal levels and instead are at moderate intensities interspersed with short bursts of high intensity activities (Bailey et al., 1995), thus using maximal tests may not provide a realistic simulation of a young person's physical capacity (Chetta et al., 2001; Rogers et al., 2003; Solway, Brooks, Lacasse, & Thomas, 2001). Secondly, maximal tests are tiring and the physiological stress of testing, as well as the possible safety risks and expense to the patient, may outweigh the information gained (Nixon et al., 1996), and many young people with CF are reluctant to perform them (Rogers et al., 2003). Thirdly, data from maximal exercise tests may not be reproducible (Stevens and Williams, 2007). Finally, these tests are usually performed by specialist respiratory personnel and require sophisticated laboratory equipment that may need to be modified for young people and may not be available in all institutions (Orenstein, 1998; McIlwaine, 2007). In view of these issues, maximal exercise testing is currently outside the scope of routine clinical physiotherapy practice (Thoracic Society of Australia and New Zealand, 2007), and is not discussed further here.

According to Braggion (1989), submaximal field tests are better tools than maximal cycle ergometry or treadmill tests to evaluate a range of parameters including cardiorespiratory adaptations to exercise, motor aspects of performance (including agility, muscle strength and range of motion), and motivation to perform. Further, while field-based exercise tests do not always determine a person's maximal exercise response, they can give valuable clinical information on factors that limit activity performance on a day-to-day basis (Noonan and Dean, 2000; Narang et al., 2003; Rogers et al., 2003). Field tests are attractive to clinicians and researchers as they provide easy to administer and inexpensive forms of exercise assessment using typical activities of daily living such as walking (Orenstein, 1998). These can be undertaken outside of formal testing laboratories which may promote a less stressful environment for the young person (Cox et al., 2006) and some are useful in the research context where portable tools can provide follow-up information without the need for repeated visits to hospital facilities. Further, there is some evidence that young people with CF prefer field tests to formal exercise tests (Selvadurai et al., 2003). However, it is important to recognize that some information which is detected by more complex exercise tests may be missed by simple field tests (Narang et al., 2003).

In summary, young people rarely engage in sustained, heavy exercise, suggesting that traditional maximal exercise tests may not represent their patterns of daily physical activity (Cooper, 1995). Submaximal tests may better simulate childhood activities and thus provide insight into their functional capacity. These performance measures must be simple and convenient to use in order to be applicable to a variety of settings, such as the clinic, the hospital bedside and in the field (Narang et al., 2003), and such tests include walk tests, step tests and jump tests.

2.4.1.1 Walk tests

A variety of walk tests exist, but the six-minute walk test (6MWT) (Butland et al., 1982) is endorsed as the safest and easiest to administer, and it is better tolerated and better reflects activities of daily living than other walk tests such as the shuttle walk test (American Thoracic Society, 2002). It is an important clinical assessment tool, since it provides a composite assessment of respiratory, cardiac and metabolic systems during exercise (Li et al., 2005). It is self-paced and assesses the submaximal level of functional capacity, where the participant chooses their own level of intensity (American Thoracic Society, 2002). This self-paced nature may more closely reflect functional performance than externally paced exercise tests such as shuttle tests (Solway et al., 2001). Further, the use of a standard time (six-minutes) rather than a predetermined distance provides a better measure of endurance (McGavin et al., 1976).

Butland et al. (1982) revised the original 12 Minute Walk Test, to better accommodate patients with respiratory disease for whom walking for 12 minutes is too exhausting. The resulting 6MWT was found to perform as well as the 12 minute walk test, and is now a widely used measure for young people with CF, as it is reproducible (Gulmans et al., 1996; Balfour-Lynn et al., 1998; Cunha et al., 2006; Mandrusiak et al., 2009a), valid (Gulmans et al., 1996) and easy to perform in young people with CF (Cunha et al., 2006). It has been studied in a range of CF cohorts including inpatients (Mandrusiak et al., 2009a) and outpatients (Butland et al., 1982; Cunha et al., 2006; Gulmans et al., 1996).

The primary measurement is distance walked in six-minutes (6MWD), but data can also be collected about oxygen saturation (SpO_2), heart rate (HR) and breathlessness (Enright, 2003). Also, 'work' can be calculated as distance walked (m) x body weight (kg) (Chuang et al., 2001) and is recommended instead of distance as it more accurately indicates true performance (Cunha et al., 2006).

As summarised by Noonan and Dean (2000), the 6MWT can be employed as a one-time measure of functional capacity, or to measure change in functional capacity over time or in response to intervention. In people with CF, the 6MWT has been validated, being compared with cycle ergometry (Gulmans et al., 1996) and the 3min step test (Balfour-Lynn et al., 1998). A significant improvement in 6MWD was found in young people with CF at completion of hospital treatment for acute respiratory infection (Upton et al., 1988). Although no minimal clinically important difference (MCID) (Guyatt et al., 2002) for 6MWD has been established for the CF population, in adults with chronic obstructive pulmonary disease an improvement of 70 meters walked after an intervention is necessary to be 95% confident that the improvement was significant (Redelmeier et al., 1997).

Li et al. (2005) found a significant correlation between the 6MWD and VO_2max on the treadmill in typical children. It was also reported that in people with CF, 6MWD correlated with VO_2max, physical work capacity and the minimum arterial oxygen saturation (SaO_2) (Nixon et al., 1996), as well as with forced expiratory volume in one second (FEV_1) (Geiger et al., 2007).

Geiger et al. (2007) presented a modified 6MWT in which the participant pushed a measuring wheel, to establish reference values of healthy young people (n=528; 3-17 years). Li et al. (2005) presented height-specific reference values from a cohort of healthy (Chinese) children (n=1445; 7-16 years). 6MWD was related to height in some studies (Nixon et al., 1996; Cunha et al., 2006) but was not in other studies (Bradley et al., 1999), and correlated with weight by Gulmans et al. (1996). Although complete data has not been developed and consensus is not reached on all issues, it is important to consider factors relating to growth when comparing repeated results for young people with CF over time, and also comparing young people with CF to normative values.

A limitation of the 6MWT is that it requires an uninterrupted corridor of at least 30 meters, so is not adaptable to all settings. Consequently, this test may not be suitable for performance at the hospital bedside or in the home, where possible space limitations may not ensure standardized administration. Hence, tests that correlate with the 6MWT but require less space may present attractive alternatives. However, where applicable, the 6MWT appears to be the preferred tool for assessing exercise capacity in young people with CF.

2.4.1.2 Shuttle tests

The modified shuttle walk test as described by Selvadurai et al. (2003) is a symptom-limited exercise test, in which the participant moves from end to end of a 10m course in time with the 'beeps' from a pre-recorded tape. This test is valid in young people with CF (Cox et al., 2006), sensitive to change after hospitalization (Bradley et al., 1999, 2000) and correlates with VO_2max (Rogers et al., 2003). It is a natural activity and easy to administer, but does require 10 meters of uninterrupted space, and its practicality in the clinic setting has been questioned (Balfour-Lynn et al., 1998). Thus, motor tasks which allow more efficient delivery, and are adaptable to a range of clinical environments such as the hospital bedside or the outpatient clinic cubicle, may provide a suitable alternative.

2.4.1.3 Step tests

The three-minute step test is an externally paced, simple and portable test which is independent of effort and validated for use in children over six-years of age (Balfour-Lynn et al., 1998). It detects improvement in exercise capacity following hospitalization (Pike et al., 2001), but its use may be limited in those with well preserved lung function and fitness levels due to a potential ceiling effect (Selvadurai et al., 2003). It is also clear that actual workload will vary according to step height and weight and height of the participant (Selvadurai et al., 2003).

2.4.1.4 Jump tests

Mandrusiak et al. (2009a) established test-retest reliability of two jump tests (Astride Jumps and Forwards-Backwards Jumps) for young people with CF in the inpatient setting, using motor measures (number of jumps, time to fatigue) and physiological measures (heart rate, oxygen saturation via pulse oximetry, Borg Rating of Perceived Breathlessness (Burdon et al., 1982), and 15 Count Breathlessness Score (Prasad et al., 2000)). These jump tests are reflective of the natural activity pattern of typical young people, which is characterized by short bursts of high intensity activity (Bailey et al., 1995), and are particularly appropriate for the clinical setting as they are portable and easy to administer in limited space environments such as at the hospital bedside or outpatient clinic room. The score is the number of jumps performed before fatigue, and this score has been shown to improve significantly after hospitalization in 33 young people with CF (7-17 years) (Wilson et al., 2005). Work is being conducted to establish references for Australian children for such simple activities used in daily life.

In summary, measures of physical performance and exercise capacity are integral to the management of young people with CF. Tests for this population should be non-invasive, simple and quick to administer, inexpensive and applicable to a variety of settings (Cooper, 1998), and reflective of typical activities of childhood. In our experience, children tolerated and enjoyed the 6MWT and jump tests, and these are user-friendly field tests.

3. Conclusion

This chapter concerns the integral role of exercise in the management of young people with CF, providing a contemporary overview of current research and practice as well as the existing limitations and gaps to direct future research. The innovative *Cystic Fibrosis Fitness Challenge* and *FitKit*TM developed by the chapter authors presented a working example of how the ICF-CY framework can direct selection of performance measures and guide development of a program, as well as assessment of effectiveness of the intervention. This contemporary information supports the evidence base for the role of exercise in the management of those with CF and is an essential aspect of the physiotherapy role within the multidisciplinary team.

4. Acknowledgment

The Authors wish to express their sincere gratitude to the staff at the Physiotherapy Department of the Royal Children's Hospital (Brisbane, Australia) and the young people with CF and their families, for their integral role in the studies on which parts of this chapter is based. Some of this work was funded by the Australian Cystic Fibrosis Research Trust PhD Studentship Grant.

5. References

Abbott, J., M. Dodd, D. Bilton, and A.K. Webb. 1994. Treatment Compliance in Adults with Cystic-Fibrosis. *Thorax*. 49:115-120.

Abbott, J., M. Dodd, and A.K. Webb. 1996. Health perceptions and treatment adherence in adults with cystic fibrosis. *Thorax*. 51:1233-1238.

American Thoracic Society. 2002. ATS statement: guidelines for the six-minute walk test. ATS Committee on Proficiency Standards for Clinical Pulmonary Function Laboratories. *American Journal of Respiratory and Critical Care Medicine*. 166:111-117.

Bailey, R.C., J. Olson, S.L. Pepper, J. Porszasz, T.J. Barstow, and D.M. Cooper. 1995. The level and tempo of children's activities: an observational study. *Medicine and Science in Sports and Exercise*. 27:1033-1041.

Baker, C., and L. Wideman. 2006. Attitudes Toward Physical Activity in Adolescents With Cystic Fibrosis: Sex Differences After Training: A Pilot Study. *Journal of Pediatric Nursing*. 21:197 - 210.

Balfour-Lynn, I.M., S.A. Prasad, A. Laverty, B.F. Whitehead, and R. Dinwiddie. 1998. A step in the right direction: Assessing exercise tolerance in cystic fibrosis. *Pediatric Pulmonology*. 25:278-284.

Bar-Or, O. 2000. Home-based exercise programs in cystic fibrosis: Are they worth it? *Journal of Pediatrics*. 136:279-280.

Baraldi, E., and S. Carraro. 2006. Exercise testing and chronic lung diseases in children. *Paediatric Respiratory Reviews*. 7 Suppl 1:S196-198.

Barker, M., A. Hebestreit, W. Gruber, and H. Hebestreit. 2004. Exercise testing and training in German CF centers. *Pediatric Pulmonology*. 37:351-355.

Behm, D.G., A.D. Faigenbaum, B. Falk, and P. Klentrou. 2008. Canadian Society for Exercise Physiology position paper: resistance training in children and adolescents. *Applied*

Physiology, Nutrition, And Metabolism = Physiologie Appliquᅢ©e, Nutrition Et Mᅢ©tabolisme. 33:547-561.

Bernard, R.S., and L.L. Cohen. 2004. Increasing adherence to cystic fibrosis treatment: A systematic review of behavioral techniques. *Pediatric Pulmonology.* 37:8-16.

Blomquist, M., U. Freyschuss, L. Wiman, and B. Strandvik. 1986. Physical activity and self-treatment in cystic fibrosis. *Archives of Disease in Childhood.* 61:362-367.

Boas, S.R., M.J. Danduran, and S.A. McColley. 1999. Parental attitudes about exercise regarding their children with cystic fibrosis. *International Journal of Sports Medicine.* 20:334-338.

Bradley, J., J. Howard, E. Wallace, and S. Elborn. 1999. Validity of a modified shuttle test in adult cystic fibrosis. *Thorax.* 54:437-439.

Bradley, J., J. Howard, E. Wallace, and S. Elborn. 2000. Reliability, repeatability, and sensitivity of the modified shuttle test in adult cystic fibrosis. *Chest.* 117:1666-1671.

Bradley, J., and F. Moran. 2008. Physical training for cystic fibrosis. *Cochrane Database of Systematic Reviews.* doi:DOI: 10.1002/14651858.CD002768.pub2.

Bradley, J., F. Moran, and J. Elborn. 2006. Evidence for physical therapies (airway clearance and physical training) in cystic fibrosis: An overview of five Cochrane systematic reviews. *Respiratory Medicine.* 100:191-201.

Braggion, C., M. Cornacchia, A. Miano, F. Schena, G. Verlato, and G. Mastella. 1989. Exercise Tolerance and Effects of Training in Young Patients with Cystic Fibrosis and Mild Airway Obstruction. *Pediatric Pulmonology.* 7:145-152.

Britto, M.T., J.M. Garrett, T.R. Konrad, J.M. Majure, and M.W. Leigh. 2000. Comparison of physical activity in adolescents with cystic fibrosis versus age-matched controls. *Pediatric Pulmonology.* 30:86-91.

Bruce, R.A. 1971. Exercise testing of patients with coronary heart disease: principles and normal standards. *Ann Clinical Research.*323-332.

Burdon, G.W., E.F. Juniper, K.J. Killian, F.E. Hargreave, and E.J.M. Campbell. 1982. The perception of breathlessness in asthma. *American Review of Respiratory Disease.* 126:825-828.

Butland, R.J.A., J. Pang, E.R. Gross, A.A. Woodcock, and D.M. Geddes. 1982. 2-Minute, 6-Minute, and 12-Minute Walking Tests in Respiratory-Disease. *British Medical Journal.* 284:1607-1608.

Carr, L., R. Smith, J. Pryor, and C. Partridge. 1996. Cystic Fibrosis Patients' Views and Beliefs About Chest Clearance and Exercise -- A pilot study. *Physiotherapy.* 82:621-627.

Cerny, F.J. 1989. Relative Effects of Bronchial Drainage and Exercise for in-Hospital Care of Patients with Cystic-Fibrosis. *Physical Therapy.* 69:633-639.

Chuang, M.L., I.F. Lin, and K. Wasserman. 2001. The body weight-walking distance product as related to lung function, anaerobic threshold and peak VO2 in COPD patients. *Respiratory Medicine.* 95:618-626.

Cooper, D.M. 1995. Rethinking Exercise Testing in Children - a Challenge. *American Journal of Respiratory and Critical Care Medicine.* 152:1154-1157.

Cooper, D.M. 1998. Exercise and cystic fibrosis: The search for a therapeutic optimum. *Pediatric Pulmonology.* 25:143-144.

Cox, N.S., J. Follett, and K.O. McKay. 2006. Modified shuttle test performance in hospitalized children and adolescents with cystic fibrosis. *Journal of Cystic Fibrosis*. 5:165-170.

Cunha, M.T., T. Rozov, R.C. de Oliveira, and J.R. Jardim. 2006. Six-minute walk test in children and adolescents with cystic fibrosis. *Pediatric Pulmonology*. 41:618-622.

Cystic Fibrosis Trust. 2001. Standards for the clinical care of children and adults with cystic fibrosis *In*, London

Cystic Fibrosis Trust. 2002. Clinical guidelines for the physiotherapy management of cystic fibrosis: Recommendations of a working group. 17-20 pp.

de Jong, W., A.A. Kaptein, C.P. vanderSchans, G.P.M. Mannes, W.M.C. vanAalderen, R.G. Grevink, and G.H. Koeter. 1997. Quality of life in patients with cystic fibrosis. *Pediatric Pulmonology*. 23:95-100.

de Jong, W., W.M.C. Van Aalderen, J. Kraan, G.H. Koeter, and C.P. van der Schans. 2001. Skeletal muscle strength in patients with cystic fibrosis. *Physiotherapy Theory and Practice*. 17:23-28.

de Meer, K., V.A.M. Gulmans, and J. van der Laag. 1999. Peripheral muscle weakness and exercise capacity in children with cystic fibrosis. *American Journal of Respiratory and Critical Care Medicine*. 159:748-754.

Dodd, M.E., and S.A. Prasad. 2005. Physiotherapy management of cystic fibrosis. *Chronic Respiratory Disease*. 2:139-149.

Enright, P.L. 2003. The Six-Minute Walk Test. *Respiratory Care*. 48:783-785.

Farbotko, K., C. Wilson, P. Watter, and J. MacDonald. 2005. Change in physiotherapy management of children with cystic fibrosis in a large urban hospital. *Physiotherapy Theory and Practice*. 21:13-21.

Gardner, L. 2004. Teaching young children about cystic fibrosis. *Pediatric Nursing*. 16:34-36.

Gudas, L.J., G.P. Koocher, and D. Wypij. 1991. Perceptions of medical compliance in children and adolescents with cystic fibrosis. *Journal of Developmental and Behavioural Pediatrics*. 12:236-242.

Gulmans, V.A.M., K. de Meer, H.J.L. Brackel, J.A.J. Faber, R. Berger, and P.J.M. Helders. 1999. Outpatient exercise training in children with cystic fibrosis: Physiological effects, perceived competence, and acceptability. *Pediatric Pulmonology*. 28:39-46.

Gulmans, V.A.M., N. vanVeldhoven, K. deMeer, and P.J.M. Helders. 1996. The six-minute walking test in children with cystic fibrosis: Reliability and validity. *Pediatric Pulmonology*. 22:85-89.

Guyatt, G.H., D. Osoba, A.W. Wu, K.W. Wyrwich, and G.R. Norman. 2002. Methods to explain the clinical significance of health status measures. . *Mayo Clinical Proc.* 77:371-383.

Higgins, L.W., D.M. Orenstein, and C.E. Baker. 2007. Development of an exercise knowledge test for children with cystic fibrosis. *Pediatric Pulmonology*. 42:359.

Hind, K., J.G. Truscott, and S.P. Conway. 2008. Exercise during childhood and adolescence: A prophylaxis against cystic fibrosis-related low bone mineral density? Exercise for bone health in cystic fibrosis. *Journal of Cystic Fibrosis*. 7:270 - 276.

Hinton, S., S. Watson, R. Chesson, and S. Mathers. 2002. Information needs of young people with cystic fibrosis. *Paediatric Nursing*. 14:18-21.

Hobbs, S.A., J.B. Schweitzer, L.L. Cohen, A.L. Hayes, C. Schoell, and B.K. Crain. 2003. Maternal attributions related to compliance with cystic fibrosis treatment. *Journal of Clinical Psychology in Medical Settings*. 10:273-277.

Holzer, F.J., R. Schnall, and L.I. Landau. 1984. The Effect of a Home Exercise Program in Children with Cystic-Fibrosis and Asthma. *Australian Paediatric Journal*. 20:297-301.

Hussey, J., J. Gormley, G. Leen, and P. Greally. 2002. Peripheral muscle strength in young males with cystic fibrosis. *Journal of Cystic Fibrosis*. 1:116-121.

Ireland, C. 2003. Adherence to Physiotherapy and Quality of Life for Adults and Adolescents with Cystic Fibrosis. *Physiotherapy*. 89:397-407.

Kettler, L.J., S.M. Sawyer, H.R. Winefield, and H.W. Greville. 2002. Determinants of adherence in adults with cystic fibrosis (Occasional Review). *Thorax*. 57:459-454.

Klijn, P.H.C., A. Oudshoorn, C.K. van der Ent, J. van der Net, J.L. Kimpen, and P.J.M. Helders. 2004. Effects of anaerobic training in children with cystic fibrosis - A randomized controlled study. *Chest*. 125:1299-1305.

Koch, C., B. Frederiksen, and N. Hoiby. 2003. Patient cohorting and infection control. *Seminars in Respiratory and Critical Care Medicine*. 24:703-716.

Lannefors, L. 2004. Influences on posture [Cystic Fibrosis Conference symposium session summary]. *Pediatric Pulmonology*. 38:155-157.

Li, A.M., J. Yin, J.T. Au, H.K. So, T. Tsang, E. Wong, T.F. Fok, and P.C. Ng. 2007. Standard reference for the six-minute-walk test in healthy children aged 7 to 16 years. *American Journal of Respiratory and Critical Care Medicine*. 176:174-180.

Li, A.M., J. Yin, C.C.W. Yu, T. Tsang, H.K. So, E. Wong, D. Chan, E.K.L. Hon, and R. Sung. 2005. The six-minute walk test in healthy children: reliability and validity. *European Respiratory Journal*. 25:1057-1060.

Mandrusiak, A., D. Giraud, J. MacDonald, C. Wilson, and P. Watter. 2010. Muscle length and joint range of motion in children with cystic fibrosis compared to matched-controls. *Physiotherapy Canada*. 62:141-146.

Mandrusiak, A., C. Maurer, J. MacDonald, C. Wilson, and P. Watter 2009a. Functional capacity tests in young people with cystic fibrosis. *New Zealand Journal of Physiotherapy*. 37:112-115.

Mandrusiak, A., J. MacDonald, and P. Watter. 2009b. The International Classification of Functioning, Disability and Health: an effective model for describing young people with cystic fibrosis. *Child: care, health and development*. 35:2-4.

Mandrusiak, A., J. MacDonald, C. Wilson., J. Paratz., P. Watter. 2009c. Effect of a targeted exercise program on function, activity and participation of young people with cystic fibrosis: using the ICF model as a basis of design. Doctoral Thesis, The University of Queensland, Australia.

Massery, M. 2005. Musculoskeletal and neuromuscular interventions: a physical approach to cystic fibrosis. *Journal of the Royal Society of Medicine*. 98:55-66.

McGavin, C.R., S.P. Gupta, and G.J.R. McHardy. 1976. 12-Minute Walking Test for Assessing Disability in Chronic-Bronchitis. *British Medical Journal*. 1:822-823.

McIlwaine, M. 2007. Chest physical therapy, breathing techniques and exercise in children with CF. *Paediatric Respiratory Reviews*. 8:8-16.

Modi, A.C., and A.L. Quittner. 2003. Validation of a Disease-Specific Measure of Health-Related Quality of Life for Children with Cystic Fibrosis. *Journal of Pediatric Psychology*. 28:535-546.

Moorcroft, A.J., M.E. Dodd, J. Morris, and A.K. Webb. 2004. Individualised unsupervised exercise training in adults with cystic fibrosis: a 1 year randomised controlled trial. *Thorax*. 59:1074-1080.

Narang, I., S. Pike, M. Rosenthal, I.M. Balfour-Lynn, and A. Bush. 2003. Three-minute step test to assess exercise capacity in children with cystic fibrosis with mild lung disease. *Pediatric Pulmonology*. 35:108-113.

Nixon, P.A., M.L. Joswiak, and F.J. Fricker. 1996. A six-minute walk test for assessing exercise tolerance in severely ill children. *Journal of Pediatrics*. 129:362-366.

Nixon, P.A., D.M. Orenstein, S.F. Kelsey, and C.F. Doershuk. 1992. The Prognostic Value of Exercise Testing in Patients with Cystic-Fibrosis. *New England Journal of Medicine*. 327:1785-1788.

Noonan, V., and E. Dean. 2000. Submaximal exercise testing: clinical application and interpretation. *Physical Therapy*. 80:782-807.

Orenstein, D.M. 1998. Exercise testing in cystic fibrosis. *Pediatric Pulmonology*. 25:223-225.

Orenstein, D.M., B.A. Franklin, C.F. Doershuk, H.K. Hellerstein, K.J. Germann, J.G. Horowitz, and R.C. Stern. 1981. Exercise Conditioning and Cardiopulmonary Fitness in Cystic-Fibrosis - the Effects of a 3-Month Supervised Running Program. *Chest*. 80:392-398.

Orenstein, D.M., and L.W. Higgins. 2005. Update on the role of exercise in cystic fibrosis. *Current Opinion in Pulmonary Medicine*. 11:519-523.

Pianosi, P., J. LeBlanc, and A. Almudevar. 2005. Peak oxygen uptake and mortality in children with cystic fibrosis. *Thorax*. 60:50-54.

Pike, S.E., S.A. Prasad, and I.M. Balfour-Lynn. 2001. Effect of intravenous antibiotics on exercise tolerance (3-min step test) in cystic fibrosis. *Pediatric Pulmonology*. 32:38-43.

Prasad, S.A., and F.J. Cerny. 2002. Factors that influence adherence to exercise and their effectiveness: Application to cystic fibrosis. *Pediatric Pulmonology*. 34:66-72.

Prasad, S.A., S.D. Randall, and I.M. Balfour-Lynn. 2000. Fifteen-count breathlessness score: An objective measure for children. *Pediatric Pulmonology*. 30:56-62.

Redelmeier, D.A., A.M. Bayoumi, R.S. Goldstein, and G.H. Guyatt. 1997. Interpreting small differences in functional status:The six-minute walk test in chronic lung disease patients. *American Journal of Respiratory and Critical Care Medicine*. 155:1278-1282.

Rogers, D., S.A. Prasad, and I. Doull. 2003. Exercise testing in children with cystic fibrosis. *Journal of the Royal Society of Medicine*. 96:23-29.

Sahlberg, M. 2008. Physical exercise in cystic fibrosis - studies on muscle strength, oxygen uptake and lung function in young adult patients. University of Gothenburg, Gothenburg, Sweden.

Salh, W., D. Bilton, M. Dodd, and A.K. Webb. 1989. Effect of Exercise and Physiotherapy in Aiding Sputum Expectoration in Adults with Cystic-Fibrosis. *Thorax*. 44:1006-1008.

Schneiderman-Walker, J., S.L. Pollock, M. Corey, D.D. Wilkes, G.J. Canny, L. Pedder, and J.J. Reisman. 2000. A randomized controlled trial of a 3-year home exercise program in cystic fibrosis. *Journal of Pediatrics*. 136:304-310.

Selvadurai, H.C., C.J. Blimkie, N. Meyers, C.M. Mellis, P.J. Cooper, and P.P. van Asperen. 2002. Randomized controlled study of in-hospital exercise training programs in children with cystic fibrosis. *Pediatric Pulmonology*. 33:194-200.

Selvadurai, H.C., P.J. Cooper, N. Meyers, C.J. Blimkie, L. Smith, C.M. Mellis, and P.P. Van Asperen. 2003. Validation of shuttle tests in children with cystic fibrosis. *Pediatric Pulmonology*. 35:133-138.

Shoemaker, M.J., and H. Hurt. 2008. The evidence regarding exercise training in the management of cystic fibrosis: A systematic review. *Cardiopulmonary Physical Therapy Journal*. 19:75-83.

Smidt, N., H.C.W. de Vet, L.M. Bouter, and J. Dekker. 2005. Effectiveness of exercise therapy: a best-evidence summary of systematic reviews. *Australian Journal of Physiotherapy*. 51:71-85.

Solway, S., D. Brooks, Y. Lacasse, and S. Thomas. 2001. A qualitative systematic overview of the meaurement properties of functional walk tests used in the cardiorespiratory domain. *Chest*. 119:256-270.

Stanghelle, J.K. 1988. Physical Exercise for Patients with Cystic-Fibrosis - a Review. *International Journal of Sports Medicine*. 9:6-18.

Stevens, D., and C.A. Williams. 2007. Exercise testing and training with the young cystic fibrosis patient. *Journal of Sports Science and Medicine*. 6:286 - 291.

Taylor, N., K. Dodd, N. Shields, and A. Bruder. 2006. APA Position Statement: Evidence regarding therapeutic exercise in physiotherapy. *In*, Australian Physiotherapy Association website. 1-5.

Thoracic Society of Australia and New Zealand. 2007. Physiotherapy for cystic fibrosis in Australia: A consensus statement. *The Thoracic Society of Australia and New Zealand*.125.

Turchetta, A., T. Salerno, V. Lucidi, F. Libera, R. Cutrera, and A. Bush. 2004. Usefulness of a program of hospital-supervised physical training in patients with cystic fibrosis. *Pediatric Pulmonology*. 38:115-118.

Upton, C.J., J.C. Tyrrell, and E.J. Hiller. 1988. 2 Minute Walking Distance in Cystic-Fibrosis. *Archives of Disease in Childhood*. 63:1444-1448.

Webb, A.K., and M.E. Dodd. 1999. Exercise and sport in cystic fibrosis: benefits and risks. *British Journal of Sports Medicine*. 33:77-78.

Webb, A.K., and M.E. Dodd. 2000. Exercise and training for adults with cystic fibrosis. *In* Cystic FIbrosis. M.E. Hodson and D.M. Geddes, editors. Arnold, London. 433-448.

Wilson, C., J. MacDonald, C. Harrison, A. Mandrusiak, A. Chang, P. O'Rourke, and P. Watter. 2005. Activity outcomes characterised within the International Classification of Functioning and Disability in young people with cystic fibrosis. *In* Sixth Australian and New Zealand Cystic Fibrosis Conference. Adelaide, Australia. 53.

World Health Organization. 2007. International classification of functioning, disability, and health—children and youth. World Health Organization, Geneva.

World Health Organization. 2001. International classification of functioning, disability, and health. World Health Organization, Geneva.

Yankaskas, J.R., B.C. Marshall, B. Sufian, and et al. 2004. Cystic fibrosis adult care: Consensus conference report. *Chest.* 125.

Permissions

The contributors of this book come from diverse backgrounds, making this book a truly international effort. This book will bring forth new frontiers with its revolutionizing research information and detailed analysis of the nascent developments around the world.

We would like to thank Dinesh D. Sriramulu, for lending his expertise to make the book truly unique. He has played a crucial role in the development of this book. Without his invaluable contribution this book wouldn't have been possible. He has made vital efforts to compile up to date information on the varied aspects of this subject to make this book a valuable addition to the collection of many professionals and students.

This book was conceptualized with the vision of imparting up-to-date information and advanced data in this field. To ensure the same, a matchless editorial board was set up. Every individual on the board went through rigorous rounds of assessment to prove their worth. After which they invested a large part of their time researching and compiling the most relevant data for our readers. Conferences and sessions were held from time to time between the editorial board and the contributing authors to present the data in the most comprehensible form. The editorial team has worked tirelessly to provide valuable and valid information to help people across the globe.

Every chapter published in this book has been scrutinized by our experts. Their significance has been extensively debated. The topics covered herein carry significant findings which will fuel the growth of the discipline. They may even be implemented as practical applications or may be referred to as a beginning point for another development. Chapters in this book were first published by InTech; hereby published with permission under the Creative Commons Attribution License or equivalent.

The editorial board has been involved in producing this book since its inception. They have spent rigorous hours researching and exploring the diverse topics which have resulted in the successful publishing of this book. They have passed on their knowledge of decades through this book. To expedite this challenging task, the publisher supported the team at every step. A small team of assistant editors was also appointed to further simplify the editing procedure and attain best results for the readers.

Our editorial team has been hand-picked from every corner of the world. Their multi-ethnicity adds dynamic inputs to the discussions which result in innovative outcomes. These outcomes are then further discussed with the researchers and contributors who give their valuable feedback and opinion regarding the same. The feedback is then collaborated with the researches and they are edited in a comprehensive manner to aid the understanding of the subject.

Apart from the editorial board, the designing team has also invested a significant amount of their time in understanding the subject and creating the most relevant covers. They scrutinized every image to scout for the most suitable representation of the subject and create an appropriate cover for the book.

The publishing team has been involved in this book since its early stages. They were actively engaged in every process, be it collecting the data, connecting with the contributors or procuring relevant information. The team has been an ardent support to the editorial, designing and production team. Their endless efforts to recruit the best for this project, has resulted in the accomplishment of this book. They are a veteran in the field of academics and their pool of knowledge is as vast as their experience in printing. Their expertise and guidance has proved useful at every step. Their uncompromising quality standards have made this book an exceptional effort. Their encouragement from time to time has been an inspiration for everyone.

The publisher and the editorial board hope that this book will prove to be a valuable piece of knowledge for researchers, students, practitioners and scholars across the globe.

List of Contributors

John M. Tomich, Urška Bukovnik, Jammie Layman and Bruce D. Schultz
Departments of Biochemistry and Anatomy and Physiology, Kansas State University, Manhattan, Kansas USA

Florian Bossard
Department of Physiology; McGill University, Montreal, Quebec, Canada

Emilie Silantieff and Chantal Gauthier
L'Institut du Thorax, INSERM UMR 1087, CNRL UMR 6291, Université de Nantes, Nantes, France

Bob Lubamba, Barbara Dhooghe, Sabrina Noël and Teresinha Leal
Louvain Centre for Toxicology and Applied Pharmacology, Université Catholique de Louvain, Brussels, Belgium

Valerie Chappe
Dalhousie University, Canada

Sami I. Said
SUNY-Stony Brook University, USA

Yifei Fan, Yeshavanth K. Banasavadi-Siddegowda and Xiaodong Wang
University of Toledo College of Medicine, USA

Gaëlle Gonzalez, Pierre Boulanger and Saw-See Hong
University of Lyon 1, France

M.C. Dechecchi
Laboratory of Molecular Pathology, Laboratory of Clinical Chemistry and Haematology, University Hospital of Verona, Verona, Italy

Rosa Patricia Arias-Llorente, Carlos Bousoño García and Juan J. Díaz Martín
Cystic Fibrosis Unit. Universitary Central Hospital of Asturias, Spain

Carlos F. Lange
Dept. of Mechanical Engineering, University of Alberta, Canada

Georgia Perpati
Adult Cystic Fibrosis Unit, Athens Hospital of Chest Diseases, Greece

Adrian H. Kendrick
Department of Respiratory Medicine, University Hospitals, Bristol, England

Allison Mandrusiak and Pauline Watter
The University of Queensland, Division of Physiotherapy, Australia

Printed in the USA
CPSIA information can be obtained
at www.ICGtesting.com
JSHW011447221024
72173JS00004B/983

9 781632 423498